Research on Diabetes II

Research on Diabetes II

Publisher: iConcept Press Ltd.
Cover design: Pineapple Design Ltd.
Interior design: iConcept Press Ltd.
Typesetting and copy editing: iConcept Press Ltd. and Pineapple Design Ltd.

ISBN: 978-1-922227-485

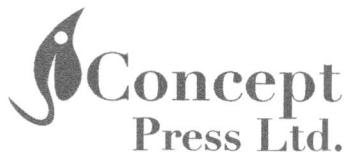

ſConcept
Press Ltd.

www.iconceptpress.com

Contents

Preface

Diabetes is a group of metabolic diseases in which a person has high blood sugar, either because the body does not produce enough insulin, or because cells do not respond to the insulin that is produced. This high blood sugar produces the classical symptoms of polyuria (frequent urination), polydipsia (increased thirst) and polyphagia (increased hunger). *Research on Diabetes II* provides the latest research and development in the area of diabetes by presenting a succinct review of the works that researchers struggling to find answers for 200 million diabetics world-wide, where the number of those afflicted is expected to double, if not triple, in coming decades.

There are totally 14 chapters in this book. Chapter 1 describes the strong relationship between diabetes (DM) and infection. Infections can elicit diabetes or make glycaemic control difficult. On the other hand; experimental models viruses appear capable of both accelerating as well as decelerating the immunological processes leading to type 1 diabetes (T1 DM). Many infections are more common in diabetic patients with increased severity and complications. Chapter 2 presents the idea of using traditional indian medicinal plants used in the traditional Ayurvedic system to treat diabetes. Specifically, the chapter discusses how the indian medicinal plants can be used as inhibitors of α-glucosidase and pancreatic α-amylase. Chapter 3 discusses the nutritional content of organic prickly pads. Findings show that different fiber quantity and mineral content along life cycle of prickly pads, suggesting that prickly pads are excellent option for people with diabetes due to the beneficial nutritional properties. Chapter 4 highlights the serious complications of diabetes mellitus, particularly oral complications. It also discusses awareness of diabetic patients towards their increased risk for oral diseases, their attitude towards maintaing good oral health and the global prevalence, pathophysiology and classifications of diabetes mellitus. Finally, it proposes a way for prevention of complications.

Chapter 5 discusses retropharyngeal abscess (RPA), a potentially serious deep space neck infection. It is an infection with abscess collection in one of the deep spaces of the neck. 95occurred in children under the age of 6. It is uncommon in adult, except adults with diabetes mellitus and those who are debilitated, older adults or immunocompromised patients. Chapter 6 addresses the issue of erectile dysfunction. It is a common health related and quality of life issue in the diabetic patients population. The chapter focuses on the surgical options to address this issue especially penile prothesis since it is well known to have a high success rate and patient satisfaction. Chapter 7 presents that fact that the presence of infection in a patient on dialysis has a substantial effect on cardiovascular mortality and morbidity, and should influence decisions regarding the use of therapies intended to minimize that risk. Chapter 8 discusses various cardiovascular effects of diabetes in the pediatric population as diabetes is a chronic disease which affects in a way or another all the stages of childhood; starting in utero, neonates, infants, children and adolescent.

Chapter 9 uses carotid intima media thickness measurement to determine significant risk factors for atherogenic vascular disease in a cohort of Nigerians with Diabetes Mellitus. This can to help in prevention of cardiovascular morbi-mortality; and they turned out to be systolic and diastolic blood pressures, 2 hour post prandial and fasting plasma glucose, total cholesterol, high density lipoprotein cholesterol, uric acid and glycosylated haemoglobin. Chapter 10 discusses diabetes mellitus, a metabolic disease which is said to cause gastrointestinal complications amongst long standing patients. This disorder, which affects the enteric nervous system that controls digestive processes, intestinal motility and nervous control, is now attracting medical attention and research with a view to designing better treatment outcome to mitigate this complication. Chapter 11 provides several important and handy tools which can be used by obstetricians, embryologists, perinatologists, forensic pathologists and clinical anthropologists for their diagnostic armamentarium so that they can arrive at highly scientific management of their patients even in areas far removed from sophisticated clinical gadgetry. Chapter 12 attempts to advance our understanding of genetic basis of autoimmunity in disease pathogenesis, facilitates determining an individual's disease status and promotes better treatment modalities against systemic lupus erythematosus. This study is very valuable and helpful in unveiling the whole complex basis of the autoimmune diseases.

Chapter 13 illustrates the complicated relationship from the pathogenetic mechanisms to the potential source of infections for humans. Convincing evidence to date indicates that viral and bacterial agents could be associated with Diabetes Mellitus development and progression. Recently, *Mycobacterium avium* subsp. *paratuberculosis* (MAP) has been postulated as the infectious agent that triggers human Diabetes Mellitus. Chapter 14 provides a brief overview of molecular level studies on neuroimmune state of patients with long-term diabetes mellitus, including those with acute ischemic stroke, and demonstrates implication of neuroimmune alterations in pathomechanisms responsible for development and progression of diabetic complications.

Editing and publishing a book is never an easy task. Each chapter in this book has gone through a peer review, a selection and an editing process so as to guarantee its quality. Without the supports and contributions of the authors and reviewers, this book can never be able to complete. We would like to thank all of the authors in this book and all of the reviewers who participated in the reviewing process: Marwan S Al-Nimer, Khalid S. Aljabri, Sandra M. Barbalho, Keshore Bidasee, Marco Matteo Ciccone, Vincenzo de Feo, Matthias Girndt, O. Huck, Anastasios J. Karayiannakis, Kwang-Won Kim, Posa Mahesh Kumar, Magdalena Labieniec-Watala, Catherine B Lawrence, Ioanna Lola, Emmanuel Mador, J.P. Majra, Milos Z Maksimovic, Abbas Ali Mansour, Gianpaolo Maso, Lampros K Michalis, Daniele Minardi, Kei Nakajima, Basil Okeahialam, T. Padma, Ravindra R. Pandharinath, N. Papanas, Yong-Ki Park, Ellen Pierce, Surya J. Prasanna, Maarten Rijpert, Kendra P. Rumbaugh, Aly Saber, V. Seshiah, Anna Södergren, Florian Szabados, Klaus Tenbrock and Sai-Ching Jim Yeung. We hope that you, the reader, will find this book interesting and useful. Any advices please feel free and are always welcome to tell us.

iConcept Press Ltd
March 2014

Diabetes and Infections: Which is the Fuel?

Nermin Kamal Saeed
Medical Microbiologist, Pathology Department
Salmaniya Medical Complex, Manama, Kingdom of Bahrain

Mohammed Al-Biltagi
Pediatric Department, Faculty of Medicine
Tanta University, Egypt

1   Introduction

There is a strong relationship between diabetes (DM) and infection. Infections can elicit diabetes or make glycaemic control difficult. On the other hand; experimental models viruses appear capable of both accelerating as well as decelerating the immunological processes leading to type 1 diabetes (T1 DM). Many infections are more common in diabetic patients with increased severity and complications. In this chapter we will discuss some of the infections that can trigger development of DM as well as the commonly encountered infections that a diabetic patient may have.

2   Diabetogenic Infections

Infection is a common trigger for many inflammatory diseases including but not only; rheumatoid arthritis, heart attacks, late-onset asthma, and Crohn's disease. Diabetes also is due to an aberrant overactive immune system exactly like the previously mentioned inflammatory diseases. Autoimmunity plays an important role in development of all types of diabetes. Type 1 diabetes is classified as either autoimmune (immune mediated or T1 DM A) or idiopathic (T1 DM B). The autoimmune type is due to a chronic autoimmune selective destruction of the pancreatic islet beta cells that leads to a marked insulin deficiency. Islet autoimmunity was also observed in adult phenotypic type 2 diabetes (T2 DM) patients. Numerous recent publications note a significant proportion of physician-diagnosed T2 DM in youth with evidence of pancreatic autoimmunity. This clinical phenomenon of antibody positivity in phenotypic T2 DM in youth, is referred to as "type 1.5 diabetes" (T1.5 DM), "double diabetes," "latent autoimmune diabetes in youth" (LADY), or "hybrid diabetes" (Badaru & Pihoker, 2012). This autoimmune-mediated DM is controlled by multiple susceptibility genes that can be modulated by various environmental factors. The role of previous viral infection to the development of T1 DM in humans is controversial. The link between T1 DM and viral infection was first noted from the epidemiological studies. Many viruses have also been shown to affect the development of DM in laboratory animals. Viruses have been appeal to explain the increasing prevalence of DM, seasonal variation in onset, and enhanced susceptibility of trans-migratory populations (Tirabassi *et al.*, 2010). Infections (especially viruses) in presence of genetic associations; may trigger the autoimmune disease process leading to DM or accelerate the already initiated disease process.

The infection can induce diabetes by different mechanisms (shown in Figure 1) including:

- Direct destruction of beta cells (e.g. parotitic pancreatitis).

- Molecular mimicry: microbial antigens share homologies with host antigens (e.g. Cytomegalovirus and Epstein-Barr virus).

- Increased processing and presentation of autoantigens during infection or epitope spreading which make the beta cells a target of the immune system and enhances autoimmunity.

- Increasing inflammation and the secretion of inflammatory cells such as cytokines.

- Increase insulin requirement during infection

- Increase insulin resistance.

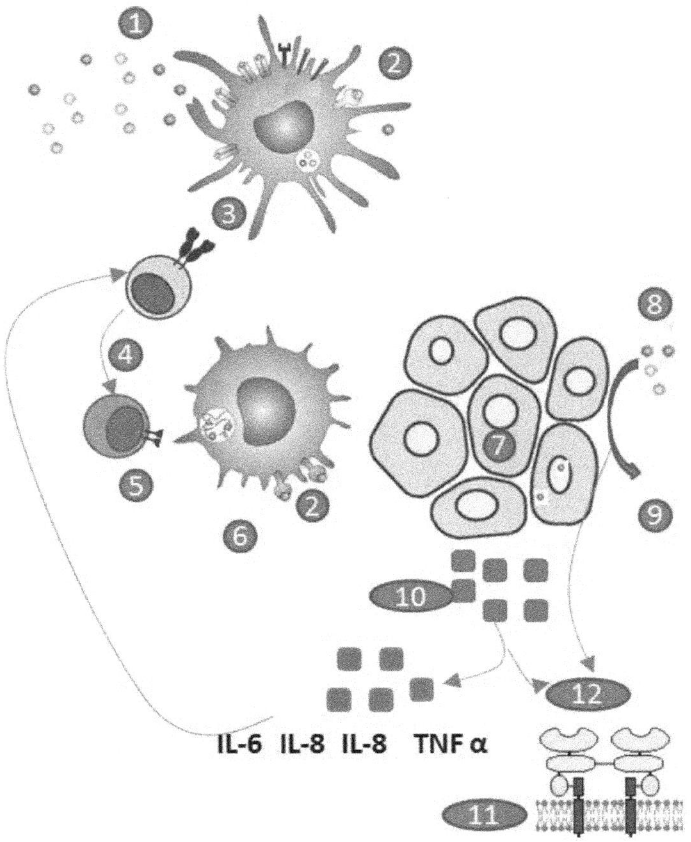

Figure 1: The mechanisms of infection induced diabetes

Figure 1 showed the mechanisms of infection induced diabetes. (1- virus, 2- Antigen presenting cell, 3- T cell receptor, 4- Activation of T cell, 5- Activated CD4+ T cell, 6- Self peptides (B-cell), 7- Pancreatic β –cells, 8- Direct viral destruction of beta cells, 9- Defective Insulin secretion, 10- β -cell autoantigens and molecular mimicry, 11- Insulin receptors,12- Insulin resistance).

2.1 Viral Infections

2.1.1 Enteroviruses

Enteroviruses are a genus of Picornaviridae family of viruses and are associated with several human and mammalian diseases. There are over 70 serotypes of enterovirus have been isolated from man and they are originally classified into five groups; polioviruses, Coxsackie A viruses (CA A1-A24), Coxsackie B viruses (CB B1-B6), echoviruses and, enterovirus. Most of the enterovirus infections are symptomatic, especially in young children, but when they do cause clinically overt disease, they can cause a wide range of disorders and can involve many of the body systems. Enteroviruses infections are one of the main environmental triggers of T1 DM and they are one of the most well studied environmental factors in relation to T1 DM sero-epidemiology, histopathology, animal studies, and in vitro experiments. Gamble *et al* were the first to report the possible link between T1 DM and enteroviral infection (Gamble *et al.*, 1969).

Higher rates of enterovirus infection (particularly with coxsackievirus B-4), defined by detection of enterovirus IgM, IgG, or both, viral RNA with reverse transcription polymerase chain reaction (RT PCR), and viral capsid protein, have been found in patients with DM at diagnosis compared with controls. Prospective studies have also shown more enterovirus infections in children who developed islet autoantibodies, subsequent DM, or both; as well as a temporal relation between infection and autoimmunity. The relation between enterovirus infection and DM is not consistent across all studies, and the subject remains controversial. Furthermore, in animal models viral infections might also protect from DM. A systematic review of coxsackie B virus serological studies did not show an association with T1 DM. Yeung *et al* showed an association between T1 DM and enterovirus infection, with a more than 9 times the risk of infection in cases of DM and three times the risk in children with autoimmunity. However, causal relation between infection and T1 DM was not possible to determine (Yeung *et al.*, 2011). Stene *et al* showed that approximately 8% of the children progressing to T1 DM had enteroviral RNA in their serum few months prior to diagnosis. They found that the presence of enterovirus RNA in serum to be a highly significant predictor of progression to clinical T1 DM. The enterovirus infection may be one of many factors that can accelerate progression to DM, e.g., through nonspecific activation of autoreactive T-cells. Also enterovirus viral infection may be able to induce insulin resistance sufficient to precipitate clinically overt DM. The most frequently implicated serotype, was coxsackievirus B4 which is responsible for 2.4% of the enterovirus infectious episodes. However, there may be differences within serotypes because enteroviruses are known to mutate rapidly (Stene *et al.*, 2010).

Enterovirus infection may cause β-cell damage and release of β-cell antigens taken up by antigen-presenting cells; activate the innate immune system; enhance the secretion of interferon-α, and perhaps up regulate the major histocompatibility complex molecules on β–cells. The "fertile field hypothesis" proposes that different viruses may increase the risk of DM in susceptible time windows after an infection, while outside this window a similar viral infection would be resolved with no further consequences for the host (Von Herrath M 2009). Enterovirus infections are more frequent during the 6-month period preceding the appearance of the first diabetes-associated autoantibodies. Enteroviral infection may also be implicated in the pathogenesis of fulminant T1 DM which results from accelerated β-cell failure and is characterized by the rapid onset of severe hyperglycemia and ketoacidosis, with subsequent poor prognosis. In such case; enterovirus initiates co-expression of interferon-γ and CXCL10 in β-cell. CXCL10 secreted from β-cell activates and attracts autoreactive T-cells and macrophages to the islets via CXCR3. These infiltrating autoreactive T-cells and macrophages release inflammatory cytokines including interferon- γ in the islets, not only damaging β-cell but also accelerating CXCL10 generation in residual β-cell and thus further activating cell-mediated autoimmunity until all β –cells have been destroyed (Tanaka *et al.*, 2009).

Coxsackie B 4 virus (CVB4) is the most common enteroviral strain observed in pre-diabetic and diabetic individuals. RNA of CVB could be detected in blood from patients at the onset or during the course of T1 DM with enhancement of the cellular immune response directed against CVB antigens in patients with T1 DM after the onset of the disease. The evidence of the CVB4 in development of T1 DM is supported by isolation of one CVB4 strain from the pancreas of a deceased diabetic child; CVB4 strain obtained from diabetic rats are able to induce diabetes after inoculation in another mice; detection of CVB4 antigens in pancreatic tissue specimens from T1 DM patients; and the ability of enterovirus isolates obtained from newly diagnosed T1 DM patients to infect and induce destruction of human islet cells in vitro (Elshebani *et al.*, 2007). CVB4 infection of islet cells induces strong inflammation mediated by natural killer (NK) cells within the islets with possible cytolysis of β-cells and release of autoantigens which activate strong immune responses. Poliovirus is one of the enteroviruses that are able to directly infect of β-cells through targeting β-cells via surface molecules such as the poliovirus receptor and integrin $\alpha_v\beta_3$. Infections by viruses that target β-cells and promote strong inflammation within the islets may thus represent the initial step in the induction of autoimmunity (Filippi & von Herrath 2008). Elevated IgA antibodies to enterovirus were observed in some patients with fulminant T1 DM which may indicate that recurrent enterovirus infection may be play a triggering role in development of fulminant T1 DM. Maternal enterovirus infections during pregnancy may increase the risk of offspring developing T1 DM during childhood. Boys of enterovirus IgM-positive mothers have approximately 5 times greater risk of developing DM as compared to boys of IgM-negative mothers. This observation suggests that gestational enterovirus infections may be related to the risk of offspring developing T1 DM in adolescence and young adulthood. Diabetes was also observed in some cases as early as 3 years of age and a case of neonatal DM with evidence of maternal enterovirus infection during pregnancy were also been reported. Maternal enterovirus infection is a significant risk factor for the development of DM in boys, but not in girls. This finding suggests that boys may be more susceptible to the diabetogenic effect of enteroviruses than girls during the prenatal period. Boys might be more susceptible to enterovirus infections, possibly due to the weaker immune system (Elfving *et al.*, 2008). T1 DM associated HLA-DR alleles (DR3 and DR4) have been associated with a stronger humoral response to enterovirus antigens compared to HLADR2. (Sadeharju *et al.*, 2003)

2.1.2   Congenital Rubella

Rubella virus has been thought to cause T1 DM, but it was conclusively associated with congenital rubella syndrome. Rubella virus has the ability to multiply in the pancreas in susceptible population. Experimental congenital rubella infection in rabbits caused histological changes in the beta-cells of the pancreatic islets similar to those found in mice made diabetic by the M variant of the encephalomyocarditis virus (Menser *et al.*, 1978). Congenital rubella syndrome (CRS) increased the risk of DM in the second and third decades of life indicating the possibility of an extensive time lag with an increased incidence of insulin-dependent DM (IDDM) in patients with CRS. Patients with CRS are at increased risk for IDDM if they have the same genetic and immunologic features seen in classic IDDM, namely the presence of HLA DR3 and the absence of HLA DR2 and if they have high prevalence of islet cell cytotoxic or surface antibodies (ICSA). This also may indicate that the genes controlling the susceptibility to T1 DM are necessary for the development of glucose intolerance in CRS patients (Ginsberg-Fellner *et al.*, 1985).

2.1.3   Mumps

Mumps virus is a paramyxovirus which has affinity for the pancreatic cells. The development of DM as a sequel of mumps pancreatitis has been reported in the literature since many decades (Harris, 1899). In most cases, symptoms of DM developed within 1-8 weeks after an infection. Several reports have discussed the relationship between mumps infection and the onset of autoimmune T1 DM with both clinical and epidemiological evidences showed the close relation between apparent or in-apparent mumps infection and DM. In vitro studies have suggested that cytokines released by mumps virus-infected beta cells may lead to an immune response against the beta cells which eventually leading to complete loss of beta cell function. The findings could suggest the presence of an association between fulminant T1 DM and mumps virus infection (Goto *et al.*, 2008). Genetic factors may also contribute to the development of fulminant T1 DM. Imagawa *et al.* reported that DR4-DQ4 haplotype is frequent in fulminant T1 DM (Imagawa *et al.*, 2005).

2.1.4   Rotavirus

Rotaviruses is dsRNA Reoviridae; responsible for a significant number of childhood gastroenteritis. It has been implicated as one of the viral triggers of diabetes-associated autoimmunity. The reason for this implication was because of demonstration of sequence analogies between T-cell epitopes within the islet antigens GAD 65 (56 kDa isoform of glutamic acid decarboxylase) and IA-2 (islet antigen-2) and rotavirus protein, suggesting potential cross-reactivity mechanisms. Rotavirus was also able to grow in monkey pancreatic islets in vitro. Honeyman *et al* reported that DM associated autoantibodies appeared in their study children concomitantly with a rise in rotavirus IgG antibody titre. Rotavirus also can change the permeability and cytokine balance in the intestinal mucosa, and may thereby enhance autoimmunity. Rotavirus gastroenteritis can initiate cytokines induced severe epithelial dysfunction that commonly associates with the disease. While the cytokine IFN-γ affects the permeability at tight junctions in the mucosa, TNF-α and IFN-γ, produced excessively during a rotavirus infection, are directly toxic to, e.g. human colonic epithelial cells (Honeyman *et al.*, 2000). On the other hand, Blomqvist *et al* and Makela *et al* could not provide any evidence supporting an association between rotavirus infections and T1 DM or the presence of T1 DM-associated autoantibodies in young children. They failed to support the hypothesis that rotaviruses are important triggers of β-cell autoimmunity in young children at increased genetic risk for T1 DM (Blomqvist *et al.*, 2005 and Makela *et al.*, 2006). Therefore, it can be concluded that the role of rotavirus in the aetiology of T1 DM is unconfirmed (Coppieters *et al.*, 2012).

2.1.5   Measles

Measles virus is one member of paramyxoviridae family. Measles infections generally occur in childhood, but infections in adolescence and adulthood can lead to major complications. Type 1 diabetes is among the various systemic disorders which have been associated with measles, with varying strengths of association. The Swedish Childhood DM Study showed significantly higher rate of T1 DM in children who developed DM among those not vaccinated against measles. The study hypothesized that measles vaccine could have a protective effect, and measles infection could have a diabetogenic effect (Blom *et al.*, 1991). Onal *et al* described a previously healthy 28 years old woman who developed T1 DM complicated with ketoacidosis following measles virus infection. Serological tests revealed significant elevation of the measles IgM and IgG titers (Onal *et al.*, 2012). However, a study done by Ramondetti *et al* showed that there was no statistical significance between the incidence of measles cases and DM rates which make the association between measles and T1 DM to be unclear (Ramondetti *et al.*, 2012).

2.1.6   Cytomegalovirus

Cytomegalovirus (CMV) is a member of the Herpesviridae family which commonly infect humans of all ages and reaches most of the population. It has a unique capacity to remain latent in tissues after recovery of the host from an acute infection. Infection with cytomegalovirus is one of the environmental factors implicated in the development of T1 DM, although the association remains unproven. Some clinical studies relate human CMV to the development of T1 DM in humans. The CMV specific viral genome was found in 22% of diabetic patients, correlating with the presence of islet cell autoantibodies in their serum. Molecular mimicry could be involved in CMV-induced diabetes by inducing islet cell autoantibodies. In addition, a CD4 T cell clone reactive to GAD65 is able to cross-reacts with a peptide of human CMV major DNA-binding protein (Alba *et al.*, 2005). Pak *et al* showed strong correlation between CMV genome and islet cell autoantibodies detected in diabetic patients suggests that persistent CMV infections may be relevant to pathogenesis in some cases of T1 DM (Pak *et al.*, 1988). The study done by Hjelmesæth *et al.*, supported the hypothesis that asymptomatic CMV infection is associated with increased risk of new-onset post-transplant DM, and suggests that impaired insulin release may involve one pathogenetic mechanism (Hjelmesæth *et al.*, 2004). The same findings were supported by the study of Zanone *et al* which showed that the association of T1 DM to cytomegalovirus infection and linked the increased risk of new onset post-transplantation DM to the associated CMV infection (Zanone *et al* 2010). On the other hand; Aarnisalo *et al* observed no association between perinatal CMV infection and progression to T1 DM. They showed that perinatal CMV infections are not associated with early serological signs of β-cell autoimmunity or progression to T1 DM in children with diabetes risk-associated HLA genotype (Aarnisalo *et al.*, 2008).

2.1.7   Influenza B

Influenza B virus is a member of Orthomyxoviridae family and is one of the viruses implicated in pathogenesis of fulminant T1 DM especially for class II HLA. A number of case reports described occurrence of fulminant T1 DM after infection with Influenza B virus. Sano *et al* described a 64 years old Japanese man who developed fulminant T1 DM following infection with influenza B virus (Sano *et al.*, 2008). Feng *et al.* also reported development of fulminant T1 DM in a 45-year-old Chinese woman who was heterozygous for HLA-DR7-DQ2 and HLA-DR9-DQ9. Yasuda *et al.*, reported occurrence of fulminant T1 DM with thrombocytopenia after influenza vaccination in a 54 years old man with HLA genotypes consistent with susceptibility to fulminant T1 DM. However, lack of well organized studies makes the role of Influenza B virus in development of fulminant T1 DM still unproven.

2.1.8   Epstein-Barr Virus

Epstein-Bar virus (EBV) is a member of the Herpesviridae family. It has been implicated in the aetiology of autoimmune diseases including autoimmune diabetes. A temporal link between EBV infection and the onset of T1 DM has been reported in a rare number of cases but without a strong association between EBV infection and development of T1 DM. However, some evidence suggests that EBV could trigger T1 DM by a mechanism of molecular mimicry. An 11 amino acid sequence in the Asp-57 region of the HLA-DQw8 beta chain is repeated 6 times in the EBV-BRF4-encoded epitope (Alba *et al.*, 2005). Some individuals who carry this sequence (GPPAA) in their HLA-DQ molecule present antibody reactivity to this epitope in EBV. As reported by Parkkonen F *et al*; two out of seven individuals who had acute EBV infection produced antibodies against an EBV-derived peptide (GPPAAGPPAAGPPAA). These two cases also contracted T1 DM immediately after the infection. This phenomenon may have potential importance in EBV-induced abnormalities, although cross-reactivity against DQ molecules could not be demonstrated in this study (Parkkonen *et al.*, 1994). Further investigation is needed to confirm a relationship between EBV and T1 DM.

2.1.9   Hepatitis C Virus (HCV)

HCV is a member of Flaviviridae family. Several studies from different parts of the world have reported that HCV infection may contribute to the development of DM, and higher prevalence of T2 DM has been observed in patients with HCV infection than in those with other forms of chronic hepatitis. Allison *et al.* were the first to link viral hepatitis C to DM in 1994. They did a retrospective study included 100 cirrhotic patients listed for transplantation. They reported that the prevalence of T2 DM was higher in patients with HCV-associated cirrhosis than in cirrhotics with other underlying liver diseases (Allison *et al.*, 1994). HCV infection is more closely related to DM than HBV infection. In a study done by Rouabhia *et al*; there was a higher prevalence of DM in patients with HCV infection (39.1%) than in those with HBV infection (5%), and DM occured at an early stage of hepatic disease. However, other factors such as metabolic syndrome, family history of DM and increased transaminases seem also to be important risk factors for the development of DM (Rouabhia *et al.*, 2010). Mehta *et al* found an increased prevalence of T2 DM among persons with HCV infection who were at least 40 years of age (Mehta *et al.*, 2000). The mechanisms by which HCV induces increased insulin resistance and the risk for development of DM has not been completely understood. Liver fibrosis progression has long been considered responsible for the appearance of insulin resistance and T2 DM in patients with chronic liver diseases. The mechanism through which HCV is associated with insulin resistance involves interference with insulin signalling, direct viral effects, pro-inflammatory cytokines, and suppressors of cytokine signalling. Excessive tumor necrosis factor alpha (TNF-α) released in HCV-infected patient's response may mediate the induction of insulin resistance. Other potential mechanisms that have been proposed include the development of insulin resistance as a consequence of elevated iron stores or fatty liver disease, both of which are associated with HCV infection. However, other studies showed that HCV infection was only associated with abnormal glucose tolerance (either impaired glucose tolerance (IGT) or frank DM) in obese participants (Howard *et al.*, 2007).

2.1.10   Hepatitis B (HBV)

HBV is one of the hepadanviridae family. There is a lower risk of DM in HBV infection which could be explained by two factors: (1) HBV infection has been controlled in most developed countries, with active HBV vaccination programme; the occurrence of chronic HBV and its complications in these countries is very low; and (2) The disease progression is rather fast in HBV infection and therefore very few patients reach the level of cirrhosis and thus DM frequency is lower in this population (Naing *et al.*, 2012).

2.1.11   Human Immune Deficiency Virus (HIV)

HIV is one of the Retroviridae family. The association between HIV infection and DM is poorly understood and complicated by the differential prevalence of risk factors for DM in HIV infected persons compared with HIV uninfected persons. While HIV infection itself is not associated with increased risk of DM, increasing age, HCV co-infection and body mass index (BMI) have a more profound effect upon the risk of DM among HIV infected persons. Further, long term anti-retroviral (ARV) treatment also increases risk (Butt *et al.*, 2009).

2.1.12   Possible Role of Other Viruses

Many other viruses had some circumstantial evidences of their role in development of DM like hepatitis A virus, varicella zoster virus, and polio virus. However, scientific evidence still needed to prove this relationship. There are also many other viruses that can induce DM in animals like *Kilham rat virus, Bovine viral diarrhoea-mucosal disease virus, Encephalomyocarditis virus, Mengovirus, Mouse hepatitis virus, Lactate dehydrogenase virus* and *Ljungan virus*. These viruses are usually used to induce experimental diabetes.

2.2   Bacterial Infections

2.2.1   *Helicobacter Pylori* (*H. pylori*)

H pylori is a gram-negative, spiral-shaped pathogenic bacterium that colonizes in the gastric mucosa and causes chronic gastritis, peptic ulcer disease, and/or gastric malignancies with a prevalence rate of about 30% in developed and up to 80% in developing countries. *H. pylori* infection has been positively related to DM prevalence in many studies (Lutsey *et al.*, 2009). *H. pylori* infection may cause dyslipidemia, because of the elevated levels of total cholesterol, low-density lipoprotein cholesterol (LDL-c), lipoprotein Lp(a), apolopoprotein apo-B, triglyceride concentrations and decreased levels of high-density lipoprotein cholesterol (HDL-C) and apolipoprotein apoA-1 concentration in the blood. In addition, plasma levels of cholesterol and LDL-c were significantly higher in *H. pylori* positive patients with ischemic stroke compared to *H. pylori* positive patients (Scharnagl *et al.*, 2004; and Kamada *et al.*, 2005). This change in lipid profile toward an atherogenic direction is due to the action of pro-inflammatory cytokines, such as IL-1 and IL-6, INF-α, and TNF-α. *H. pylori* infection can promote platelet activation and aggregation and increase various proatherogenic factors including homocysteine, which is a risk factor for T2 DM, obesity, and CVD. It also can increase reactive oxygen free radicals and increases circulating concentrations of lipid peroxides, also associated with DM and CVD. Finally, *H. pylori* infection influences the apoptosis. This may play an important role in development of metabolic syndrome, and insulin resistance; suggesting a possible mechanistic relationship between *H. pylori* and DM (Polyzos *et al.*, 2011). Jeon *et al.* demonstrated in a prospective cohort study that *H. pylori* infection leads to an increased rate of incident DM. They found that the seropositive for *H. pylori* at enrolment were 2.7 times more likely at any given time to develop DM than seronegative individual (Jeon *et al.*, 2012). However a previous study by Xia *et al* showed that *H. pylori* infection appears not to be associated with DM or upper gastrointestinal symptoms in DM (Xia *et al.*, 2005). However; there is a great need for further studies on the potential causative role of *H. pylori* on DM that could be used to inform effective prevention strategies for DM.

2.2.2   Other Bacteria

The role of other bacteria in pathogenesis of DM is controversial. Bacterial meningitis can induce hyperglycaemic blood glucose levels in majority of patients on admission. Hyperglycemia may be caused by the physical stress reaction, abnormal blood-glucose regulation mechanisms as a result of central nervous system insults, and preponderance of diabetics for pneumococcal meningitis. Patients with DM and bacterial meningitis are at high risk for unfavorable outcome (Schut *et al.*, 2009). Other bacterial infections like scarlet fever or typhoid fever were implicated in development of fulminant T1 DM but still need to be investigated.

3   Diabetes-preventing Infections

Despite that the viruses can be strong inducers of inflammation; the viral infections and other types of infectious diseases would actually prevent T1 DM. According to the "hygiene hypothesis"; viruses invoke immune mechanisms that help in elimination of auto aggressive T-cells attacking the β-cells, ultimately leading to their immediate but temporally limited amelioration. Instead of enhancing immune function and exerting effector functions such as killing of infected cells or inducing interferon production, the viral infection can turn immune responses off through distinct immunoregulatory mechanisms, involving both the innate and adaptive immune system, that protect against the development of T1 DM. Many of these mechanisms involve the secretion of immune modulatory cytokines such as IL-10, IL-4, or transforming growth factor (TGF)-β (Herrath, 2009). Invariant NKT cells (iNKT cells) are non-conventional T lymphocytes restricted by the CD1d molecule, which presents glycolipid antigens. Many studies have shown the protective role of iNKT cells against the development of autoimmune diseases, including T1 DM. Although iNKT cells inhibit autoimmune responses, they also promote immune responses against viruses. When stimulated; the iNKT cells promptly secrete copious amounts of various cytokines, and they can provide activation/maturation signals to other immune cells such as DCs, NK cells, T cells, and B cells. With certain viral infections; these cells also can promote plasmacytoid DC (pDC) function locally in the pancreatic islets, leading to enhanced type-I IFN production and low viral burden (Nishio *et al.*, 2010 and Diana *et al.*, 2009). So that restoration of efficient regulatory T cell (T reg cell) populations is therefore a promising therapeutic approach to prevent and even cure disease with the ultimate goal is to tackle the disease at its root, to eliminate the cause for T1 DM (Nishio *et al.*, 2010).

Infections with several pathogens such as *lymphocytic choriomeningitis virus* (LCMV), some *enteroviruses, helminths* or *Salmonella* have been shown to significantly decrease DM incidence. Most of the studies were performed in animal models because of the limited availability of relevant human samples in T1 DM research. Pierce *et al* showed that specific areas in some viral genomes can help to decrease the incidence of autoimmune DM. Autoimmune T1 DM is inhibited in non-obese diabetic (NOD) mice transgenically expressing all early region 3 (E3) genes of the adenovirus genome under control of a rat insulin promoter (RIPE3/NOD). Genes in E3 of the adenovirus genome allow the virus to evade host immune responses by interfering with MHC class I-mediated antigen presentation and TNF-α or Fas-induced apoptosis of infected cells. These findings indicate that all E3 genes must be expressed to inhibit the diabetogenic potential of NOD immune cells. They also demonstrate that the antiapoptotic E3 genes most effectively protect pancreatic β-cells from diabetogenic immune responses (Pierce *et al*; 2003). Filippi *et al* showed that viruses that do not inflict damage on β-cells provided protection from T1 DM by triggering immune-regulatory mechanisms. They showed that infection of pre-diabetic NOD mice with Coxsackie virus B3 or LCMV delayed DM onset and reduced disease incidence. This delay was due to transient up-regulation of programmed cell death-1 ligand 1 (PD-L1) on lymphoid cells, which prevented the expansion of diabetogenic CD8+ T cells expressing programmed cell death-1 (PD-1). Reduced T1 DM incidence was caused by increased numbers of invigorated CD4+CD25+ Tregs, which produced TGF-β and maintained long-term tolerance. Full protection from T1 DM resulted from synergy between PD-L1 and CD4+CD25+ Tregs (Filippi *et al.*, 2009).

Not only the viral infection could prevent development of DM but also other microbes may have similar effects. Silva *et al* showed that immune-stimulation with Q fever complement-fixing antigen (QFA) can prevent the development of autoimmune DM. However, the mechanism whereby QFA protects against DM currently is not known (Silva *et al.*, 2003). Infection, commencing across a wide age range, with a live, attenuated strain of *Salmonella typhimurium*, will halt the development of T1 DM in the NOD mice. Zaccone *et al* showed that infection of NOD mice with attenuated, but not killed, *Salmonella typhimurium* can reduce the incidence of T1 DM, even if infection occurs after the development of a peri-islet pancreatic infiltrate. Functional diabetogenic effector T cells were still present, as demonstrated by the initiation of DM in NOD-scid recipients of transferred splenocytes. High levels of IFN-γ were secreted by splenocytes of infected mice, but there was no evidence of involvement of IL-10 in the protective effect of the infection (Zaccone *et al.*, 2004). The protective mechanism appears to involve the regulation of autoreactive T cells in a manner associated with long lasting changes in the innate immune compartment of these mice. The autoreactive T cells priming and trafficking were altered in mice that had been infected previously by *S. typhimurium*. These changes were associated with sustained alterations in patterns of chemokine expression. There was small numbers of dendritic cells from mice that had been previously infected with, but cleared all trace of a *S. Typhimurium;* which were able to prevent the development of DM in the highly synchronized and aggressive cyclophosphamide-induced model. The effects observed on autoreactive T cell trafficking were recapitulated by the immunomodulatory dendritic cell transfers in the cyclophosphamide model (Raine *et al*., 2006). Ola *et al* showed that the intranasal treatment with the B-subunit of *Escherichia coli* heat labile enterotoxin (EtxB), a protein that binds GM1 ganglioside (as well as GD1b, asialo-GM1 and lactosylceramide with lower affinities), protected NOD mice from developing DM in a receptor-binding dependent manner. Protection was associated with a significant reduction in the number of macrophages, CD4(+) T cells, B cells, and major histocompatibility complex class II (+) cells infiltrating the islets (Ola *et al*.,2006).

Infection with *Mycobacteria* or immunization of mice with *Mycobacteria*-containing adjuvant was able to prevent DM in NOD mice. Infection of NOD mice with *Mycobacterium avium*, done before the mice show overt DM, resulted in permanent protection of the animals from DM and this protective effect was associated with increased numbers of CD4þ T cells and B220þ B cells. The protective effect of *M. avium* infection against DM of NOD mice may be achieved by peripheral deletion of autoreactive T lymphocytes via Fas–FasL. The event may result from molecular mimicry between mycobacterial antigen and pancreatic autoantigens, leading to deletion of lymphocytes reactive to β-cells as a consequence of the immune response directed to *Mycobacteria*, or simply deletion of bystander autoreactive lymphocytes. The regulatory role of Fas up-regulation on activated lymphocytes could then be able to suppress unintended activation of autoreactive clones, thereby protecting against the initiation of the autoimmune aggression of the pancreatic islets of NOD mice (Martins & Aguas; 1999). Bergerot *et al* showed that oral intake of small amounts (2-20 µg) of human insulin conjugated to cholera toxin B subunit (CTB) can effectively suppress β-cell destruction and clinical DM in adult NOD mice. The protective effect could be transferred by T cells from CTB-insulin-treated animals and was associated with reduced lesions of insulitis. Furthermore, adoptive co-transfer experiments involving injection of Thy-1,2 recipients with diabetogenic T cells from syngeneic mice and T cells from congenic Thy-1,1 mice fed with CTB-insulin demonstrated a selective recruitment of Thy-1,1 donor cells in the peripancreatic lymph nodes concomitant with reduced islet cell infiltration. These results suggest that protection against autoimmune DM can be achieved by feeding minute amounts of a pancreas islet cell autoantigen linked to CTB and appears to involve the selective migration and retention of protective T cells into lymphoid tissues draining the site of organ injury (Bergerot *et al*., 1997).

Helminth infestation can modulate the immune response. Intestinal nematode parasites can produce strong polarized Th2-type responses in mice. Helminth infection can enhance susceptibility to certain infectious diseases, like TB and viral hepatitis but also have protective effects in murine models of asthma, multiple sclerosis, and inflammatory bowel disease. Inoculation of NOD with *Trichinella spiralis*, *Heligmosomoides polygyrus*, or *Schistosoma mansoni* markedly reduced the rate of T1 DM and suppressed lymphoid infiltration in the islets. Injection of whole eggs or soluble antigens from the schistosome egg antigen or the schistosome worm antigen in NOD mice was able to prevent T1 DM. Qian *et al* showed that the *H. polygyrus* strongly reduced the spontaneous onset of DM in NOD mice when given as late as 12 weeks of age and even prevented the much more aggressive Cyp-induced T1 DM in NOD mice. *H. Polygyrus* induced Th2-type response markedly increases in IL-10, FoxP3+ Tregs, and AAMɸs (Liu *et al* 2009). Jim´enez *et al* showed that *T. crassiceps* infection protects against Multiple Low Dose

Streptozotocin- Induced DM, independently of the genetic background of the host (Espinoza-Jiménez *et al.*, 2010).

4   Effects of Diabetes on Infections

Individuals with DM can have any infection that affects the general population with more increased risk of mortality and morbidity of a variety of specific infectious complications than in normal population. This increased risk is due to both the effect of DM on the immune system as well as the higher prevalence of pre-existing chronic conditions, such as cardiovascular disease or chronic kidney disease (CKD). The immune abnormalities in DM are due to higher pro-inflammatory pro-coagulant, and anti-fibrinolytic activity, depression of the antioxidant system, and humoral immunity as well as higher expression of pathogen recognition cell-surface receptors. There are also defects in leukocyte function, especially migration, phagocytosis, intracellular killing, chemotaxis; and complement dysfunction due to decreased polymorph nuclear (PMN) membrane fluidity. These changes occur especially with poor glycemic control, and microvascular and macrovascular angiopathy which increase soft tissue and organ infections in diabetic patients. There is also a decrease in the antibacterial activity of urine, gastrointestinal and urinary dysmotility, and greater number of medical interventions in these patients. Peripheral sensory neuropathy may result in unawareness of lower extremity trauma and inadequate attention to minor wounds with increased incidence of infection. The higher mortality of infection in diabetic patients is also due to the increased risk of acute organ dysfunction due to higher chronic disease burden (Yende *et al.*, 2010).

The infections affect all organs and systems. There is an increased frequency and severity of many infections among diabetic patients which include foot infections; rhinocerebral mucormycosis; cystitis; complicated urinary tract infections, including pyelonephritis; intrarenal abscesses; perinephric abscesses; pneumonia; lower-extremity soft tissue infection, including polymicrobial gangrene; emphysematous or gangrenous cholecystitis; and malignant otitis externa. There is also increased carrier state rate of *Staphylococcus aureus* among those patients which raises risk for infection with this organism. There are different risk factors which may act alone or in combination in favour of certain infections. Hyperglycemia is nearly a constant risk factor for most infections. Male sex is a risk factor for emphysematous cholecystitis caused by *Clostridium perfingens* while the female sex is a risk factor for urinary tract infection. Insulin injection is a risk factor for infections with *Staphylococcus aureus*. Angiopathy is a risk factor for polymicrobial soft tissue infection especially with *Streptococci*, *anaerobes*, and *gram-negative bacteria*. Age is very important risk factor for both pneumonia and emphysematous cholecystitis (Schaberg & Norwood; 2002).

4.1   Respiratory Tract Infections

4.1.1   Effects on Pneumonia

Pneumonia is a major cause of morbidity and mortality among diabetic patients with a higher risk of death following pneumonia than in non diabetics. About 20% of subjects with community acquired pneumonia (CAP) have DM with an increased incidence of pneumonia due to different pathogens in diabetic patients. There is an increase in *S. aureus* caused pneumonia secondary to nasal carriage, particularly among recently hospitalized diabetic patients. There is also increased incidence of pneumonia due to both *gram-negative* organisms and fungi among those patients. Diabetes was present in 69% of patients with *Escherichia coli* pneumonia. The most frequent respiratory infections associated with DM are caused by *Streptococcus pneumoniae* and influenza virus. Despite that the incidence of pneumococcal infection was virtually identical in diabetic and non-diabetic subjects; however, the diabetic subjects are 15.8-25.6 times more likely to be hospitalized for pneumonia during the first 13 weeks of the influenza season. The relative risk of hospitalization for influenza is 5.7-6.2 times greater in diabetic than non-diabetic subjects. The severity of *Streptococcus pneumonia* and influenza was more aggressive in diabetic patients than that found in the general population. This increased rate of hospitalization may be due to the lower threshold for hospitalization for treatment of complicated pneumonia in diabetic subjects (Bouter *et al.*, 1991). Pneumonia was a contributing factor in 25% of the fatal cases of diabetic ketoacidosis. *Klebsiella pneumonia* and *S. aureus* were the most frequent causes. The mortality due to pneumonia and influenza in diabetic patients who were diagnosed at age of 30 years was 1.7 times higher than for non-diabetic subjects. Younger-onset patients with DM (age <30 years) were 7.6 times more likely to die from these infections over an average follow-up period of 8.5 years (Wheat; 1980). The increase in mortality is not only due to an altered immune response, but may be due to worsening of pre-existing cardiovascular and kidney disease (Yende *et al.*, 2010).

4.1.2 Tuberculosis (TB)

Diabetes is a high risk factor for infection with TB with higher risk for development of multi-resistant TB and that treatment failures and death in diabetic than in non diabetic patients. Tuberculosis developed most frequently in patients with poor glycaemic control. Diabetic patients who needed more than 40 units of insulin per day are twice as likely to develop TB as those using lower doses, thus linking severity of DM with risk of TB (Dooley & Chaisson; 2009). DM depresses the immune response (impairing chemotaxis, phagocytosis, and antigen presentation in response to *Mycobacterium tuberculosis* infection and affecting T-cell function and proliferation) facilitating infection and progression to symptomatic disease. The American Thoracic Society includes patients with DM in their list of patients who are considered immunosuppressed enough to require isoniazid for a positive purified protein derivative (PPD). Diabetic TB has been described as an acute, exudative, rapidly caseating disease that progresses to a toxic downhill course. Patients with DM also present with more advanced disease and are more liable to have lower lobe disease. TB infection and treatment also might induce glucose intolerance and complicate the glycemic control i.e. rifampicin increasing the metabolism of oral antidiabetic drugs. Diabetic patients with positive tuberculin reactions who have never been treated should receive isoniazid and pyridoxine for 1 yr regardless of their age or radiographic findings due to potentially greater severity of TB in diabetic individuals (Dooley & Chaisson 2009; Ruslami *et al.*, 2010; Wheat; 1980).

4.1.3 Influenza and H1N1

Influenza increases frequency of medical consultation, hospitalization, ICU admission, and risk of death in diabetic population. About 14-21% of the hospitalized patients due to influenza A (H1N1) are diabetics. Conversely, the risk of respiratory illness and of hospitalization within 14 days of a diagnosis of influenza in patients with DM may be reduced by oseltamivir.

4.2 Urinary Tract Infections

Urinary tract infections are among the more common infection in diabetic patients especially in women. There is higher incidence of urinary tract infections especially in upper tract in diabetic patients than in non diabetics. Although the majority of urinary tract infections in diabetic patients are asymptomatic, DM also may lead to a predisposition to more severe infections. The most common organisms involved are *E. coli*, followed by other gram-negative bacteria. This increased incidence in DM is due to several predisposing factors. Diabetic neuropathy can cause neurogenic bladder and dysfunction which is probably the most important predisposing factor. The neurogenic bladder causes obstruction of normal urine flow. Obstruction of the lower urinary tract enhances the development of urinary tract infections especially pyelonephritis. Diabetes-associated angiopathy correlates with the increased incidence of urinary tract infection in diabetic patient. The glucosuria and the high concentrations of urinary glucose impair phagocytic function of polymorph nuclear leukocytes. Also the higher rate of urologic procedures and manipulation is also an important predisposing factor in some cases. The common renal infections in diabetic patients include pyelonephritis, renal carbuncles (intra-renal abscesses caused by hematogenous spread of *S. aureus*), renal corticomedullary abscesses, perinephric abscesses, and the rare but devastating emphysematous pyelonephritis. Nosocomial urinary tract infections are also more common in diabetic individuals.

Acute pyelonephritis was found to be four-to fivefold higher in diabetic than in non-diabetic individuals. A possible explanation for this increased rate may be reflected in the studies that show lower urinary tract obstruction. It is associated with risk of bacteraemia, long hospitalization, and mortality especially in elderly diabetics (Kofteridis *et al.*, 2009). However, Rhee *et al* found that an older age and DM were not found to be independently associated with hospital admission in women with acute pyelonephritis (Rhee *et al.* 2011). The presence of small vessel disease superimposed on renal parenchymal infection may account for the high incidence of renal papillary necrosis in diabetic persons. Presence of bacteraemia indicates severe infection. Most infections are caused by *Escherichia coli* or *Proteus sp.* The clinical presentation is similar to that of non-diabetic individuals, except for the bilateral renal involvement. Additionally, persons with DM are at increased risk for complications such as perinephric and/or renal abscesses, emphysematous pyelonephritis, and renal papillary necrosis (Peleg *et al.*, 2007).

Emphysematous pyelonephritis (EPN) is a severe necrotizing kidney infection characterized by gas production in or around the kidneys (in perinephric tissue). It is a rare and often life threatening condition that commonly occurs in diabetics and may require life-saving urgent nephrectomy. Over 70% of reported cases have occurred in diabetic patients. The enteric *gram-negative bacilli* such as *Escherichia coli* and *Enterobacter aerogenes* are the most frequent pathogens, followed by *Klebsiella sp., Proteus sp., Candida and Streptococcus* with *E. coli* accounting for 60%. Gas formation in EPN is due to pathogenic bacteria causing mixed acid fermentation in a hyperglycemic environment in tissues that are ischemic. This results in tissue destruction and encourages purulent infection and inhibition of removal of locally produced gas. Fever and flank pain are nearly always present, and a renal mass can be felt in 45% of cases. Crackles in the flank or thigh are less frequent. Abdominal radiographs frequently show mottled lucencies overlying the kidneys. Abdominal computerized tomography allows the identification of gas in the urinary tract. Survival is higher in patients managed with antibiotics plus surgery (67%) than with antibiotic therapy alone (30%). Surgery is recommended for patients who do not improve after a few days of antibiotic therapy (Laway *et al.*, 2012).

Renal carbuncles (intrarenal abscesses) are caused by the hematogenous spread of *S. Aureus* while renal corticomedullary abscesses are intrarenal foci of infection associated with reflux and obstruction caused by the same organisms that typically cause pyelonephritis. Perinephric abscesses may be more common in diabetic patients. DM is present in about one-third of patients with perinephric abscesses. Perinephric abscesses are caused either by the rupture of intrarenal abscesses into tissue surrounding the kidney or by the hematogenous or lymphatic deposition of organisms into that tissue. *E. coli* or other organisms are usually isolated, but a wide variety of organisms, such as *S. aureus, fungi, anaerobes, and mycobacteria*, have been reported. *Staphylococci* cause about 10% of cases. The onset typically is insidious. Symptoms have been present for more than 5 days in the majority of patients with perinephric abscesses compared with only about 10% of patients with pyelonephritis. It should be suspected in patients with urinary tract infections and an abdominal or flank mass or persistent fever after 4 days of antimicrobial therapy. Effective treatment requires surgical drainage of the abscess in addition to specific antibiotics. Papillary necrosis is another important complication of urinary tract infections in diabetic patients. DM has been present in over 50% of patients with papillary necrosis. Papillary necrosis was found to be about five times more frequent in diabetic than non-diabetic individuals. It should be suspected if patients with urinary tract infections responds poorly to antimicrobial therapy or develops renal insufficiency (Casqueiro *et al.*; 2012).

Cystitis emphysematosa is less severe and is usually cured by antibiotics alone. It is characterized by the presence of gas vesicles in the bladder wall. It is associated with infection by *coliform* organisms in patients with glycosuria. A history of pneumoturia may be obtained although the diagnosis is made radiographically. Its course is benign (Schaberg & Norwood; 2002). Asymptomatic bacteriuria (ASB) refers to the presence of bacteria in bladder urine in an asymptomatic individual. It is a significant risk factor for pyelonephritis and renal dysfunction in diabetic patients. The most commonly isolated microorganism was *Escherichia coli*. The duration of DM, high HbA1c, glucosuria and pyuria are risk factors for ASB in diabetic patients. Bacteriuria may be a marker for bladder neuropathy indicating more severe DM. Also; new retinopathy appeared in 21% of diabetic patients with persistent bacteriuria compared with only 4% of diabetic patients whose bacteriuria cleared. It is more in the diabetic women than in diabetic men. Some studies reported progression to pyelonephritis, whereas other suggested that this does not lead to serious complications. Thus, routine recommendation of antibiotic therapy for asymptomatic bacteriuria in diabetic women remains controversial (Casqueiro *et al.*; 2012).

Urinary fungal infections are more common in diabetic patients than non-diabetics; the majority of which are clinically insignificant. Diabetes is present in 20%- 90% of patients with *Torulopsis glabrata* urinary tract infections. *Candida* was cultured from the urine of 35% of glycosuric diabetic persons in one study. Both *Candida* and *T. glabrata* can cause cystitis, pyelonephritis, renal or perinephric abscesses, fungus balls, and a clinical picture identical to gram-negative sepsis. Several factors may explain the predisposition of diabetic patients to fungal infections of the urinary tract. Glycosuria has been shown to be important. Yeast is present in the urine of 35% of diabetic patients with glycosuria compared with only 9% of diabetic patients without glycosuria. Fungal cystitis may result in the formation of "fungal balls" which may cause urinary tract obstruction. Unfortunately, some *Candida* and *T. glabrata* are initially resistant to 5-fluorocytosine and others become resistant during therapy (Segireddy *et al.*, 2011).

4.3   Gastrointestinal and Hepatic Infections

The regularity of gastrointestinal motility and sensitivity are important mechanisms of defence against infections. Diabetes is responsible for about one quarter of gastroparesis. Both chronic hyperglycemia and gastrointestinal dysmotility contribute to increase the risk of gastrointestinal infectious processes. Common gastrointestinal and liver infection in diabetic patients include; *H. pylori*; oesophageal *candidiasis*; emphysematous cholecystitis; *Hepatitis C*; and *Hepatitis B* infection.

4.3.1   H. Pylori Infection

Many studies evaluated the prevalence of *H. pylori* infection in diabetic patients and the possible role of this infection in their metabolic control. Some studies found a higher prevalence of the infection in diabetic patients and reduced glycemic control while others did not support any correlation between metabolic control and *H. pylori* infection. Infection with *H. pylori* is common in diabetic patients who have inadequate metabolic control as such individuals are colonized by *H. pylori* in the gastric antrum, probably because of chemotactic factors such as tumor necrotic factor (TNF), interleukins-IL1, IL2, and IL8 which are present in gastric epithelium. These cytokines induce a number of changes in the gastric epithelium that promote inflammation and epithelial damage thus leading to increased risk of aberrant repair giving the picture of gastric atrophy or epithelial cell metaplasia. Infection with *H. pylori* is an important factor for diabetes-associated dyspepsia. The role of *H. pylori* infection in diabetic dyspepsia is mainly related to blood glucose concentration. Hyperglycemia may induce infection by *H. pylori* or the silent infection may get reactivated and produce symptoms of dyspepsia in DM (Saluja *et al.*, 2002; Devrajani *et al.*, 2010).

4.3.2   Oral Eosophageal Candidiasis

Candida albicans is the most common etiological agent. The increased frequency of oro-esophageal candidiasis is due to both the increase in its virulence and the production of extracellular enzymes such as proteinase and phospholipase. It can be manifested as median rhomboid glossitis or central papillary atrophy, atrophic glossitis, denture stomatitis, pseudomembranous candidiasis, and angular cheilitis. Oesophageal candidiasis needs high suspicion and endoscopy is required (Menezes *et al.*, 2007).

4.3.3   Emphysematous Cholecystitis

Emphysematous cholecystitis is a rare but severe infection associated with gas-forming organisms such as *Clostridial* species and other anaerobes. It occurs more frequently in male diabetics. However, nowadays; *Salmonella enteritidis* and *Campylobacter* are the main pathogens. It presented with the same clinical presentation of non-complicated cholecystitis with right upper quadrant abdominal pain, vomiting, and fever. However, patients with this illness are usually more ill and crackles can be felt on abdominal palpation which may denote with a worse prognosis. Clinical signs of peritonitis are usually not observed. The diagnosis is made by the detection of gas inside the gall bladder, demonstrated in radiograph or computerized tomography imaging of the abdomen. Treatment is by a combined surgical intervention and antibiotic therapy (Calvet & Yoshikawa; 2001).

4.3.4   Hepatitis C (HCV)

As mentioned before that infection with *hepatitis C* increases the risk of having DM. About one third of patients with *HCV* infection have DM, mostly T2 DM. Patients with HCV are 3 times more likely to develop DM than individuals who are *HCV* negative. Association of DM with *hepatitis C* infection increases the severity of the liver disease and degree of fibrosis compared to non-diabetic *HCV* patients. The frequency of DM increased along with pathological staging. The fibrosis score was higher in diabetic *HCV* patients. Liver biopsy specimens of diabetic HCV patients showed higher inflammatory activity defined by histological activity index score than the nondiabetic *HCV* group for moderate and severe stages. Individuals with T2 DM have a higher incidence of liver function test (LFT) abnormalities than individuals who do not have DM (Elhawary *et al.*, 2011).

4.3.5   Hepatitis B (HBV)

HBV infection outbreaks have been reported among diabetic patients who received routine finger sticks. Transmission was attributed to the use of shared equipment and lapses in aseptic technique or infection control practices associated with blood glucose monitoring (Perz & Fiore, 2005).

4.4   Skin and Soft Tissue Infections

Diabetes mellitus is associated with increased frequency of skin and soft tissue infections such as folliculitis, furunculosis, and subcutaneous abscesses. Incidence ranges from 20-50%, mostly in T2 DM. The major underlying cause is hyperglycemia and ketoacidosis leading to immune dysfunction. Recurrent furunculosis and folliculitis especially of the back may be the first sign of DM presentation. Pyodermic infections such as impetigo, folliculitis, carbuncles, furunculosis, ecthyma, and erysipelas if present can be more severe and widespread in diabetic patients. Soft tissue infections of the lower extremities and gangrene are among the most dreaded complications associated with DM. Patients with DM clearly have an elevated risk of infected lower-extremity ulceration and subsequent amputation (Lipsky *et al.*, 2010). Fungal skin infection especially mucocutaneous *Candida* occurs more frequently in diabetic patients, especially those with poorly controlled disease. Candidal infection can be an early sign of undiagnosed DM. Perlèche is a classic sign of DM in children, and localized candidal infection of the female genitalia (vulvovaginitis) has a strong association with DM. It is important to remember that in men, Candida balanitis, and intertrigo (axillary, inguinal web space), can be the presenting signs of DM. Paronychia, onychomycosis and glossitis are also common (Mujtaba, 2009). Association of dermatophyte infection with DM is controversial but recent data shows a statistically significant relationship. Common superficial infections are caused by *Trichophyton rubrum, T mentagrophytes,* and *Epidermophyton floccosum.* In diabetic patients, onychomycosis or tinea pedis should be monitored and treated, as it can be a port of entry for infection. This is especially true for patients with neurovascular complications and intertrigo (Hattemn *et al.*; 2008).

4.4.1   Foot Infection

Diabetic foot infections are common, and serious. They are diverse, and can range from cellulitis of a toe to gangrene of the foot. Diagnostic and treatment strategies are correspondingly varied. Foot ulcers usually occur in patients with sensory polyneuropathy who develop skin breakdown after unrecognized trauma. These infections can be monomicrobial but usually polymicrobial. *S. aureus* and *S. epidermidis* are isolated from around 60% of all the infected ulcers. *Enterococci, streptococci,* and *enterobacteria* are less frequent, and 15% of the infected ulcers have strict anaerobic bacteria. Infection in a very recently acquired superficial ulcer is likely to be monomicrobial due to aerobic *gram-positive cocci*, such as *staphylococci*, while a long duration of ulceration and increased depth are likely to increase the chances of the wound, yielding both polymicrobial growth and resistant organisms (Nicolau & Stein; 2010). Infection easily occurs in tissue with an inadequate microvascular or macrovascular blood supply. Uncontrolled soft tissue infection can then lead to necrotizing processes and systemic sepsis. The clinical presentations of these infections are very variable and poor, often leading to delayed diagnosis especially with less pain sensation due to diabetic neuropathy. The diabetic foot infections are usually classified into moderate or "non-limb threatening" and serious or "limb-threatening". Moderate infections are defined as superficial, with cellulitis less than 2.0 cm in the largest diameter, without evidence of serious ischemia, systemic toxicity, or bone and/or articular involvement. Serious infections are defined as deep ulceration, with celullitis equal to or greater than 2.0 cm in the largest diameter, with evidence of serious ischemia, systemic toxicity, or bone and/or joint involvement (Joseph & Lipsky; 2010). Chronic infection, such as osteomyelitis, can also occur in conjunction with cutaneous ulcers. Treatment of these infections involves a combination of early surgical intervention for debridement or amputation and any necessary vascular repair, antibiotic therapy, and local wound care.

4.4.2   Necrotizing Fasciitis

Necrotizing fasciitis is characterized by fast and progressive necrosis of the fascia and subcutaneous tissue, causing fulminant local tissue destruction, microvascular thrombosis, and systemic signs of toxicity. About 10-60% of all cases of necrotizing fasciitis occur in patients with DM. It is a life threatening bacterial infection of the soft tissue with spread along facial planes; with a mortality of approximately 40% of the cases. The perenium, trunk, abdomen and upper extremities are most commonly involved. In DM fasciitis; although most cases result from polymicrobial facultative *gram negative bacilli* such as *Escheracia coli* and *anaerobes* such as *bacteroids, peptoptreptococcus* and *clostridium species*, approximately 10% cases are monomicrobial often due to *streptococcal species*. Type I fasciitis is caused by the combination of an anaerobic microorganism with one or more facultative aerobic microorganisms, and type II fasciitis is caused by a *group A streptococcus* with or without the involvement of *staphylococci*. The initial symptoms are fever and intense local pain, followed by areas of skin necrosis with small ulcers that drain a colourless fluid and have unpleasant smell. Degree of pain and toxicity are out of proportion to the severity of the findings. Air in the soft tissues can be better detected by radiograph. Treatment includes urgent surgical debridement and appropriate antibiotics (Shimizu & Tokuda, 2010; Oncul *et al.*, 2008)

4.4.3   Fournier Gangrene

Fournier gangrene is a fasciitis that affects the male genitalia causing fulminant gangrene of the penis and scrotum in young men. It can however occur at any age, women may be susceptible, but the disease predominantly affects men. Up to 70% of the patients with this infection have DM. It usually involves the scrotum, but can be extend to the penis, perineum, and abdominal wall. Contrary to the general belief, the testicles are usually spared. It is a life-threatening emergency with a mortality rate of up to 40%. Predisposing factors include DM, alcoholism, intravenous drug use, *HIV* and malignancy. Fournier's gangrene is caused by normal skin commensals of the perineum and genitalia which act synergistically to cause infection. The most common etiologic agents are *E. coli, Klebsiella sp., Proteus sp.,* and *Peptostreptococcus*. The etiology can also be polymicrobial, involving *Clostridium, aerobic* or *anaerobic streptococci,* and *Bacteroides*. Treatment involves vigorous antibiotic therapy, surgical debridement and treatment of identified predisposing factors.

4.5   Head and Neck Enfections

The two most serious head and neck infections in diabetic patients are invasive external otitis and rhinocerebral mucormycosis. Periodontal infection is also a common infection in diabetic patients.

4.5.1   Malignant Otitis Externa

Malignant otitis externa is a unique infection occurs almost exclusively in diabetic individuals, and usually seen in elderly persons. Recently, however, cases have been described in patients without diabetes. It is a severe, necrotizing infection of the external auditory canal that can extend to the skull base, adjacent regions, and central nervous system with high morbidity and mortality. It is caused almost exclusively by *Pseudomonas aeruginosa* but rarely by *Aspergillius*. *Pseudomonas aeruginosa* is not a part of the normal flora of the ear. The presence of that organism is thought to be increased in the presence of hot, humid conditions or following irrigation of the ear with non-sterile water. The organism is thought to penetrate the cartilage in the external auditory canal through the naturally occurring fissures of Santorini. A necrotizing cellulitis exacerbated by microvascular disease then occurs. Infection then involves mastoid air cells and the temporal bone. Subsequently, the base of the skull becomes involved. The infection begins insidiously, but it is characterized by a gradually worsening, excruciating pain, purulent discharge associated with a polypoid mass of granulation tissue. Signs of systemic infection such as fever and leukocytosis are absent. The soft tissues around the ear are swollen and tender. A polypoid mound of granulation tissue is seen in the ear canal at the osseus-cartilaginous junction in 90% of patients (Carfrae & Kesser, 2008).

Facial nerve paralysis complicates 50% of cases. Skull base osteomyelitis and cranial nerve involvement may occur. So, paralysis of other cranial nerves indicates extension to the bones of the skull. Meningitis and sigmoid sinus thrombosis are rare complications. Radiographs of the ear and mastoid are usually normal; thus, the diagnosis must be made on clinical grounds. The best diagnostic method is the magnetic resonance imaging. The diagnosis is confirmed by the isolation of *Pseudomonas aeruginosa* from cultures of drainage from the ear in cases in which patients have severe ear pain, with granulation tissue present in the external auditory canal with or without radiographic evidence of disease. Other organisms rarely cause this disease e.g. *Staphylococci* or facultative *gram-negative bacilli*. *P. aeruginosa* may also be found in the ear canal of patients with uncomplicated otitis externa, culturing pseudomonas is not diagnostic of malignant otitis externa. The predisposition of diabetic patients may be due to the diabetic microangiopathy. Blood vessels in the infected tissues show marked intimal proliferation, leading some to speculate that vascular insufficiency resulting from diabetic microangiopathy may predispose to this infection. Therapy should include debridement and antibiotic therapy. Traditionally, standard therapy has been a combination of extended spectrum penicillin and an aminoglycoside given for 4–8 weeks, depending on the severity of illness. Use of a single drug, such as ciprofloxacin given orally or ceftazidime given intravenously for 6 weeks, has shown success in less severely ill patients. Early initiation of antibiotic therapy and surgical intervention are important for optimal outcomes. Without prompt recognition and therapy, the mortality may approach 40 percent (Rubin & Yu, 1988; Schaberg & Norwood; 2002).

4.5.2 Rhinocerebral Mucormycosis

Mucormycosis (also referred to as zygomycosis or phycomycosis) is a rare opportunistic, extremely difficult to treat, invasive and often fatal infectious disease that is usually associated with diabetic ketoacidosis. Mucormycosis is caused by fungi of the class *Zygomycetes*. The genus most commonly associated with human infections is *Rhizopus*, followed by *Mucor*, *Absidia* and *Cunninghamella*. Several distinct patterns of infection occur, including rhinocerebral infection and invasive pulmonary or gastrointestinal disease. The ubiquitous organisms invade through nasal passages producing black necrotic tissue and black pus. More than 50% of cases with mucormycosis are diabetics. This is because the acidic pH associated with diabetic ketoacidosis decreases the serum inhibitory activity against the *Rhizopus*. Ketosis also impairs the inflammatory response and permits tissue invasion in experimental mucormycosis. Acidosis and high concentrations of glucose increase the growth rate of *phycomycetes*. There is also over expression of some host receptors that mediate the invasion and damage to human epithelial cells by *Rhizopus* (Liu *et al.*, 2010). Mucormycosis is usually acute but occasionally chronic. Clinical features of this infection are distinctive with classical triad of paranasal sinusitis, ophthalmoplegia with blindness, and unilateral proptosis with cellulitis, bloody nasal discharge, unilateral headache, eyelid swelling, and lacrimation. Facial or eye pain and necrotic wound of the palate and nasal mucosa may occur. Ischemic nasal turbinates become necrotic. Black necrotic eschar in the nasal cornet is a characteristic sign. Jugular tenderness may be present with thrombophlebitis of the internal jugular vein. Paralysis of cranial nerves II-V, seizures, hemiparesis, coma, or other findings of meningoencephalitis appear as a result of vascular thrombosis and extension of the infection through the orbit and cribriform plate to the meninges and brain. Unilateral proptosis, chemosis, and retinal vein engorgement suggest that cavernous sinus thrombosis has occurred. Papilledema and retinal hemorrhages may develop later. Untreated patients frequently die within a week of onset of the infection. Thus, clinicians must be familiar with this rare but life-threatening infection (Severo *et al.*, 2010).

4.5.3   Periodontal Infection

Periodontitis ranks sixth among all complications of DM and is four times more common in persons with DM. It is a chronic inflammatory disease characterized by the formation of a periodontal pocket, loss of connective tissue, and alveolar bone resorption, which may sometimes result in tooth loss. DM and periodontitis are common multi-genetic and multifactorial chronic diseases with a higher incidence at increased age. Both of the morbidities negatively affect periodontal health and systemic health, thus affecting the quality of life. There is a bidirectional correlation between DM and periodontitis. Periodontitis starts or disseminates insulin resistance, thus worsening glycemic control. Persistent poor glycemic control has been associated with a greater incidence and progression of gingivitis and periodontitis, producing a vicious circle.

4.6   Other Infections

4.6.1   Malaria

Co-occurrence of T2 DM and malaria may have substantial implications. An increased risk for *P. falciparum* infection in persons with DM might become clinically relevant (and microscopically detectable) under several conditions. The impact of semi-immunity on controlling parasitemia may weaken with advancing T2 DM and immune dysfunction as suggested by the observed risk increase with increasing glucose concentration. Conversely, children who lack semi-immunity but have more severe T1 DM may be particularly prone to malaria. Such vulnerability is also conceivable for women with gestational DM whose immune systems are relatively naive with regard to pregnancy-specific *P. falciparum*. Moreover, low-level infections in patients with T1 DM may constitute an unrecognized infectious reservoir in areas where malaria is endemic. The lowered *P. falciparum* prevalence under metformin medication is due to biguanides' antimalarial efficacy (Danquah *et al.*, 2010; Okell *et al.*, 2009).

4.6.2   Bacteraemia

There is increased morbidity and mortality rate due to bacteremia in the diabetic patients which exceeded that of the non-diabetic patients. In NHDS study (1989 to 1991); the prevalence of bacteremia caused by

S. aureus and enteric organisms in diabetic subjects exceeded that in non-diabetic subjects by a large margin. Bacteremia is found in a 1.9-fold higher proportion of diabetic versus non-diabetic hospitalizations. The greatest difference was seen in the youngest age group (18-44 years, relative frequency = 2.0), with a gradual decline as age increased. However, the improved management of diabetic patients with acute illnesses in recent years may account for the absence of an effect of DM on outcomes in these patients (Leibovici *et al.*, 1991; Peralta *et al.*, 2009).

4.6.3 Surgical Site Infection (SSI)

Surgical site infections continue to constitute a challenge for surgeons. Protocols are now in place to reduce the rate of post operative infection. DM is a known major risk factor for SSI. Complications of DM, specifically peripheral neuropathy, have been shown to increase the risk of developing a post-operative infection. Gram-negative wound infections are three times more frequent in diabetic than in non-diabetic individuals. Postoperative hyperglycemia is the most important risk factor for surgical site infection. Aggressive early postoperative glycemic control should reduce the incidence of SSI (Ata *et al.*, 2010).

5   Effects of Infection on Diabetes

Maintaining good glycemic control is not easy. Infection or an illness such as a cold or flu, for instance, can cause high blood sugars, loss of DM control, and may induce ketoacidosis especially in T1 DM. Infection stimulates the release of stress hormones such as cortisol and adrenaline. Cortisol binds to receptors on the fat cells, liver and pancreas, which increases glucose levels available for muscles to use. Cortisol also antagonizes insulin effects. Adrenaline enhances release of glucose from glycogen as well as the release of fatty acids from adipose tissue. These hormones work against the action of insulin and, as a result, the body's production of glucose increases, which results in high blood sugar levels. Persistent hyperglycemia associated with low insulin release or effects can induce development of ketoacidosis. Hyperglycemia weakened immune system and can lead to more serious conditions. There are contradictory reports on *H pylori* prevalence and its relationship to late complications of DM. Interestingly, diabetics with *H. pylori* infection had a higher incidence of neuropathy, although there was no association between the duration and regulation of DM, retinopathy, nephropathy and *H. pylori* status. Some data indicate a possible association of *H. pylori* infection with coronary insufficiency and/or cerebral occlusive vascular disease in adults with DM. Another consequence of this infection is the increase in insulin requirements in children with T1 DM. The efficiency of *H. pylori* eradication is lower in persons with DM, whereas the re-infection rates are seen to be higher. Periodontitis starts or disseminates insulin resistance, thus worsening glycemic control. Periodontal therapy and proper care produced a significant improvement in the clinical condition, but did not affect metabolic control (Liz *et al.*, 2011). *HCV* infection is strongly associated with development of insulin resistance and T2 DM. *HCV* is able to induce insulin resistance (IR) directly and the role of specific viral genotypes responsible for such effect is disputed. IR has consistently been found to be closely linked to fibrosis in *HCV* infection, although also typically associated with T2 DM in pre-fibrotic stages (Lonardo *et al.*, 2009). DM is a particular co-morbid illness that warrants attention as a threat to HIV-infected patients. Both *HIV* infection and use of antiretroviral medications to treat *HIV* may be risk factors for DM. Patients with *HIV* should be screened for diabetes at diagnosis, at the onset, and during HAART therapy. An oral glucose tolerance test is recommended to assess the insulin resistance. The treatment of DM in *HIV* poses some limitations. For example, although metformin is the drug of choice, its use may not be tolerated by cachectic patients or by those with lypo-atrophy. The side effects of thiazolidinediones (e.g. higher cardiovascular morbidity, osteoporosis) may prevent their use in *HIV* patients with DM. Glinides and sulfonylureas may not be effective due to insulin resistance. Therefore, insulin is the drug of choice for *HIV*-associated DM (Satlin *et al.*, 2011).

6   Diabetes and Vaccination

6.1   Effect of Vaccines on Diabetes

The induction or exacerbation of autoimmune diseases is a potential adverse effect of immune-stimulating drugs. Some studies has raised the possibility that immunisation by vaccines can influence the pathogenesis of T1 DM. A link between childhood vaccinations and the development of T1 DM has been proposed for several reasons. First, there is a temporal association between the widespread introduction of general childhood immunizations and the increase in the incidence of T1 DM in developed countries. Second, it has been observed that specific vaccines prevent T1 DM in murine models and others induce it. And third, some findings suggest an association between infections and T1 DM (Hviid *et al.*, 2004). Epidemiological studies, however, have so far failed to demonstrate any causal relationship between vaccination and autoimmune diseases, including T1 DM. Few studies claimed the role of some vaccines may share in pathogenesis of autoimmune DM. However, a study done by Wahlberg *et al*, showed that *hemophilus influenza B* (HIB) vaccination may have an unspecific stimulatory polyclonal effect increasing the production of GADA and IA-2A; an immune process that later may lead to T1 DM. This might be of importance under circumstances when the beta cell-related immune response is activated by other mechanisms (Wahlberg *et al.*, 2003).

Some reports have suggested that natural mumps or mumps vaccinations can induce islet cell autoimmunity, but there is no evidence that mumps-measles-rubella mass vaccination programmes have changed the incidence of DM in any population. An independent protective role of measles virus has been suggested in one study. Recent studies have indicated that *enterovirus* infections may induce beta cell autoimmunity and clinical DM. The only currently available *enterovirus* vaccine is the poliovirus vaccine which, in theory, could modulate the protection against other *enteroviruses* by inducing cross-reactive T cell immune responses; however, this hypothesis has not been tested so far (Hiltunen *et al.*, 1999). There are some sporadic reports of preserving β-cell function when BCG vaccination is administered soon after diabetes onset. A study done by Zhu *et al* showed that intranasal vaccination with HSP65 gene was derived from *Mybobacterium tuberculosis var. bovis* NOD mice could prevent the development of DM. Their results demonstrated that intranasal vaccination with HSP65 reduced significantly the inflammatory process associated with auto-immune diabetes. They suggested that this approach may offer novel therapeutic avenues for the treatment for of T1 DM (Zhu *et al.*, 2011). However, a previous study done by Allen *et al.* showed that vaccination with BCG at the time of onset of type T1 DM does not increase the remission rate or preserve beta-cell function (Allen *et al.*, 1999). However, repeated BCG vaccination is safe and may be more effective than a single dose in preventing T1 DM in NOD mice (Shehadeh *et al.*, 1997). Ravel *et al* showed that the incidence of autoimmune diabetes was slightly reduced by the DTaP-IVP vaccine with significant reduction of blood glucose level treated with the DTaP-IVP vaccine relative to the untreated control mice (Ravel *et al.*, 2003). There were no solid causal relation between childhood vaccination and T1 DM. Larger epidemiological studies are still needed to obtain more reliable data in most suggested associations (Salemi & D'Amelio, 2010).

6.2   Effects of Diabetes on Vaccine

Enhancement of personal DM management and increased media messages about DM could improve DM knowledge or awareness and hence increase the patient awareness about the need for proper vaccination. Adhesiveness to vaccination is affected by several factors that may include race, gender, patient's knowledge, socioeconomic status, vaccine availability, the access to and the quality of the medical service available. Dunlap & Rudenko reported that the diabetic patients who are younger than 65 years tend to be more likely to recognize that they are at high risk of complications from influenza and pneumococcal disease; however, their vaccination rates tend to be lower than those of patients who are over 65. Patients aged 65 and over have a higher rate of vaccination, but are vaccinated because of their age, not recognizing that having diabetes and being older puts them into a high-risk category. Many patients are not receiving the influenza vaccine because they fear becoming ill or experiencing adverse effects. They also found that a large proportion of patients are not receiving the pneumococcal vaccine because they were unaware that it is needed or their physician had not recommended it to them (Dunlap & Rudenko, 2012). Younossi & Stepanova found that despite the vaccination rates in diabetic cohorts are increasing, they remain low and there is a need for a better implementation of the vaccination recommendations for these populations is warranted (Younossi ZM, Stepanova M, 2011).

The Immune response induced by the vaccines in diabetic patients may be not equal to that induced by healthy controls. Leonardi *et al* studied the efficacy of *HBV* vaccine in diabetic children. They observed a reduced seroprotection rate for *HBV* vaccination in diabetics. They found significantly-lower mean antibody titre against HBV in IDDM children than healthy controls. However, there was no correlation found between antibody titre, age, duration of disease and HbA1c. They did not find any difference of gender, age, years of onset of the disease and metabolic control, between diabetics with anti-HBs antibodies and those without (Leonardi *et al.*, 2012). A similar finding was observed with inactivated influenza A (H1N1) 2009 monovalent vaccine. Kostinov & Tarasova found that intensity of immunity after HBV vaccination in children with T1 DM decreased with increasing number of diabetic complications. If number of T1 DM-associated complications exceeds 3, especially in children living in rural area, serologic monitoring is essential for deciding whether booster vaccination against HBV is needed (Kostinov MP, & Tarasova AA, 2008). The same was observed for pneumococcal vaccine. Tarasova *et al*, found lower intensity of immune response and antibody titres to polysaccharide pneumococcal vaccine in children with DM compared to children with respiratory diseases (Tarasova *et al.*, 2007). Nam *et al* noted low cross-reactive antibody carrying rate and low seroconversion rate in adult patients with DM who were vaccinated with single-dose adjuvanted, inactivated, pandemic H1N1 influenza vaccination. This finding stimulated them to recommend two-dose vaccination or to have antibody titres measured after the first vaccination to ensure the protective efficacy of the vaccine.

6.3   Recommendations

It should be emphasized that vaccination in diabetic patients is free of any risk; provided that there are no other contraindications, e.g. allergy to vaccine components or severe acute febrile illness. In case of unstable glycaemia and significantly impaired immune system due to DM, vaccination with live attenuated vaccines should be carefully considered and measured against the risks of exposure to each and every specific infectious agent. There is no reason to be afraid of vaccination in diabetic patients provided that general contraindications are respected. On the contrary, this risk group can benefit from vaccination more remarkably since it may have some life-saving potential (Mad'ar *et al*, 20111). For example; adults with T2 DM, like other individuals from recognized risk groups, can benefit considerably from influenza vaccination, and no difference in vaccine effectiveness was observed between first-time and repeat vaccination (Looijmans-Van den *et al.*, 2006). Effective DM management, including self-care, healthcare provider-care, and getting vaccinated against influenza and pneumonia, is vital in reducing DM morbidity and mortality. Providing directed education to patients about the importance of vaccination and discussing with them the expected adverse effects may improve rate of vaccination.

The basic vaccinations recommended for diabetics include immunizations against influenza, pneumococcal infections, tetanus and viral hepatitis B. Other vaccines are administered only after individual assessment of benefits and risks for the diabetic patient. Most often, these are vaccinations against viral hepatitis A, tick-borne encephalitis, meningococcal infections and other infections that put risk in diabetic patients travelling abroad (Beran J, 2006). Because serum levels of tetanus antibody decreased in diabetic patients older than 50 years of age, whereas this period of time is prolonged to 65 years in healthy individuals; it is recommended that all individuals over 65 years should be vaccinated against tetanus. However, vaccination over 50 years of age might be considered for diabetic patients (Tamer *et al.*, 2005). According to the Centers for Disease Control and Prevention (CDC) guidelines for vaccination of adults with diabetes; the following vaccines are recommended:

- **Pneumococcal Vaccine:** All adults ≥ 65 years of age and Adults < 65 years of age with diabetes; it is recommended to give 1 dose once in their life with 1 additional dose at ≥ 65 and ≥ 5 years from first dose.

- **Influenza Vaccine:** should be given for all adults 1 dose annually. The best time to get is between October and mid-November, before the flu season begins.

- **Hepatitis B vaccine:** It should be administered to unvaccinated adults with DM who are aged 19 through 59 years. Hepatitis B vaccination may be administered at the discretion of the treating clinician to unvaccinated adults with diabetes mellitus who are aged ≥60 years. Although the HBV vaccination series traditionally consists of doses at 0, 1, and 6 months, the CDC recommends incorporating the series into regular visit intervals, as effectiveness is comparable even when the intervals between doses are longer than those stated above (CDC, 2011). Early vaccination against HBV is indicated in patients likely to progress to end-stage kidney disease.

- **Tetanus/Diphtheria (Td) Toxoid Vaccine/Tdap:** Most people get Td toxoid as part of their routine childhood vaccinations, but all adults need a Td booster shot every 10 years with Tdap in place of one Td vaccine. Other vaccines may be given at the same time as Td toxoid.

- **Shingles:** All adults should have 1 dose at ≥ 60 years of age.

- **HPV:** it is given for all women up to age 26, unless immunized earlier and all men up to age 21 (may be vaccinated up to age 26), unless immunized earlier. Three doses are given at 0, 2, 6 months.

References

Badaru A, Pihoker C. (2012) Type 2 diabetes in childhood: clinical characteristics and role of β-cell autoimmunity. Curr Diab Rep. Feb; 12(1):75-81.

Aarnisalo J, Veijola R, Vainionpää R, Simell O, Knip M, Ilonen J. (2008) Cytomegalovirus infection in early infancy: risk of induction and progression of autoimmunity associated with type 1 diabetes. Diabetologia. 51(5):769-72.

Alba A, Planas R, Verdaguer J, Vives-Pi M. (2005) Viral infections and autoimmune diabetes. INMUNOLOGÍA. 24(1): 33-43.

Allen HF, Klingensmith GJ, Jensen P, Simoes E, Hayward A, Chase HP. (1999) Effect of Bacillus Calmette-Guerin vaccination on new-onset type 1 diabetes. A randomized clinical study. Diabetes Care. 22(10):1703-7.

Allison ME, Wreghitt T, Palmer CR, Alexander GJ. (1994) Evidence for a link between hepatitis C virus infection and diabetes mellitus in a cirrhotic population. J Hepatol. 21:1135-1139.

Ata A, Lee J, Bestle SL, Desemone J, Stain SC. (2010) Postoperative Hyperglycemia and Surgical Site Infection in General Surgery Patients. Arch Surg. 145(9):858-864.

Beran J. (2006) Diabetes mellitus and immunization. Vnitr Lek. 52(5):438-42.

Bergerot I, Ploix C, Petersen J, Moulin V, Rask C, Fabien N, Lindblad M, Mayer A, Czerkinsky C, Holmgren J, Thivolet C. (1997) A cholera toxoid-insulin conjugate as an oral vaccine against spontaneous autoimmune diabetes. Proc Natl Acad Sci U S A. 29;94(9):4610-4.

Blom L, Nyström L, Dahlquist G. (1991) The Swedish childhood diabetes study. Vaccinations and infections as risk determinants for diabetes in childhood. Diabetologia. 34(3):176-81.

Blomqvist M, Juhela S, Eekkila S, Korhonen S, Simell T, Kupila A, Vaarala O, Simell O, Knip M, Ilonen J. (2005) Rotavirus infections and development of diabetes-associated autoantibodies during the first 2 years of life. Rev Diabet Stud. 2(4): 192–207.

Bouter KP, Diepersloot RJ, Romunde LK van, Uitslager R, Masurel N, Hoekstra JB, Erkelens DW. (1991) Effect of epidemic influenza on ketoacidosis, pneumonia and death in diabetes mellitus: A hospital register survey of 1976-79 in the Netherlands. Diabetes Res Clin Pract 12:61-68.

Butt AA, McGinnis K, Rodriguez-Barradas MC, Crystal S, Simberkoff M, Matthew Goetz B, Leaf D, Justice AC, For the Veterans Aging Cohort Study. (2009) HIV Infection and the Risk of Diabetes Mellitus. AIDS. 19; 23(10): 1227–1234.

Calvet HM, Yoshikawa TT. (2001) Infections in diabetes. Infect Dis Clin North Am. 15:407–20.

Carfrae MJ, Kesser BW. (2008) Malignant otitis externa. Otolaryngol Clin North Am.41:537–49.

Casqueiro J, Casqueiro J, Alves C. (2012) Infections in patients with diabetes mellitus: A review of pathogenesis. Indian J Endocrinol Metab. 16: S27–S36.

Centers for Disease Control and Prevention (CDC). (2011) Use of hepatitis B vaccination for adults with diabetes mellitus: recommendations of the Advisory Committee on Immunization Practices (ACIP). MMWR Morb Mortal Wkly Rep. 60:1709–1711.

Coppieters KT, Boettler T, von Herrath M. (2012) Virus Infections in Type 1 Diabetes. Cold Spring Harb Perspect Med. 2 (1): a007682.

Danquah I, Bedu-Addo G, Mockenhaupt FP. (2010) Type 2 Diabetes Mellitus and Increased Risk for Malaria Infection. Emerg Infect Dis. 16(10): 1601–1604.

Demir M, Gokturk HS, Ozturk NA, Kulaksizoglu M, Serin E, Yilmaz U. (2008) Helicobacter pylori prevalence in diabetes mellitus patients with dyspeptic symptoms and its relationship to glycemic control and late complications. Dig Dis Sci. 53(10):2646-9.

Devrajani BR, Shah SZA, Soomro FA, Devrajani T. (2010) Type 2 diabetes mellitus: A risk factor for Helicobacter pylori infection: A hospital based case-control study. Int J Diabetes Dev Ctries. 30(1): 22–26.

Diana, J., and A. Lehuen. 2009. NKT cells: friend or foe during viral infections? Eur. J. Immunol. 39:3283–3291.

Dooley KE, Chaisson RE. (2009) Tuberculosis and diabetes mellitus: Convergence of two epidemics. Lancet Infect Dis. 9:737–46.

Dunlap AM, Rudenko AW. (2012) Evaluating the difference in preventive vaccination uptake in patients with diabetes mellitus. Ann Pharmacother. 46(4):609-10.

Elfving M, Svensson J, Oikarinen S, Jonsson B, Olofsson P, Sundkvist G, Lindberg B, Lernmark A, Hyöty H, Ivarsson SA. (2008) Maternal Enterovirus Infection during Pregnancy as a Risk Factor in Offspring Diagnosed with Type 1 Diabetes between 15 and 30 Years of Age. Exp Diabetes Res. 2008:271958.

Elhawary EI, Mahmoud GF, El-Daly MA, Mekky FA, Esmat GG, Abdel-hamid M. (2011) Association of HCV with diabetes mellitus: an Egyptian case-control study. Virol J. 2011; 8: 367.

Elshebani A, Olsson A, Westman J, Tuvemo T, Korsgren O, Frisk G. (2007) Effects on isolated human pancreatic islet cells after infection with strains of enterovirus isolated at clinical presentation of type 1 diabetes. Virus Res 124:193–203.

Espinoza-Jiménez A, Irma Rivera-Montoya, Roberto Cárdenas-Arreola, Liborio Morán, Luis I. Terrazas. (2010) Taenia crassiceps Infection Attenuates Multiple Low-Dose Streptozotocin-Induced Diabetes. J Biomed Biotechnol. 2010: 850541.

Feng Y, Yao M, LI O, SUN Y, LI C, Shen J. (2010) Fulminant type 1 diabetes in China: a case report and review of the literature. J Zhejiang Univ-Sci B (Biomed & Biotechnol) 11(11):848-850.

Filippi CM, Estes EA, Oldham JE, von Herrath MG. (2009) Immunoregulatory mechanisms triggered by viral infections protect from type 1 diabetes in mice. J Clin Invest. 119(6):1515-23.

Filippi CM, von Herrath MG. (2008) Viral Trigger for Type 1 Diabetes: Pros and Cons. Diabetes. 57(11): 2863–2871.

Gamble D, Kinsley M, Fitzgerald M, Bolton R, Taylor K. (1969) Viral antibodies in diabetes mellitus. BMJ.3:627.

Ginsberg-Fellner F, Witt ME, Fedun B, Taub F, Dobersen MJ, McEvoy RC, Cooper LZ, Notkins AL, Rubinstein P. (1985) Diabetes mellitus and autoimmunity in patients with the congenital rubella syndrome. Rev Infect Dis. 7 (1):S170-6.

Goto A, Takahashi Y, Kishimoto M, Nakajima Y, Nakanishi K, Kajio H, Noda M. (2008) A case of fulminant type 1 diabetes associated with significant elevation of mumps titers. Endocr J. 55(3):561-4.

Gulinuer Awuti, Kurexi Younusi, Linlin Li, Halmurat Upur, Jun Ren. (2012). Epidemiological Survey on the Prevalence of Periodontitis and Diabetes Mellitus in Uyghur Adults from Rural Hotan Area in Xinjiang. Exp Diabetes Res. 2012: 758921.

Harris, H. F. (1899). A case of diabetes mellitus quickly following mumps. Boston Medical and Surgical Journal, 140, 465.

Hattemn SV, Boots MA, Thio HB. (2008) Skin menifestations of diabetes. Cleveland Clin J Med. 75: 772-87.

Hiltunen M, Lönnrot M, Hyöty H. (1999) Immunisation and type 1 diabetes mellitus: is there a link? Drug Saf. 20(3):207-12.

Hjelmesæth J, • Sagedal S, Hartmann A, Rollag H, Egeland T, Hagen M, Nordal KP, Jenssen T. (2004) Asymptomatic cytomegalovirus infection is associated with increased risk of new-onset diabetes mellitus and impaired insulin release after renal transplantation. Diabetologia . 47:1550–1556.

Honeyman MC, Coulson BS, Stone NL, Gellert SA, Goldwater PN, Steele CE, Couper JJ, Tait BD, Colman PG, Harrison LC. (2000) Association between Rotavirus Infection and Pancreatic Islet Autoimmunity in Children at Risk of Developing Type 1 Diabetes. Diabetes. 49(8):1319-24.

Howard AA, Lo Y, Floris-Moore M, Klein RS, Fleischer N, Schoenbaum EE.(2007) Hepatitis C virus infection is associated with insulin resistance among older adults with or at risk of HIV infection. AIDS. 12; 21(5): 633–641.

Hviid A, Stellfeld M, Wohlfahrt J, Melbye M. (2004) Childhood Vaccination and Type 1 Diabetes. N Engl J Med. 350:1398-404.

Imagawa A, Hanafusa T, Uchigata Y, Kanatsuka A, Kawasaki E, Kobayashi T, Shimada A, Shimizu I, Maruyama T, Makino H. (2005) Different contribution of class II HLA in fulminant and typical autoimmune type 1 diabetes mellitus. Diabetologia. 48(2):294-300.

Jeon CY, Haan MN, Cheng C, Clayton ER, Mayeda ER, Miller JW, Aiello AE. (2012) Helicobacter pylori infection is associated with an increased rate of diabetes. Diabetes Care. 35 (3):520-5.

Joseph WS, Lipsky BA. (2010) Medical therapy of diabetic foot infections. J Vasc Surg. 52 (3) :67S–71.

Kamada T, Hata J, Kusunoki H, Ito M, Tanaka S, Kawamura Y, Chayama K, Haruma K. (2005) Eradication of Helicobacter pylori increases the incidence of hyperlipidaemia and obesity in peptic ulcer patients. Dig Liver Dis. 37:39–43.

Kofteridis DP, Papadimitraki E, Mantadakis E, Maraki S, Papadakis JA, Tzifa G, Samonis G. (2009) Effect of diabetes mellitus on the clinical and microbiological features of hospitalized elderly patients with acute pyelonephritis. J Am Geriatr Soc. 57(11):2125-8.

Kostinov MP, Tarasova AA. (2008) Intensity of immunity in children with type 1 diabetes mellitus vaccinated against hepatitis B. Zh Mikrobiol Epidemiol Immunobiol. (5):61-5.

Laway BA, Bhat MA, Bashir MI, Ganie MA, Mir SA, Daga RA. (2012) Conservative management of emphysematous pyelonephritis. Indian J Endocrinol Metab. 16(2): 303–305.

Leibovici L, Samra Z, Konisberger H, Kalter-Leibovici O, Pitlik SD, Drucker M. (1991) Bacteremia in adult diabetic patients. Diabetes Care 14:89-94.

Leonardi S, Giovanna V, Teresa GM, Michele MD, Gianluigi M, Mario LR. (2012) Hepatitis B vaccination failure in children with Diabetes Mellitus? The debate continues. Hum Vaccin Immunother. 1;8(4).

Li Z, Sha YQ, Zhang BX, Zhu L, Kang J. (2011) Effect of community periodontal care intervention on periodontal health and glycemic control in type 2 diabetic patients with chronic periodontitis. Beijing Da Xue Xue Bao. 18;43(2):285-9.

Lipsky BA, Tabak YP, Johannes RS, Vo L, Hyde L, Weigelt JA. (2010) Skin and soft tissue infections in hospitalized patients with diabetes: Culture isolates and risk factors associated with mortality, length of stay and cost. Diabetologia. 53:914–23.

Liu M, Spellberg B, Phan QT, Fu Y, Fu Y, Lee AS, Edwards JE, Filler SG, Ibrahim AS. (2010) The endothelial cell receptor GRP78 is required for mucormycosis pathogenesis in diabetic mice. J Clin Invest. 120:1914–24.

Liu Q, Sundar K, Mishra PK, Mousavi G, Liu Z, Gaydo A, Alem F, Lagunoff D, Bleich D, Gause WC. (2009) Helminth Infection Can Reduce Insulitis and Type 1 Diabetes through CD25- and IL-10-Independent Mechanisms. Infect Immun. 77(12): 5347–5358.

Lonardo A, Adinolfi LE, Petta S, Craxì A, Loria P. (2009) Hepatitis C and diabetes: the inevitable coincidence? Expert Rev Anti Infect Ther. 7(3):293-308.

Looijmans-Van den Akker I, Verheij TJ, Buskens E, Nichol KL, Rutten GE, Hak E. (2006) Clinical effectiveness of first and repeat influenza vaccination in adult and elderly diabetic patients. Diabetes Care. 29(8):1771-6.

Lutsey PL, Pankow JS, Bertoni AG, Szklo M, Folsom AR. (2009). Serologic Evidence of Infections and Type 2 Diabetes: The MultiEthnic Study of Atherosclerosis. Diabet Med. 26(2): 149–152.

Mad'ar R, Benesová D, Brandejská D, Cermáková M, Dvorková A, Gazárková O, Jakubalová S, Kochová I, Lastovicková J, Nebáznivá D, Orolinová M, Polomis K, Rehka V, Sattranová L, Schejbalová M, Slámová A, Skalleová D, Sevcíková H, Tkadlecová H, Tmejová M, Trmal J, Turková D. (2011) Vaccination of patients with diabetes mellitus--a retrospective study. Cent Eur J Public Health. 19(2):98-101.

Makela M, Oling V, Marttila J, Waris M, Knip M, Simell O, Ilonen J. (2006) Rotavirus-specific T cell responses and cytokine mRNA expression in children with diabetesassociated autoantibodies and type 1 diabetes. Clin Exp Immunol 145: 261–270.

Martins TC, Aguas AP. (1999) Mechanisms of Mycobacterium avium-induced resistance against insulin-dependent diabetes mellitus (IDDM) in non-obese diabetic (NOD) mice: role of Fas and Th1 cells. Clin Exp Immunol. 115(2):248-54.

Mehta SH, Brancati FL, Sulkowski MS, Strathdee SA, Szklo M, Thomas DL. (2000) Prevalence of Type 2 Diabetes Mellitus among Persons with Hepatitis C Virus Infection in the United States. Ann Intern Med. 17;133(8):592-9.

Menezes EA, Augusto KL, Freire CC, Cunha FA, Montenegro RM, Montenegro-Júnior RM. (2007) Frequency and enzymatic activity of Candida spp.oral cavity of diabetic patients of the service of endocrinology of a hospital of Fortaleza-CE. J Bras Patol Med Lab. 43:241–4.

Menser MA, Forrest JM, Bransby RD. (1978) Rubella infection and diabetes mellitus. Lancet. 14;1(8055):57-60.

Mujtaba SG. (2009) Review Article: Diabetic's skin; a storehouse of infections. J Pak Ass Dermato. 19: 34-37.

Naing C, Mak JW, Ahmed SI, Maung M. (2012) Relationship between hepatitis C virus infection and type 2 diabetes mellitus: Meta-analysis. World J Gastroenterol. 14; 18(14): 1642–1651.

Nam JS, Kim AR, Yoon JC, Byun Y, Kim SA, Kim KR, Cho S, Seong BL, Ahn CW, Lee JM. (2012) The humoral immune response to the inactivated influenza A (H1N1) 2009 monovalent vaccine in patients with Type 2 diabetes mellitus in Korea. Diabet Med. 28(7):815-7.

Nicolau DP, Stein GE. (2010) Therapeutic options for diabetic foot infections: a review with an emphasis on tissue penetration characteristics. J Am Podiatr Med Assoc. 100:52–63.

Nishio, J., M. Feuerer, J. Wong, D. Mathis, and C. Benoist. (2010) Anti-CD3 therapy permits regulatory T cells to surmount T cell receptor–specified peripheral niche constraints. J. Exp. Med. 207:1879–1889.

Okell LC, Ghani AC, Lyons E, Drakeley CJ. (2009) Submicroscopic infection in Plasmodium falciparum–endemic populations: a systematic review and meta-analysis. J Infect Dis. 200:1509–17.

Ola TO, Williams NA. (2006) Protection of non-obese diabetic mice from autoimmune diabetes by Escherichia coli heat-labile enterotoxin B subunit. Immunology. 117(2):262-70.

Onal ED, Polat B, Balkan F, Kaya G, Ersoy R, Cakır B, Deniz O. (2012) Positive measles serology and new onset of type 1 diabetes presented with bilateral facial paralysis: a case report. Braz J Infect Dis. 16(3):305-6.

Oncul O, Erenoglu C, Top C, Küçükardali Y, Karabudak O, Kurt Y, Akin ML, Cavuslu S, Celenk T. (2008) Necrotizing fasciitis: A life-threatening clinical disorder in uncontrolled type 2 diabetic patients. Diabetes Res Clin Pract. 80: 218-23.

Pak CY, Eun HM, McArthur RG, Yoon JW. (1988) Association of cytomegalovirus infection with autoimmune type 1 diabetes. Lancet. 2; 2(8601):1-4.

Parkkonen P, Hyöty H, Ilonen J, Reijonen H, Yla-Herttuala S, Leinikki P. (1994) Antibody reactivity to an Epstein-Barr virus BERF4-encoded epitope occurring also in Asp-57 region of HLA-DQ8betas chain. Clin Exp Immunol. 95: 287–293.

Peleg AY, Weerarathna T, McCarthy JS, Davis TM. (2007) Common infections in diabetes: Pathogenesis, management and relationship to glycaemic control. Diabetes Metab Res Rev. 23:3–13.

Peralta G, Sánchez MB, Roiz MP, Garrido JC, Teira R, Mateos F. (2009) Diabetes does not affect outcome in patients with Enterobacteriaceae bacteremia. BMC Infect Dis. 13; 9:94, 1-9.

Perz JF, Fiore AE. (2005) Hepatitis B virus infection risks among diabetic patients residing in long-term care facilities. Clin Infect Dis. 1; 41 (5):760-1.

Pierce MA, Chapman HD, Post CM, Svetlanov A, Efrat S, Horwitz M, Serreze DV. (2003) Adenovirus early region 3 antiapoptotic 10.4K, 14.5K, and 14.7K genes decrease the incidence of autoimmune diabetes in NOD mice. Diabetes. 52(5):1119-27.

Polyzos SA, Kountouras J, Zavos C, Deretzi G. (2011) The association between Helicobacter pylori infection and insulin resistance: a systematic review. Helicobacter. 16:79–88.

Raine T, Zaccone P, Mastroeni P, Cooke A. (2006) Salmonella typhimurium infection in nonobese diabetic mice generates immunomodulatory dendritic cells able to prevent type 1 diabetes. J Immunol. 15;177(4):2224-33.

Ramondetti F, Sacco S, Comelli M, Bruno G, Falorni A, Iannilli A, d'Annunzio G, Iafusco D, Songini M, Toni S, Cherubini V, Carle F; RIDI Study Group. (2012) Type 1 diabetes and measles, mumps and rubella childhood infections within the Italian Insulin-dependent Diabetes Registry. Diabet Med. 2012 Jun;29(6):761-6.

Ravel G, Christ M, Liberge P, Burnett R, Descotes J. (2003) Effects of two pediatric vaccines on autoimmune diabetes in NOD female mice. Toxicol Lett. 15;146(1):93-100.

Rhee JE, Kim K, Lee CC, Kang J, Lee JW, Shin JH, Suh G, Singer AJ. (2011) The lack of association between age and diabetes and hospitalization in women with acute pyelonephritis. J Emerg Med. 41(1):29-34.

Robert Allard, Pascale Leclerc, Claude Tremblay, Terry-Nan Tannenbaum. (2010) Diabetes and the Severity of Pandemic Influenza A (H1N1) Infection. Diabetes Care. 33(7): 1491–1493.

Rouabhia S, Malek R, Bounecer H, Dekaken A, Amor FB, Sadelaoud M, Benouar A. (2010) Prevalence of type 2 diabetes in Algerian patients with hepatitis C virus infection. World J Gastroenterol. 21; 16(27): 3427-3431.

Rubin J, Yu VL. (1988) Malignant external otitis: insights into pathogenesis, clinical manifestations, diagnosis, and therapy. Am J Med 85:391–98.

Ruslami R, Aarniutse RE, Alisjahbana B, van der Ven AJ, van Crevel R. (2010) Implications of the global increase of diabetes for tuberculosis control and patient care. Trop Med Int Health. 15:1289–99.

Sadeharju K, Knip M, Hiltunen M, Akerblom HK, Hyöty H. (2003) The HLA-DR phenotype modulates the humoral immune response to enterovirus antigens. Diabetologia. Aug; 46(8):1100-5.

Salemi S, D'Amelio R. (2010) Could autoimmunity be induced by vaccination? Int Rev Immunol. 29(3):247-69.

Saluja JS, Ajinkya M, Khemani B, Khanna S, Jain R. Helicobacter pylori and diabetes mellitus. (2002) Bombay Hosp J. 44:57–60.

Sano H, Terasaki J, Tsutsumi C, Imagawa A, Hanafusa T. (2008) A case of fulminant type 1 diabetes mellitus after influenza B infection. Diabetes Res Clin Pract. 79(3):e8-9.

Satlin MJ, Hoover DR, Glesby MJ. (2011) Glycemic control in HIV-infected patients with diabetes mellitus and rates of meeting American Diabetes Association management guidelines. AIDS Patient Care STDS. 25(1):5-12.

Schaberg DS, Norwood JM. (2002) Case Study: Infections in Diabetes Mellitus. Diabetes Spectrum. 5(1): 37-40.

Scharnagl H, Kist M, Grawitz AB, Koenig W, Wieland H, Marz W. (2004) Effect of Helicobacter pylori eradication on high-density lipoprotein cholesterol. Am J Cardiol. 15;93(2):219-20.

Schut ES, Westendorp, Jan de Gans WF, Kruyt ND, Spanjaard L, Reitsma JB, van de Beek D. (2009) Hyperglycemia in bacterial meningitis: a prospective cohort study. BMC Infect Dis. 9: 57.

Segireddy M, Johnson LB, Szpunar SM, Khatib R. (2011) Differences in patient risk factors and source of candidaemia caused by Candida albicans and Candida glabrata. Mycoses. 54(4):e39-43.

Sehmi S, Osaghae S. (2011) Type II diabetes mellitus: new presentation manifesting as Fournier's gangrene. JRSM Short Rep. 2(6): 51.

Severo CB, Guazzelli LS, Severo LC. (2010) Zigomicose. J Bras Pneumol. 36:134–41.

Shehadeh N, Etzioni A, Cahana A, Teninboum G, Gorodetsky B, Barzilai D, Karnieli E. (1997) Repeated BCG vaccination is more effective than a single dose in preventing diabetes in non-obese diabetic (NOD) mice. Isr J Med Sci. 33(11):711-5.

Shimizu T, Tokuda Y. (2010) Necrotizing fasciitis. Intern Med J. 49:1051–7.

Silva DG, Charlton B, Cowden W, Petrovsky N. (2003) Prevention of autoimmune diabetes through immunostimulation with Q fever complement-fixing antigen. Ann N Y Acad Sci. 1005:423-30.

Stene LC, Oikarinen S, Hyöty H, Barriga KJ, Norris JM, Klingensmith G, Hutton JC, Erlich HA, Eisenbarth GS, Rewers M. (2010) Enterovirus Infection and Progression From Islet Autoimmunity to Type 1 Diabetes The Diabetes and Autoimmunity Study in the Young (DAISY). Diabetes. 59(12): 3174–3180.

Tamer A, Karabay O, Ekerbicer H, Tahtaci M, Selam B, Celebi H. (2005) Impaired immunity against tetanus in type 2 diabetes. Med Sci Monit. 11(12):CR580-4.

Tanaka S, Nishida Y, Aida K, Maruyama T, Shimada A, Suzuki M, Shimura H, Takizawa S, Takahashi M, Akiyama D, Arai-Yamashita S, Furuya F, Kawaguchi A, Kaneshige M, Katoh R, Endo T, Kobayashi T. (2009) Enterovirus Infection, CXC Chemokine Ligand 10 (CXCL10), and CXCR3 Circuit A Mechanism of Accelerated β-Cell Failure in Fulminant Type 1 Diabetes. Diabetes. 58(10): 2285–2291.

Tarasova AA, Kostinov MP, Iastrebova NE, Skochilova TV. (2007) *Effect of vaccination against pneumococcal infection in children with type 1 diabetes mellitus. Zh Mikrobiol Epidemiol Immunobiol. (6):45-9.*

Tirabassi RS, Guberski DL, Blankenhorn EP, Leif JH, Woda BA, Liu Z, Winans D, Greiner DL, Mordes JP. (2010) *Infection with Viruses From Several Families Triggers Autoimmune Diabetes in LEW.1WR1 Rats: Prevention of Diabetes by Maternal Immunization. Diabetes. 59(1): 110–118.*

von Herrath M. Can we learn from viruses how to prevent type 1 diabetes? (2009) *The role of viral infections in the pathogenesis of type 1 diabetes and the development of novel combination therapies. Diabetes. 58:2–11.*

Wahlberg J, Fredriksson J, Vaarala O, Ludvigsson J; Abis Study Group. (2003) *Vaccinations may induce diabetes-related autoantibodies in one-year-old children. Ann N Y Acad Sci. 1005:404-8.*

Wheat LJ. (1980) *Infection and Diabetes MellitusD1ABETES CARE, 3(1):187-197.*

Xia HH-X, Talley NJ, Kam EPY, Young LJ, Hammer J, Horowitz M. (2001) *Helicobacter pylori infection is not associated with diabetes mellitus, nor with upper gastrointestinal symptoms in diabetes mellitus. Am J Gastroenterol. 96:1039–1046.*

Yasuda H, Nagata M, Moriyama H, Kobayashi H, Akisaki T, Ueda H, Hara K, Yokono K. (2012) *Development of fulminant Type 1 diabetes with thrombocytopenia after influenza vaccination: a case report. Diabet Med. 29(1):88-9.*

Yende S, van der Poll T, Lee M, Huang DT, Newman AB, Kong L, A Kellum JA, Harris TB, Bauer D, Satterfield S, Angus DC. (2010) *The influence of pre-existing diabetes mellitus on the host immune response and outcome of pneumonia: analysis of two multicenter cohort studies. Thorax. 65(10): 870–877.*

Yeung W G, Rawlinson WD, Craig ME. (2011) *Enterovirus infection and type 1 diabetes mellitus: systematic review and meta-analysis of observational molecular studies. BMJ. 342: d35.*

Younossi ZM, Stepanova M. (2011) *Changes in hepatitis A and B vaccination rates in adult patients with chronic liver diseases and diabetes in the U.S. population. Hepatology. 54(4):1167-78.*

Zaccone P, Raine T, Sidobre S, Kronenberg M, Mastroeni P, Cooke A. (2004) *Salmonella typhimurium infection halts development of type 1 diabetes in NOD mice. Eur J Immunol. 34 (11):3246-56.*

Zanone MM, Favaro E, Quadri R, Miceli I, Giaretta F, Romagnoli R, David E, Perin PC, Salizzoni M, Camussi G. (2010) *Association of cytomegalovirus infections with recurrence of humoral and cellular autoimmunity to islet autoantigens and of type 1 diabetes in a pancreas transplanted patient. Transpl Int. 1;23(3):333-7.*

Zhu AH, Jin L, Liu JJ, Liu MY, Lv AJ, Zheng YL. (2011) *Intranasal vaccination with mycobacterial 65-kD heat-shock protein can prevent insulitis and diabetes in non-obese diabetic mice. Xi Bao Yu Fen Zi Mian Yi Xue Za Zhi. 27(11):1165-8.*

Traditional Indian Antidiabetic Medicinal Plants as Inhibitors of Pancreatic α-Amylase and α-Glucosidase

Sudha Ponnusamy
Institute of Bioinformatics and Biotechnology
University of Pune, Maharashtra, India

Ameeta RaviKumar
Institute of Bioinformatics and Biotechnology
University of Pune, Maharashtra, India

1 Introduction

Diabetes mellitus is a carbohydrate metabolism disorder resulting in abnormally high blood sugar level (hyperglycemia). It can be caused by hereditary, increasing age, poor diet, imperfect digestion, obesity, sedentary lifestyle, stress, drug-mediated, infection in pancreas, hypertension, high serum lipid and lipo-proteins, less glucose utilization and other factors (Alberti & Zimmet, 1998). The World Health Organi-zation (WHO) estimates that worldwide, 346 million people have diabetes with more than 80% of diabet-ics living in low- and middle-income countries. The number is expected to grow to double by 2030 (WHO, 2012). Of the two main forms of diabetes, type 2 accounts for over 90 % of the cases globally. It is characterized by insulin resistance or abnormal insulin secretion, either of which may predominate (WHO, 1999; Zimmet *et al.*, 2001). The primary aim of managing type 2 diabetes is to delay, or even prevent, the complications of the disease by achieving good glycemic control. In addition to drug therapy, this often involves changes in lifestyle, such as diet and exercise. The main groups of oral synthetic drugs available along with their mechanism of action and side effects are listed in Table 1. Insulin is increasing-ly considered part of a treatment regimen in type 2 diabetics, particularly the use of long-acting prepara-tions to provide a constant basal insulin release (Hall & Nicholson, 2009). Increasedside effects, lack of curative treatment for several chronic diseases, high cost of new drugs, are some reasons for renewed public interest in complementary and alternative medicines (Humber, 2002).

1.1 Complementary and Alternative Medicine in Diabetes Mellitus

Ayurveda, the traditional Indian medicine (TIM) as well as the traditional Chinese medicine (TCM) re-main the most ancient yet living traditions in complementary and alternative therapy (Humber, 2002). Use of indigenous drugs of natural origin forms a major part of such therapies with more than 1500 herb-als sold as dietary supplements or ethnic traditional medicines (WHO, 2001).Pharmaceutical companies have renewed their strategies in favor of natural product drug development and discovery (Seidl, 2002). Ethnobotanical studies of traditional herbal remedies used for diabetes around the world have identified more than 1200 species of plants with hypoglycemic activity. These plants are broadly distributed throughout 725 different genera. The pharmacopoeia of India is especially rich in herbal treatments for diabetes (Shekelle *et al.*, 2005). While plant derivatives with purported hypoglycemic properties have been used in folk medicine and traditional healing systems, very few of these traditional anti-diabetic plants have received proper scientific or medical scrutiny despite recommendations by (WHO). Ayurveda and other Indian traditional approaches have described more than 800 plants in the Indian subcontinent, known to possess antidiabetic potential. These require to be effectively studied and in fact only few of them have been characterized for their mechanistic actions (Grover *et al.*, 2002; Mukherjee *et al.*, 2006; John *et al.*, 2009).

1.2 Targets of Action: Pancreatic α-amylase and α-glucosidase

Type 2 diabetes is a multifactorial disease caused by oligo- and polygenic genetic factors as well as non-genetic factors that result from a lack of balance between the energy intake and output and other life style related factors. Understanding of diabetes pathogenesis is essential to the development of new methods for treatment and strategies of this disease (Hansen, 2002). Of the many targets for antidiabetic agents, pancreatic α-amylase and α-glucosidase are discussed in this chapter.

Oral Hypoglycemic Agent	Mechanism of Action	Side Effects
Sulphonylurea	Stimulates release of Insulin from β-cell of pancreas	Increase in appetite and weight gain (Kelle, 1995). Increase in occurrence of cardiovascular risk (Feinglos & Bethel, 1999; Sheehan, 2003).
Meglitinides	Stimulate release of insulin from β-cell of pancreas by binding to ATP-sensitive potassium ion channels. Short acting and meal adjusted dosing.	High cost, gastrointestinal disturbances, hypersensitivity reactions including pruritus, rashes and urticaria (Bastaki, 2005).
Biguanides Metformin	Improves insulin sensitivity in skeletal muscles, decrease hepatic gluconeogensis, inhibits glycogneolysis, and reduces plasma triglyceride of low density lipoprotein. In liver, stimulates AMP-protein kinase to enhance fatty acid oxidation with inhibition of lipogenesis and glucose production (Stumvoll et al., 2007).	No effect on insulin secretion, hypoglycemia occurs in monotherapy so always should be used in combinatorial therapy with other hypoglycemic agents. Gastrointestinal disturbances, metallic taste, nausea, abdominal pain and diarrhea, severe lactic acidosis (Stumvoll et al., 1995; Bolen et al., 2007)
Thiazolidinediones (TZD)	TZDs are selective agonists for nuclear peroxisome proliferator-activated receptor-gamma. The TZDs bind to PPAR-γ, which activates insulin-responsive genes that regulate carbohydrate and lipid metabolism. TZDs lower insulin resistance in peripheral tissue, but an effect to lower glucose production by the liver. Enhances the insulin sensitivity in adipocytes and muscles by increasing efficiency of glucose transporters. TZDs activate genes that regulate free fatty-acid (FFA) metabolism in peripheral tissue, thus lowering triglycerides and non-esterified fattyacid levels and inducing differentiation of adipocytes (Bastaki, 2005).	Weight gain, edema, and increase risk of cardiovascular death. Increases risk of mortality when used in intensive therapy (ACCORD et al., 2007)
α-Glucosidase Inhibitors	α-Glucosidase inhibitors competitively block small intestine brush border enzymes that are necessary to hydrolyze oligo and polysaccharides to monosaccharide. Inhibition of this enzyme slows the absorption of carbohydrates; the postprandial rise in plasma glucose is blunted in both normal and diabetic subjects (Bischoff, 1995).	Dose-related flatulence, diarrhea, and abdominal bloating, high cost. Hypoglycemia (Reabasa-Lhoret&Chiasson, 1998).

Table 1: Current synthetic oral hypoglycemic drugs for Type 2 diabetes with their side effects

Pancreatic α-amylase (E.C. 3.2.1.1), and α-glucosidase (E.C, 3.2.1.20) are the enzymes in the digestive system responsible for the break down of the carbohydrates from diet. Digestion of carbohydrates, about 5 %is initiated by salivary amylases, which gets destroyed in the gut due to the high acid environment. When the food enters the intestine, the acidic pH from the gut is neutralized by bicarbonate from pancreas and mucous that lines the walls of the intestine. Pancreatic α-amylase is secreted into the small intestines by the pancreas and α-glucosidase enzymes are located in the brush border of the small intestines. Pancreatic α-amylase breaks down the carbohydrates into oligosaccharides, which are subsequently broken down to monosaccharide by α-glucosidase. Further, glucose and other monosaccharide are transported via the hepatic portal vein to the liver. Monosaccharides not immediately utilized for energy are stored as glycogen in the liver or as fat (triglycerides) in adipose tissue, liver and plasma. Carbohydrates that are resistant to digestion in the intestine enter the colon, where they are fermented by colonic bacteria to produce short-chain fatty acids, carbon dioxide and methane (Barrett & Udani, 2011).

In Type 2 diabetic patients, degradation of this dietary starch proceeds rapidly and leads to elevated post prandial hyperglycemia (PPHG). Hence retardation of starch digestion by inhibition of these enzymes viz., pancreatic α-amylase and α-glucosidase would play a key role in the control of diabetes. However, the discovery of safe, specific high-affinity inhibitors of these digestive enzymes for the development of therapeutics has remained elusive (Bhat *et al.*, 2008; Sudha *et al.*, 2010; Sudha *et al.*, 2011) (Figure 1).

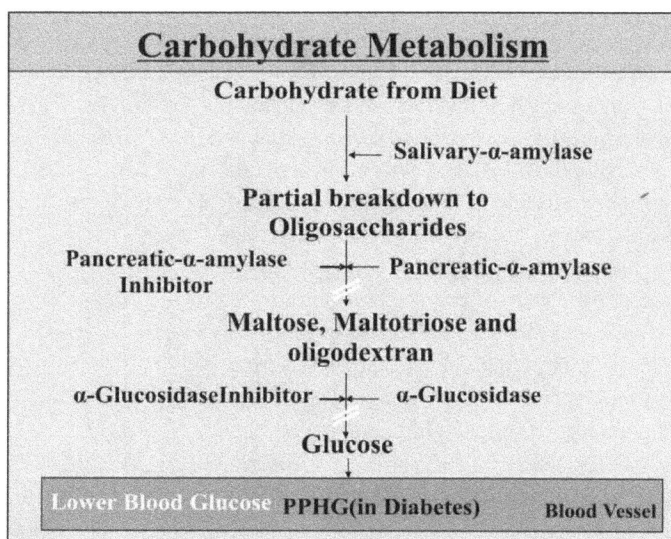

Figure1: Carbohydrate from diet is partially broken down to oligosaccharides by salivary α-amylase, which further catalyzed by pancreatic α-amylase in gut to maltose, maltotriose and oligodextrans. α-glucosidase acts on maltose and maltotriose to form monosaccharide (glucose), which enters the blood vessels. In case of Type 2 diabetics, carbohydrate digestion after meals leads to a condition called as post prandial hyperglycemia (PPHG). Double bar marks (///) indicate inhibition of pancreatic α-amylase and α-glucosidase activity leading to a reduction of maltose, oligosaccharide and glucose concentration and finally lowers the blood glucose level.

2 Pancreatic α-amylase and α-glucosidase Inhibitors from Indian Medicinal Plants

Indian medicinal plants have been an exemplary source of medicine. Research conducted in last few decades on plants mentioned in ancient literature or used traditionally for diabetes has shown antidiabetic property (Grover *et al.*, 2002). Very few of these plants have been characterized for their mechanistic action on varying antidiabetic targets. Plants are known to posses enzyme inhibitors as a defensive mechanism against the predating insects. The enzyme inhibitors act on key insect gut digestive hydrolases, the α-amylases and proteinases. Several kinds of α-amylase and proteinase inhibitors, present in seeds and vegetative organs, act to regulate numbers of phytophagous insects. This defensive mechanism has been acquired by plants over a period of time due to evolution. Pancreatic α-amylases and α-glucosidases are potent targets for antidiabetic agents (amylase and glucosidase inhibitors). These inhibitors would retard the starch digestion (Figure 1) in type 2 diabetic patients subsequently lowering post prandial hyperglycemia (PPHG). The presence of amylase inhibitors naturally in plants for their defenses has thus therapeutic implication as antidiabetic agents (Franco *et al.*, 2002; Bhat *et al.*, 2008).

2.1 Objective

The major work discussed in this chapter is screening and identification of lead pancreatic α-amylase and α-glucosidase inhibitors form known hypoglycemic Indian plants. The plants screened are listed in Table 2.

Plant Name	Family Name	Parts Used	Hypoglycemic and Medicinal Property
Adansoniadigitata L.	Bombacaceae	Leaves	Lowers blood glucose level due to insulin like effect on peripheral tissues; by promoting glucose uptake and metabolism or by inhibiting hepatic Gluconeogenesis (Tanko et al., 2008).
Allium sativum L.	Alliaceae	Rhizomes	Lowers blood pressure and improves lipid profile, decreases serum glucose, triglycerides, cholesterol, urea, uric acid, increases serum insulin levels (Eidia et al., 2006).
Aloe vera (L.) Burm.F.	Liliace	Leaf Gel	Hypoglycemic activity, decreases fasting glucose levels, hepatic transaminases, plasma and liver cholesterol, triglycerides, free fatty acids and phospholipids. Improves plasma insulin level. Restores normal levels of LDL and HDL and cholesterol Reduces levels of hepatic phosphatidylcholine hydroperoxide and have hypocholesterimic efficacy, diminishes degenerative changes in kidney tissues (Yagi et al., 2009)
Azadirachta indica A. Juss.	Meliaceae	Leaves	Antihyperglycemic activity, increase in glucose uptake and glycogen deposition, inhibits activity of epinephrine on glucose metabolism resulting in utilization of peripheral glucose. Does not alter cortisol concentration (Modak et al., 2007; Chattopadhyay, 1999)
Bixaorellana L.	Bixaceae	Leaves	Hypoglycemic activity by lowering blood glucose by

			stimulating peripheral utilization of glucose (Russell et al., 2005)
Bougainvillea spectabilis Willd.	Nyctaginaceae	Leaves	Hypoglycemic effect is by D-pinitol which exerts insulin-like effect and inhibits α-glucosidase (Narayanan et al., 1987).
Casia fistula L.	Caesalpiniaceae	Leaves	Hypoglycemic activity decreases blood glucose level (Rizvi et al., 2009).
Catharanthus roseus (L.). G. Don	Apocynaceae	Leaves	Reduces blood glucose by enhancing secretion of insulin from b-cells of Langerhans or through extra pancreatic mechanism (Nammi et al., 2003).
Cinnamomum verum J.S.Presl	Lauraceae	Leaves, Bark	Hypoglycemic activity is by enhancing insulin activity, increasing lipid metabolism and antioxidant status, capillary function. Reduces the blood glucose and elevates the plasma insulin level (Khan et al., 2003; Verspohl et al., 2005).
Coccinia grandis (L.) Voigt.	Cucurbitacea	Fruit	Reduces blood glucose and glycosylated hemoglobin content. C. *indica* extracts lowers blood glucose by depressing its synthesis, depression of glucose 6-phosphatase and fructose1,6, bisphosphatase and enhancing glucose oxidation by shunt pathway through activation of glucose 6-phosphate dehydrogenase (Shibib et al., 1993)
Curcuma longa L.	Zingiberaceae	Rhizome	Hypoglycemic, hypolipidemic, and antioxidant property. Decreased influx of glucose in polyol pathway, increasing NADPH/NADP ratio and increased activity of glucose peroxidase (Arun&Nalini, 2002).
Ficus bengalensis L.	Moraceae	Leaves, Bark	Stimulates insulin secretion from beta cells inhibits insulin degradative process (Achrekar et al., 1991).
Ficus recemosa L.	Moraceae	Fruit pulp	Hypoglycemic activity by β-sitosterol isolated was found to lower the blood glucose level (Paarakh, 2009).
Linum usitatisumum L.	Linaceae	Seeds	Reduces fasting blood sugar levels, total cholesterol; reduces carbohydrate absorption from gut and clinical symptoms of diabetes associated with dyslipidamia (Thakur et al., 2009).
Mangifera indica L.	Anacardiaceae	Fruit, Leaves	Reduces glucose absorption in type 2 diabetes. Stimulates glycogenesis in liver causing reduction in blood glucose level (Bhowmik et al., 2009).
Momordica charantia L.	Cucurbitaceae	Leaves, fruit, seeds	Hypoglycemic effect by inhibition of glucose-6-phosphatase and fructose-1-6-biphosphatase in liver and stimulation of hepatic glucose-6-phosphate dehydrogenase (Shibib et al., 1993).
Murraya koenigii L. Spreng	Rutaceae	Leaves	Increases glucogenesis and decreases glycogenolysis and gluconeogenesis (Khan et al., 1995).

Morus alba L.	Moraceae	Leaves	Antiphlogistic, diuretic, expectorant and antidiabetic. Increases b-cell number in diabetic islets. Reduces levels of glycosylated hemoglobin. Decreases triglycerides, cholesterol and VLDL to normal levels in type II DM. Restores elevated levels of blood urea (Mohammadi&Naik, 2008).
Nerium oleander L.	Apocynaceae	Leaves	Clorogenic acid, querecetin and cathechin induce post prandial hyperglycemia by acting as α-glucosidase inhibitors (Ishikawa et al., 2007).
Ocimumtenuiflorum L.	Laminaceae	Leaves	Lowers blood glucose level, modulates cellular antioxidant defense system. Improves b cell function and enhances insulin secretion. Inhibits absorption of glucose from the intestine (Sethi et al., 2004)
Piper nigrum L.	Piperaceae	Seeds	Reduces glucose and serum lipid levels (Kaleem et al., 2005).
Syzygiumcumini L. Skeels (Jamun)	Myrtaceae	Seeds	Reduces blood glucose level, increase in serum insulin level, exhibits insulinase activity. Hypoglycemic activity mediated through insulin release mechanism, glycogen content and hepatic glucokinase, hexokinase, glucose-6-phosphate, and phosphofructokinase levels in diabetic mice (Modak et al., 2007)
Terminaliachebula Retz.	Combretaceae	Fruit	Decreases blood glucose levels by enhancing secretion of insulin from b cells of Langerhans or through extra pancreatic mechanism. Inhibits advanced glycosylation end products, which contribute to renal damage (Rao & Nammi, 2006).
Tinosporacordifolia (Willd.) Miers	Menispermaceae	Stem	Decreases blood glucose level through glucose metabolism. It exhibits inhibitory effect on adrenaline-induced hyperglycemia (Singh et al., 2003).
Trigonellafoenum-graceum L.	Fabaceae	Seeds	Decreases post prandial blood glucose level (Ismail, 2009).
TribulusterrestrisL.	Zygophyllaceae	Seeds	Hypoglycemic activity by inhibiting oxidative stress (Kostova & Dinchev, 2005).
ZingiberofficinaleRosc.	Zingiberaceae	Rhizome	Lowers plasma glucose level, (Agoreyo et al., 2006)

Table 2: Indian Medicinal plant sources and their traditional uses.

Screening is initiated by amylase and glucosidase inhibition assays of plant extracts prepared by solvent extraction protocol. The positive extracts are further subjected to bioactivity guided isolation of lead inhibitor components by varying chromatographic techniques. Enzyme inhibition kinetics performed would reveal the mode of inhibition of the lead purified inhibitor.

2.2   Extraction Protocols

Extraction, as the term is used pharmaceutically, involves the separation of medicinally active portions of plant or animal tissues from the inactive or inert components by using selective solvents in standard extraction procedures. The extract thus obtained can be further fractionated to isolate individual lead bioactive entities. Thus, standardization of extraction procedures contributes significantly to the final quality of the herbal drug (Reichardt, 2003).

Sequential solvent extraction is one such extraction protocol used to extract the desired components from plants based on their solubility in solvents varying in polarity. In Ayurveda, the herbal formulations prepared are generally aqueous in nature. Moreover, aqueous extracts contain peptides, proteins, or glycans, which would otherwise be denatured by organic solvents and high-temperature extraction. The recommended sequential solvent extraction is from a higher polar solvent (water) sequentially to a nonpolar solvent based on their relative polarity (Sudha *et al.*, 2010; Sudha *et al.*, 2011). The values for relative polarity are normalized from measurements of solvent shifts of absorption spectra (Reichardt, 2003). The extraction scheme is represented in Figure 2. Twenty-seven hypoglycemic plants listed in Table 2 yielded 217 extracts.

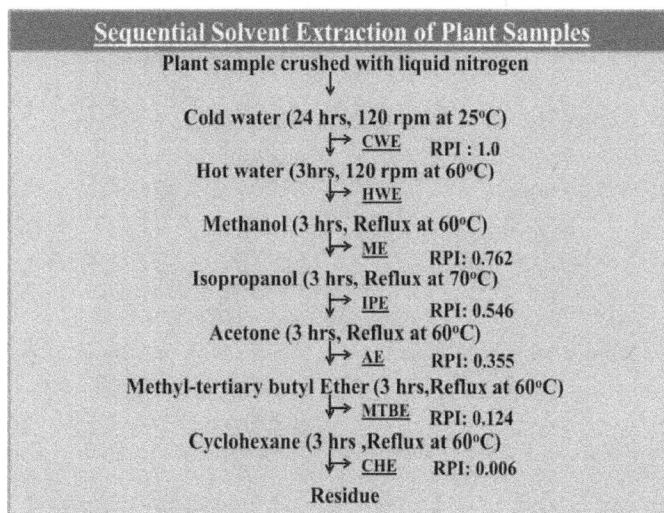

Figure 2: Plant samples are crushed with liquid nitrogen and sequentially extracted with solvents of decreasing polarity, initiating with water (Relative Polarity RP) of 1.0 and ending with cyclohexane (RP:0.006). CWE: Cold water extract; HWE: Hot water extract; ME: Methanol extract; IPE: Isopropanol extract; AE: Acetone extract; MTBE: Methyl-tertiary Butylether extract; CHE: Cyclohexane extract.

2.3   Biochemical Assay Protocols

Enzyme assays are experimental protocols that make enzyme-catalyzed chemical transformations visible. Such assays are very important for high-throughput screening in the context of drug discovery (Goddard & Reymond, 2004). One Unit (U) is defined as the amount of the enzyme that catalyses the conversion of 1 micromole of substrate or formation of 1 micromole of product per minute under the given assay conditions (Lehninger, 4th edition).

2.3.1 Pancreatic α-amylase Assay

There are mainly two types of assays that are used to determine the activity of α-amylase. One is based on measuring the amount of product formed i.e maltose a reducing sugar by the dinitrosalicylic acid (DNS) assay or the Nelson–Somogyi (Miller, 1959; Somogyi, 1952) method, whereas the other is based on the decreased staining value of blue starch–iodine complexes i.e measurement of substrate depletion (Fuwa, 1954).There are many chlorogenic substrates which are been approved by IFCC (International Federation for Clinical Chemistry) to determine the α-amylase activity.

Starch-iodine assay: The assay followed for screening of 126 extracts (Sudha *et al.*, 2011) of the 217 extracts initially was microtitre plate based on the starch-iodine test (Xiao *et al.*, 2006). Acarbose, was used a positive control. Appropriate controls were kept. A dark-blue color indicates the presence of starch; a yellow color indicates the absence of starch while a brownish color indicates partially degraded starch in the reaction mixture. In the presence of inhibitors from the extracts the starch added to the enzyme assay mixture is not degraded and gives a dark blue color complex whereas no color complex is developed in the absence of the inhibitor, indicating that starch is completely hydrolyzed by α-amylase.

3, 5-dinitrosalicylic acid assay: The positively screened 21extracts of the 126 by starch-iodine test along with the remaining 91 extracts (Sudha *et al.*, 2010) were quantitatively assayed for pancreatic α-amylase inhibition by chromogenic DNSA method. In this method, in presence of the free carbonyl group (C=O), present in the reducing sugars, (maltose formed due to amylase activity on starch) 3,5-dinitrosalicylic acid (DNSA) is reduced to 3-amino,5-nitrosalicylic acid under alkaline conditions:

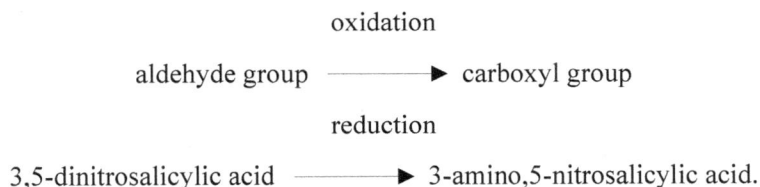

$$\text{aldehyde group} \xrightarrow{\text{oxidation}} \text{carboxyl group}$$

$$\text{3,5-dinitrosalicylic acid} \xrightarrow{\text{reduction}} \text{3-amino,5-nitrosalicylic acid.}$$

Appropriate enzyme and extract controls were kept.

One unit of enzyme activity is defined as the amount of enzyme required to release one micromole of maltose from starch per min under the assay conditions.

% Relative enzyme activity = (enzyme activity of test / enzyme activity of control) ×100;

% Inhibition in the *α*-amylase activity = (100 − % Relative enzyme activity).

The extracts are evaluated in terms of their IC_{50} value. The IC_{50} values were defined as the concentration of the extract, containing the *α*-amylase inhibitor that inhibited 50% of the pancreatic-*α*-amylase activity.

Structurally as well as mechanistically, porcine pancreatic α-amylase is closely related to human pancreatic-α-amylase (Brayer *et al.*, 1995). The enzyme used for screening is porcine pancreatic α-amylase. Further work is carried on human pancreatic α-amylase. Aqueous extracts (both hot and cold water) of *F. bengalensis* bark, *S. cumini*, methanol extracts of *B. orellana*, *C. longa*, *C. verum*, isopropanol extracts of *C. longa*, *C. verum*, *M. koenigi*, *L. usitatisumum*, *M. alba* and, *O. tenuiflorum*, and acetone extracts of *C. longa* and *T. terrestris* exhibited significant porcine pancreatic-α-amylase inhibition ≥ 50 % at a concentration ranging from 9.4 and 1900 μgmL^{-1}. On comparing the IC_{50} values of extracts against PPA and HPA with that of the positive control Acarbose (IC_{50} value both against PPA and HPA is 10.2 μgmL^{-1}), and the stability of the extracts over a period of time, except methanol extracts of *C. longa* and *C. verum* the remaining 13 extracts listed in Table.3 were taken further to isolate the lead inhibitor components. Of these, the 4 extracts, highlighted in red, exhibited a concentration independent inhibition whereas the other 8 extracts exhibited concentration dependent inhibition. *C.longa* isopropanol extract exhibited the least IC_{50} value of $0.16 \, \mu gmL^{-1}$ on HPA.

2.3.2   α-glucosidase Assay

α-Glucosidase catalyzes the hydrolysis of terminal α-1,4- and α-1,6-glucosidic linkages of glycogen. There are a few enzyme assays. The fluorescence assay uses 4-methylumbelliferyl-a-D-glucopyranoside (4MU-α-glc) as the fluorogenic substrate. The product of this substrate, 4-methylumbelliferone (4MU), emits at a peak of 440 nm in the fluorescence spectra. Chromogenic assays that use p-nitrophenyl-α-D-glucopyranoside and 2-naphthyl-α-D-glucopyranoside as substrates are also available for α-glucosidase assay. In addition, p-nitrophenyl-α-D-maltoheptaoside has been used for compound screening, but the screen throughput was relatively low (Motabar *et al.*, 2009). The α-glucosidase assay performed used the fluorescence assay with 4-MU-α-Glc as the substrate. One unit of enzyme activity is defined as the amount of enzyme required to release one micromole of 4-MU from 4-MU-α-Glc per min under the assay conditions (Sudha *et al.*, 2012).

% Relative enzyme activity = (enzyme activity of test / enzyme activity of control) *100;

% Inhibition in the *α*-amylase activity = (100 − % Relative enzyme activity)

2.4   Isolation of Lead Inhibitor Component

Natural products remain a prolific source of discovery of newer drugs and drug leads from vedic period. The conventional drug discovery process aims in identifying single pure active constituent from an active extract and a method to estimate it in the crude drug (Bhutani *et al.*, 2010). Bioassay-guided fractionation of medicinal plants is a routine feature in the attempt to isolate bioactive components from natural sources. Bioassay-guided fractionation linked to chromatographic separation techniques leads to the isolation of biologically active molecules whose chemical structures can readily be determined by modern spectroscopic methods (Phillipson *et al.*, 2001).

Bioactive guided purification of lead human pancreatic α-amylase inhibitor from the 13 extracts listed in Table 3 initiated with a qualitative phytochemical analysis of the extract, revealing the possible class of phytoconstituents present in these crude extracts. Alkaloids, proteins, tannins, cardiac glycosides, flavonoids, saponins and steroids are the class of compounds qualitatively detected in the extracts. GCMS analysis of the extracts revealed the probable compounds present.

Of these, *C.longa* isopropanol extract which exhibited the most potent human pancreatic α-amylase inhibition with the least IC_{50} value was worked on initially for the lead inhibitor compound. Preliminary phytochemical and GCMS analysis of this crude *C. longa* isopropanol extract suggested the presence of curcuminoids, sesquiterpenes and cinnamic acid as the components present. Bioactivity guided isolation of the lead inhibitor component with solvent fractionation and chromatographic techniques with characterization with HPLC and NMR in comparison with the standards revealed bisdemethoxycurcumin as a lead small molecule inhibitor of porcine and human pancreatic α-amylase with an IC_{50} value of 0.026 and 0.025 mM, respectively. The crude extract from rat gut was also checked for inhibition of α-amylase and α-glucosidase activity with BDMC at the HPA IC_{50} value (0.025 mM). The α-glucosidase from Baker's yeast and rat intestinal crude extract exhibited weaker inhibition of 16.4% and 21.0%, respectively, as compared to 53% for α-amylase from rat intestine, suggesting that BDMC is a better pancreatic α-amylase inhibitor as compared to α-glucosidase (Sudha *et al.*, 2012).

Plants	Extracts	Name of Compound	Molecular Formula	Molecular Wt	IC_{50} (μg/ml)value HPA
B. orellana L.(Leaves)	Methanol	β-tocopherol	$C_{28}H_{48}O_2$	416	49.0 ± 5.4E-3
		Vitamin E	$C_{29}H_{50}O_2$	430	
C. longa (Rhizomes)	Isopropanol	Podocarpic acid	$C_{17}H_{22}O_3$	274	0.16 ± 4.0E-5
		Curlone	$C_{15}H_{22}O$	218	
		Cinnamic-acid	$C_9H_8O_2$	148	
C. longa (Rhizomes)	Acetone	3-Cyano-7-hydroxy-4-methylcoumarin	$C_{11}H_7NO_3$	201	7.4 ± 1.0E-4
		Curlone	$C_{15}H_{22}O$	218	
		5-amino-2-hydroxybenzoic acid	$C_7H_7NO_3$	153	
C. verum (Leaves)	Isoporpanol	Naphthalene,1,2,3,4- tetrahydro-1,1,6-trimethyl	$C_{13}H_{18}$	174	1.0 ± 1.0E-4
		Eugenol	$C_{10}H_{12}O_2$	164	
		4-acetoxycinnamic acid	$C_{11}H_{10}O_4$	206	
F.bengalensis (Bark)	Cold water	ND			4.4 ± 2.3E-4
F.bengalensis (Bark)	Hot water	ND			125 ± 1.0E-3
L.usitatisumum (Seeds)	Isopropanol	2-cyclopentene-1-undecanoic acid	$C_{16}H_{28}O_2$	252	540 ± 2.0E-3*
		cyclopentane undecanoic acid	$C_{16}H_{30}O_2$	254	
M. alba (Leaves)	Isopropanol	Napthelene	$C_{10}H_8$	128.6	1440 ± 6.0E-3*
		Hexadeconoic acid	$C_{16}H_{32}O_2$	256.4	
		9, 12-octadecadienic acid	$C_{17}H_{31}COOH$	280.44	
M. koenigii L.(Leaves)	Isopropanol	Cyclohexanone, 2-methyl-5-(1-methylethenyl)	$C_{10}H_{16}O$	152	127 ± 4.0E-3
		2,3,5,6-tetrachlorohydroquinone	$C_6H_2Cl_4O_2$	247	
		Vitamin E	$C_{29}H_{50}O_2$	430	
Ocimum tenuiflorum L.(Leaves)	Isopropanol	Camphene	$C_{10}H_{16}$	136.24	8.9 ± 3.5E-3*
		Methyleugenol	$C_{11}H_{14}O_2$	178.23	
		2-heptanol, 5-ethyl	$C_9H_{20}O$	144.25	
S. cumini (Seeds)	Cold water	ND			42.1 ± 2.6E-3
S. cumini (Seeds)	Hot water	ND			4.1± 2.8E-4
T. terrestris L. (Seeds)	Acetone	Sorbinose	$C_6H_{12}O_6$	180	511 ± 5.0E-3
		Ethyl crotonate	$C_6H_{10}O_2$	114	

Table 3: GCMS analysis of extracts exhibiting ≥ 50% inhibition on α-amylase activity. ND: Not determined. * IC_{50} (μg /ml) for PPA.

2.5   Enzyme inhibition kinetics

Enzyme inhibition is defined as a reduction in enzyme activity through the binding of an inhibitor to a catalytic or regulatory site on the enzyme, or in the case of uncompetitive inhibition, to the enzyme–substrate complex. Inhibition can be reversible which involves non covalent bonding irreversible involving covalent binding. Inhibitors differ in the mechanism by which they decrease enzyme activity. There are three basic mechanisms of inhibition–competitive, noncompetitive, and uncompetitive inhibition. A competitive inhibitor is usually a close analogue of the substrate. It binds at the catalytic site but does not undergo catalysis. A noncompetitive inhibitor does not bind to the catalytic site but binds to a second site on the enzyme and acts by reducing the turnover rate of the reaction. An uncompetitive inhibitor does not bind to the enzyme but only the enzyme–substrate complex. Enzyme kinetics is principally concerned with the measurement and mathematical description of the enzyme reaction rate and its associated constants. The Michaelis–Menten equation, as presented by Michaelis and Menton and further developed by Briggs and Haldane (Briggs & Haldane, 1925; Michaelis & Menton, 1913) is fundamentally important to enzyme kinetics.

$$v = v_{max}[A] / (K_m + [A])$$

where [A] is the substrate concentration; K_m is an inverse measure of the affinity or strength of binding between the enzyme and its substrate. The lower the K_m, the greater the affinity (so the lower the concentration of substrate needed to achieve a given rate).The k_{cat}, is the turnover number of the enzyme, is a measure of the maximum catalytic production of the product under saturating substrate conditions per unit time per unit enzyme. The larger the values of k_{cat}, the more rapidly catalytic events occur. The v_{max} is the maximum velocity that an enzyme could achieve. The measurement is theoretical because at given time, it would require all enzyme molecules to be tightly bound to their substrates.

Evaluating enzyme kinetics using a nonlinear plot Michaelis and Menten is avoided by using one of the three common linearization methods, Lineweaver–Burke, Eadie–Hofsteeplots; Hanes plots to obtain estimates for K_m and v_{max}. In case of competitive inhibitor, an increase in the inhibitor concentration will increase the apparent K_m of the enzyme. However, since an infinite substrate concentration will exclude the competitive inhibitor, there is no effect on v_{max}. Whereas, in case of a simple noncompetitive inhibitor K_m is not altered, but v_{max} reduces as inhibitor concentration increases. In case of an uncompetitve inhibitor, sequestration of the enzyme–substrate complex will reduce the apparent k_{cat} because the inhibited enzyme is less catalytically effective. Apparent v_{max} is reduced (and apparent K_m increased) because binding of the inhibitor cannot be prevented by increasing the substrate concentration.

Enzyme inhibition kinetics in other words reveals the mechanism of inhibition. The kinetics alters with respect to purity of the inhibitor and the substrate worked on. The effect of bisdemethoxycurcumin on the kinetics of HPA catalyzed hydrolysis of starch was studied at differing inhibitor concentrations. The double reciprocal LB plots revealed that the mode of bisdemethoxycurcumin inhibition is uncompetitive for starch as a substrate with an apparent K_i of 3.0 µM and decrease in both the apparent K_m and v_{max}values. Thus bisdemethoxycurcumin binds to the enzyme at a site other than the active site. Stoichiometry in enzyme inhibition kinetics accounts for the ratio in which the inhibitor molecules bind to an enzyme molecule to exhibit enzyme inhibition. The stoichiometry of bisdemethoxycurcumin:HPA when calculated at varying concentration of inhibitor to a fixed concentration of enzyme accounts for one molecule of bisdemethoxycurcumin binding to one molecule of HPA, thus exhibiting a stiochiometry1:1 (Sudha *et al.*, 2012).

3   Conclusion

Many different plants have been used individually or in formulations for treatment of diabetes and its complications due to their advantages over current drug therapy. One of the major problems with this herbal formulation is that the active ingredients are not well defined. It is important to know the active component and their molecular interaction, which will help to analyze therapeutic efficacy of the product and also to standardize the product. In this limelight, target based drug discovery would reveal the mode of action of the drug on the antidiabetic targets. Human pancreatic α-amylase and α-glucosidase are the preliminary enzymes in carbohydrate metabolism, the retardation of their activities by inhibitors would play a key role in management of diabetes. Plants are a good source of glycosidase inhibitors as a key defensive mechanism against insects. This property has been exploited for its therapeutic implication against diabetes mellitus for retarding the activities of these glycosidases. With this rationale, in our research work carried out, 217 plant extracts from 27 different hypoglycemic plants have been screened for α-amylase and α-glucosidase inhibitors. The screening finally concluded with *C.longa* isopropanol extract exhibiting potent pancreatic α-amylase inhibition at an IC_{50} value of $0.16\mu gml^{-1}$. Bioactivity guided isolation and characterization of lead inhibitor compound from *C.longa* isopropanol extract resulted inbisdemethoxycurcumin as the potent lead inhibitor component with an IC_{50} value of 0.025 mM. HPA inhibition kinetics revealed its mode of inhibition to be uncompetitive with a stoichiometry of 1:1(Sudha *et al.*, 2012).Thus, an inactivator of HPA *viz.*, BDMC isolated from *C. longa* functioning via uncompetitive inhibition could be developed as a lead anti-diabetic compound. Knowledge gained in this study would help future developments of functional foods for controlling starch digestion and postprandial hyperglycemia. As per the drug discovery module, *in vivo* preclinical studies would reveal the pharmacokinetic and pharmacodynamic parameters for the drug to be an eligible lead for clinical studies.

Acknowledgement

The authors thank University Grants Commission, New Delhi for financial support.

References

ACCORD Study Group, Buse, J. B., Bigger, J. T., Byington, R. P., Cooper, L. S., Cushman, W. C., Friedewald, W. T., Genuth, S., Gerstein, H. C., Ginsberg, H. N., Goff, D. C. Jr, Grimm, R. H. Jr, Margolis, K. L., Probstfield, J. L., Simons-Morton, D. G., & Sullivan, M. D. (2007). Action to control cardiovascular risk in diabetes (ACCORD) trial. Design and methods.American Journal of Cardiology, 99, S21-S33.

Achrekar, S., Kaklij, G. S., Pote, M. S., & Kelkar, S. M. (1991). Hypoglycemic activity of Eugenia jambolana and Ficusbengalensis: mechanism of action. In Vivo, 5(2), 143-147.

Agoreyo, F. O., Agoreyo, B. O., & Onuorah, M. N. (2006). Effect of aqueous extracts of Hibiscus sabdariffa and Zingiber Officinale on blood cholesterol and glucose levels of rats. Phytotherapy Research, 20, 764.

Arun, N. & Nalini, N. (2002). Efficacy of turmeric on blood sugar and polyol pathway in diabetic albino rats. Plant Foods for Human Nutrition, 57(1), 41-52.

Alberti, K. G., & Zimmet, P. Z. (1998). Definition, diagnosis and classification of diabetes mellitus and its complications. Part 1: diagnosis and classification of diabetes mellitus. Report of a WHO Consultation.Diabetic Medicine, 15(7), 539-553.

Barrett, M. L.,&Udani, J. K. (2011). A proprietary alpha-amylase inhibitor from white bean (Phaseolus vulgaris): A review of clinical studies on weight loss and glycemic control, Nutrition Journal, 10(24), 1-10.

Bastaki, S. (2005). Diabetes mellitus and its treatment. International Journal of Diabetes & Metabolism, 13, 111-134.

Bhat, M., Zinjarde, S. S., Bhargava, S.Y. RaviKumar, A. & Joshi, B. N. (2008).Antidiabetic Indian Plants: A good source of potent amylase inhibitors. Evidence based Complementary and Alternative Medicine, 2011, 1-6. doi:10.1093/ecam/nen040.

Bhowmik, A., Khan, L. A., Akhter, M., & Rokeya, B. (2009). Studies on the antidiabetic effects of Mangifera indica stembarks and leaves on nondiabetic, type 1 and type 2 diabetic model rats. Bangladesh Journal of Pharmacology, 4,110-114.

Bhutani, K. K., & Ghoil, V. M. (2010). Natural products drug discovery in India: Status and appraisal. Indian Journal of Experimental Biology, 48, 199-207.

Bischoff, H. (1995). The mechanism of α-glucosidase inhibition in the management of diabetes. Clinical and Investigative Medicine, 18, 303-311.

Bolen, S., Feldman, L., Vassy, J., Wilson, L., Yeh, H. C., Marinopoulis, S., Wiley, C., Selvin, E., Wilson, R., Bass, E. B., &Brancati, F. L. (2007). Systematic review: comparative effectiveness and safety of oral medications fortype 2 diabetes mellitus. Annals Internal Medicine.147, 386-99.

Brayer, G. D., Luo, Y., & Withers, S. G. (1995).The structure of human pancreatic α- amylase at 1.8 A° resolution and comparisons with related enzymes. Protein Science, 4, 1730-1742.

Briggs, G., & Haldane, J. (1925). A note on the kinetics of enzyme action. Biochemical Journal, 19, 338-339.

Chattopadhyay, R.R. (1999). Possible mechanism of antihyperglycemic effect of Azadirachta indica leaf extract: part V. Journal of Ethnopharmacology, 67(3), 373-376.

Eidia, A., Eidib, M., & Esmaeillia, E. (2006). Antidiabetic effect of garlic (Allium sativum L.) in normal and streptozotocininduced diabetic rats. Phytomedicine, 13, 624-629.

Feinglos, M. N., & Bethel, M. A. (1999). Therapy of type 2 diabetes, cardiovascular death, and the UGDP. American Heart Journal, 138, 346-352.

Franco, O. L., Rigden, D. J., Melo, F. R., & Grossi-de-SaÂ, M. F. (2002). Plant α-amylase inhibitors and their interaction with insect α-amylases: Structure, function and potential for crop protection. European Journal of Biochemistry, 269, 397-412.

Fuwa, H. (1954). A new method of micro determination of amylase activity by the use of amylose as the substrate. The Jorunal of Biochemistry, 41, 583-603.

Goddard, J. P., & Reymond, J. L. (2004). Recent advances in enzyme assays, TRENDS in Biotechnology, 22(7), 363-370.

Grover, J. K., Yadav, S., & Vats, V.(2002). Medicinal plants of India with anti-diabetic potential. Journal of Ethnopharmacology, 81(1), 81-100.

Hall, G. M., & Nicholson, G. (2009). Current therapeutic drugs for type 2 diabetes, still useful after 50 years? Anesthesia & Analgesia, 108(6), 1727-1730.

Hansen, T. (2002). Type 2 diabetes mellitus--a multifactorial disease. Annales Universitatis Mariae Curie-Sklodowska. Section D: Medicina, 57(1), 544-549.

Humber, J. M. (2002). The role of complementary and alternative medicine: accommodating pluralism. Journal of American Medical Association, 288, 1655-1656.

Ishikawa, A., Yamashita, H., Hiemori, M., Inagaki, E., Kimoto, M., Okamoto, M., Tsuji, H., Memon, A. N., Mohammadi, A., & Natori, Y. (2007). Characterization of inhibitors of post prandial hyperglycemia from the leaves of Nerium indicum. Journal of Nutritional Science and Vitaminology, 53, 16-173.

Ismail, M. Y. M. (2009). Clinical evaluation of antidiabetic activity of Trigonella seeds and Aegle marmelos leaves. World Applied Sciences Journal, 7(10), 1231-1234.

John, Z. L. & Luguang, L. (2009). Ginseng on hyperglycemia: effects and mechanisms. Evidence-Based Complementary and Alternative Medicine, 6, 423–427.

Kaleem, M., Sarmad, H., & Bano, B. (2005). Protective effects of Piper nigrum and Vinca rosea in alloxan induced diabetic rats. Indian Journal of Physiology and Pharmacology, 49(1), 65-71.

Kelle, D.E.(1995). Effects of weight loss on glucose homeostasis in NIDDM. Diabetes Reviews, 3, 366-377.

Khan, B. A., Abraham, A., & Leelamma, S. (1995). Hypoglycemic action of Murraya koenigii (curry leaf) and Brassica juncea (mustard): mechanism of action. Indian Journal of Biochemistry and Biophysics, 32(2), 106-108.

Khan, A., Safdar, M., Khan, M. M. A., Khattak, K. N.,& Anderson, R. A.(2003). Cinnamon improves glucose and lipids of people with type 2 diabetes. Diabetes Care, 26(12), 3215-3218.

Kostova, I., &Dinchev, D. (2005). Saponins in Tribulus terrestris-chemistry and bioactivity. Photochemistry Reviews, 4, 111–137.

Lehninger, Principles of Biochemistry, page 94, 4th Edition.

Michaelis, L., & Menton, M. (1913). Die kinetik der invertinwirkung. Biochemische Zeitschrift, 49, 333-369.

Miller, G.L. (1959). Use of dinitrosalicylic acid reagent for determination of reducing sugar. Analytical Chemistry, 31,426-428.

Modak, M., Dixit, P., Londhe, J., Ghaskadbi, S., & Devasagayam, T.P.A. (2007). Indian herbs and herbal drugs used for the treatment of diabetes. Journal of Clinical Biochemistry and Nutrition, 40(3), 163-173.

Mohammadi, J., & Naik, P. R. (2008). Evaluation of hypoglycemic effect of Morus alba in an animal model. Indian Journal of Pharmacology, 40(1), 15-18.

Motabar, O., Shi, Z. D., Goldin, E., Liu, K., Southall, N., Sidransky, E., Austin, C. P., Griffiths, G. L., Zheng, W. (2009). A new resorufin-based α-glucosidase assay for high-throughput screening. Analytical Biochemistry, 390, 79-84.

Mukherjee, P. K., Maiti, K., Mukherjee, K., & Houghton, P. J. (2006). Leads from Indian medicinal plants with hypoglycemic potentials. Journal of Ethnopharmacology, 106(1), 1-28.

Nammi, S., Boini, M. K., Lodagala, S., & Behara, R. B. S.(2003). The juice of fresh leaves of Catharanthus roseus Linn. reduces blood glucose in normal and alloxan diabetic rabbits. BMC Complementary and Alternative Medicine, 3(4),1-4.

Narayanan, C. R., Joshi, D. D., Mujumdar, A. M., & Dhekne, V. V. (1987). Pinitol-a new anti-diabetic compound from the leaves of Bougainvillea spectabilis. Current Science, 56, 139-141.

Paarakh, P. M. (2009). Ficus racemosa linn.—an overview. Natural Product Radiance, 8(1), 84-90.

Phillipson, J. D. (2001). Phytochemistry and medicinal plants.Phytochemistry, 56, 237-243.

Rao, N. K., & Nammi, S. (2006). Antidiabetic and renoprotective effects of the chloroform extract of Terminalia chebula Retz. seeds in streptozotocin induced diabetic rats. BMC Complementary and Alternative Medicine, 6(17), 1-6.

Reabasa-Lhoret, R., & Chiasson, J. L. (1998). Potential of α-glucosidase inhibitors in elderly patients with diabetes mellitus and impaired glucose tolerance. Drug Aging, 3, 131-143.

Reichardt, C. (2003). Solvents and solvent effects in organic chemistry, Wiley-VCH Publishers, 3rd Edition.

Rizvi, M. M. A., Irshad, M., Gamal El Hassadi, G., &Younis, S. B. (2009). Bioefficacies of Cassia fistula: An Indian labrum. African Journal of Pharmacy and Pharmacology, 3(6), 287-292.

Russell, K. R. M., Morrison, E. Y. St. A., & Ragoobirsingh, D. (2005). The effect of annatto on insulin binding properties in the dog. Phytotherapy Research, 19(5), 433-436.

Seidl,P.R.(2002). Pharmaceuticals from natural products: current trends. Annals of the Brazilian Academy of Sciences, 74,145-150.

Sethi, J., Sood, S., Seth,S., & Talwar, A.(2004). Evaluation of hypoglycemic and antioxidant effect of Ocimum sanctum. Indian Journal of Clinical Biochemistry, 19(2), 152-155.

Sheehan, M. T. (2003). Current therapeutic opinion in type 2 diabetes mellitus: a practical approach. Clinical Medicine & Research, 1, 189-200.

Shekelle, P. G., Hardy, M., Morton, S. C., Coulter, I., Venuturupalli, S., Favreau, J., Hilton, L. K (2005). Are Ayurvedic herbs for diabetes effective? The Journal of Family Practice, 54(10), 876-886.

Shibib, B.A., Khan, L A., & Rahman, R. (1993). Hypoglycaemic activity of Coccinia indica and Momordica charantia in diabetic rats: depression of the hepatic gluconeogenic enzymes glucose-6-phosphatase and fructose-1,6- bisphosphatase and elevation of liver and red-cell shunt enzyme glucose-6-phosphate dehydrogenase. Biochemical Journal, 292(1), 267-270.

Singh, S. S., Pandey, S. C., Srivastava, S., Gupta, V. S., Patro, B., & Ghosh, A. C. (2003). Chemistry and Medicinal Properties of Tinospora cordifolia (Guduchi). Indian Journal of Pharmacology, 3, 83-91.

Somogyi, M. (1952). Notes on sugar determination. Journal of Biological Chemistry, 195, 19-23.

Stumvoll, M., Nurjhan, N., Perriello, G., Dailey, G., & Gerich, J.E. (1995).The metabolic effects of metformin in non-insulin-dependent diabetes mellitus. The New England Journal of Medicine, 333, 550-554.

Stumvoll, M., Ha¨ring, H. U., &Matthaei, S. (2007). Metformin. Endocrinology Research, 32, 39-57.

Sudha, P.,Ravindran, R., Zinjarde, S Bhargava, S.,& Ravi Kumar, A.(2010). Evaluation of traditional Indian antidiabeticmedicinal plants for human pancreatic amylase inhibitory effect in vitro.Evidence-Based Complementary and Alternative Medicine, 2011, 1-10.

Sudha, P., Zinjarde, S., Bhargava, S., & Ravi Kumar, A. (2011). Potent α-amylase inhibitory activity of Indian Ayurvedic medicinal plants. BMC Complementary and Alternative Medicine, 2011, 11(5), 1-10.

Sudha , P., Zinjarde. S., Bhargava, S., Rajamohanan, P.R., & RaviKumar, A. (2012). Discovering Bisdemethoxycurcumin from Curcuma longa rhizome as a potent small molecule inhibitor of human pancreatic α-amylase, a target for type-2 diabetes. Food Chemistry, 2012, 135(4), 2638-2642.

Tanko, Y., Yerima, M., Mahdi, M. A., Yaro, A.H., & Mohammed A. (2008). Hypoglycemic activity of methanolicstem bark of Adansonnia digitata extract on blood glucose levels of streptozocin-induced diabetic wistar rats. International Journal of Applied Research in Natural Products, 1(2), 32-36.

Thakur, G., Mitra, A., Pal, K., & Rousseau, D. (2009). Effect of flaxseed gum on reduction of blood glucose & cholesterol in type 2 diabetic patients. International Journal of Food Sciences and Nutrition, 60(S6), 126-136.

Verspohl, E. J., Bauer, K., & Neddermann, E.(2005). Antidiabetic effect of Cinnamomum cassia and Cinnamomum zeylanicumin vivo and in vitro. Phytotherapy Research, 19(3), 203-206.

World Health Organization (WHO), Diabetes Programme, 2012, http//www.who.Int/diabetes/en/.

World Health Organization. (1999). Definition, diagnosis and classification of diabetes mellitus and its complications. Part 1:Diagnosis and classification of diabetes mellitus (Department of noncommunicable disease surveillance, Geneva)

Legal status of traditional medicine, complementary/alternative medicine: a worldwide review World Health Organization, Geneva, 2001.

Xiao, Z., Storms, R., & Tsang, A. (2006). A quantitative starch-iodine method for measuring α-amylase and glucoamylase activities. Analytical Biochemistry, 351(1),146-148.

Yagi, A., Hegazy, S., Kabbash, A., & Abd-El Wahab, E. (2009). Possible hypoglycemic effect of Aloe vera L. high molecular weight fractions on Type 2 Diabetic patients. Saudi Pharmaceutical Journal, 17(3),210-218.

Zimmet, P., Alberti, K. G. M.,& Shaw, J. (2001). Global and societal implications of the diabetes epidemic. Nature, 414, 782-787.

Nutritional Content of Organic Prickly Pads (Opuntia ficus indica) Could be Cure to Different Disease Conditions

Esther Pérez-Torrero, Margarita I. Hernández-Urbiola
Departamento de Posgrado e Investigación, Facultad de Ingeniería
Universidad Autónoma de Querétaro, Querétaro, México

Mario E. Rodríguez-García
Departamento de Nanotecnología, Centro de Física Aplicada y Tecnología Avanzada
Universidad Nacional Autónoma de México, Querétaro, México

1 Introduction

Prickly pads nutritional content is good option between food recommendations for human nutrition and health care maintaining. This requires the use of the best available scientific evidence nutraceutical properties to achieve the goals an expertise team who plays the leading role in providing nutrition in order to prevent degenerative disease such as diabetes (Luo *et al.*, 2010; Musabayane, 2012). Diabetes is a serious degenerative diseases related to metabolic disorder; diabetes mellitus has been defined as a chronic disease of carbohydrate metabolism, but lipid and protein metabolism are also affected (Bailey, 2002; Bennet, 2004).

The consumption of *Opuntia* cactus is a popular herbal remedy among Mexican American patients in their management of type 2 diabetes mellitus. Animal and human studies have demonstrated the hypoglycemic properties of the Opuntia (prickly pear) cactus that are likely attributable to both its fiber content and specific hypoglycemic molecular agents. Reduction in serum glucose levels are best observed when the cactus cladodes are consumed in cooked form, alluding to heating as a necessary step in attaining its hypoglycemic properties (López, 2007). The *Opuntia* spp. cladodes and fruits serve as a source of varied number of phytoconstituents, mainly sugar, phenolics and pigments. Although the reported evidences provide the effectiveness of Opuntia spp., active constituents, bioavailability, pharmacokinetics and physiological pathways for various biological actions are not well known in sufficient detail or with confidence. Still more attention is required toward the development of simple, feasible and cost-effective pharmaceutical preparations of Opuntia spp. cladodes and fruit juice, as well as the ethnobotanical approach, if combined with mechanism of action, biochemical and physiological methods, would provide useful pharmacological leads (Chauhan *et al.*, 2012). Other study propose antihyperglycemic effect by protecting the liver from peroxidation damage and by maintaining tissue function, thereby improving the sensitivity and response of target cells in diabetic mice to insulin (Zhao *et al.*, 2011).

The traditional liquefied extract of the cladode of *Opuntia streptacantha* produces an anti-hyperglycemic effect when administered before a glucose challenge, and this anti-hyperglycemic effect is maintained after filtering the extract. Administration of both plants can improve glycemic control by blocking the hepatic glucose output, especially in the fasting state (Andrade-Cetto & Wiedenfeld, 2010).

The chronic hyperglycemia of diabetes is associated with long term damage, dysfunction and failure of various organs, especially the eyes, kidneys, nerves, heart and blood. At present, the treatment of diabetes mainly involves the use of plants with hypoglycemic properties. However, due to unwanted side effects the efficacies of these compounds are debatable and there is a demand for new compounds for the treatment of diabetes (Moller, 2001). Hence, plants have been suggested as a rich, as yet unexplored source of potentially useful antidiabetic drugs. These efforts may provide treatment for all and justify the role of novel traditional medicinal plants having anti-diabetic potentials (Kavishankar *et al.*, 2011).

Previous studies reported that the main constituents of dietary fiber or unavailable carbohydrate are non-starch polysaccharides, having physiological actions on gastrointestinal tract and inhibit absorption of glucose and its uptake, also studied the role of viscous and fermentable fibers in the treatment of diabetes mellitus (Cameron-Smith *et al.*, 1994, Eastwood & Morris, 1992 Galibois *et al.*, 1994, Gallaher *et al.*, 1995, Jackson *et al.*, 1999, Johnson & Gee 1986, Moharib, 2000). An increased dietary intake of plant fiber is currently being recommended for lowering of plasma lipids in persons with hyperlipidemia and improving the control (Easwaran *et al.*, 1994).

Dietary fiber has been defined previously as the plant polysaccharides and lignin, which are resistant to hydrolysis by digestive enzymes of man. Dietary fiber has been one of the most enduring dietary interests of this decade worldwide. It is a mixture of variety of polysaccharides, cellulose, hemicelluloses, pectin, gums, mucilage, algal polysaccharides and lignin has been found to have hypoglycemic effect (Lafrance et al., 1998, Prasad et al., 1995).

As for the general population, people with diabetes are encouraged to choose a variety of fiber-containing foods such as legumes, fiber-rich cereals (≥5 g fiber/serving), fruits, vegetables, and whole grain products because they provide vitamins, minerals, and other substances important for good health. Moreover, there are data suggesting that consuming a high-fiber diet (50 g fiber/day) reduces glycemia in subjects with type 1 diabetes and glycemia, hyperinsulinemia, and lipemia in subjects with type 2 diabetes (Franz et al., 2002). Palatability, limited food choices, and gastrointestinal side effects are potential barriers to achieving such high-fiber intakes. However, increased fiber intake appears to be desirable for people with diabetes, and a first priority might be to encourage them to achieve the fiber intake goals set for the general population of 14 g/1,000 kcal (Institute of Medicine, 2002).

2   Prickly Pads Characteristics

Organic natural plants are good alternative food sources because they often contribute to human health and its maintenance. It has been demonstrated in several studies that transgenic and cultivated crops have the potential to directly endanger or damage health because of pesticides and insecticide treatments used to enhance and protect these crops many of these foods are generally associated with health issues or for example, the development of allergies from the toxic effects from fertilizers used to enhance such crops nutritional value and also the microbiological safeness of these foods (OMS, 2005).

In Mexico, cactus *Opuntia ficus indica* have been used since prehispanic times, as an important component of diets and for the agricultural economy. They have also been accompanied with other products such as maize, amaranth and agave to name but a few (Betancourt-Domínguez et al., 2006). Prickly pads are grown throughout Mexico and in all North and South American. This cactus grows in many other regions of the world such as: Africa, Australia and in the Mediterranean (Piga, 2004). Cactus pads are commonly called "*nopales*" or "nopalitos" when they are fresh young prickly pads from 3-4 weeks of age. Traditionally "nopales" have been consumed in Mexico and Unites States, using several different preparations or cooking methods. Furthermore, the older stage pads are frequently used as forage, especially when there is shortage of fresh forage due to droughts. This plant is cheap, plentiful and sometimes it has also been used for erosion control (Le Houérou, 1996).

3   Health Benefits of Prickly Pads

Dietary fiber is composed of several chemical components that are resistant to digestive enzymes such as cellulose, hemicelluloses, pectin, lignin, gums, etc. (Periago et al., 1993). The fiber content of a food varies according to the species of the plant and its maturity stage. It is noteworthy that plant seeds, berries, fruit skins and the bran layers of cereal grains generally contain large amounts of fiber (Saénz, 1997). The benefits associated with fiber content are well known, especially for the prevention of illnesses such as: diabetes, treatment of gastrointestinal disorders, illnesses associated with low dietary fiber intake, reduction of glucose values in the blood, anti-hyperlipidemic and anti-hypercholesterolemic effects (Palumbo et al., 2003, Feugang et al., 2006, Gebremariam, 2006, Saénz, 1997). Age related differences within the species can be attributed to the type of *Opuntia*, the climatic conditions where the plants grow as a result of factors such as pluvial precipitation or availability of irrigation.

Regarding the benefit of fiber content in the prickly pads powders, is interesting to remark the relationship between the intake of carbohydrates and the current epidemic of obesity and diabetes as a subject of present interest. Ever since glucose is an essential source of energy, with limited body stores, maintenance of blood levels and changes in its metabolism are strongly determined by the intake of carbohydrates in the diet. Depending on the individual genetic susceptibility and the impact of other risk factors, these metabolic changes can deteriorate and induce abnormalities which increase the risk to develop diseases (Manuel-y-Keenoy & Perez-Gallardo, 2012).

The existing obesity epidemic is becoming a major public health burden for both countries developed and developing. More than ten years ago the World Health Organization estimated that 90% of diabetes mellitus type 2 and 30-40% of cardiovascular disease cases are directly caused by obesity (WHO, 1998). Because has been reported that even small changes in body weight (5 kg) have an impact on health. In particular, a fat excess of abdomen in contrast than peripheral fat, for example, with increases of 5 cm in waist circumference, is associated with increased risk to lead disease. These changes are the inevitable result of an imbalance between energy intake and the expenditure. This imbalance reflects life habits, which include a diet with a caloric content that is excessive for the often low levels of physical activity (Hill & Prentice, 1995; Saris, 2003).

Previous studies demonstrated that young prickly pads are rich in calcium and this increases according to the age of the pads. Most current literature addresses the usefulness of young pads, but does not include data concerning prickly pads in advanced maturity stages (Rodríguez-García *et al.*, 2007, Sáenz, 2000, Stintzing & Schieber, 2001).

Opuntia prickly pads are an important source of several nutritional elements like pectin, mucilage and minerals. Currently there is only information related to young stage pads and .precious little relating to the nutritional value of older maturity stage pads. The fresh young pads also know as cladodes are an excellent source of proteins including essential amino acids, and vitamins. Several studies have reported that high levels of amino acids especially proline, taurine and serine can also be found in prickly pads (Moreno-Alvarez *et al.*, 2008, Piga, 2004, Stintzing & Carle, 2005 Stintzing & Schieber, 2001). In contrast, not much information is available about the older prickly pads regarding amino acids profile. Also noteworthy, is that there is a gap in studies that have already been published regarding the nutritional and mineral content of the advanced stage pads.

The tannins are amorphous solids, quite soluble in water and alcohol, are virtually insoluble in ether where produce precipitates with alkaloids, jellies and salts of many heavy metals of the group of the alkaline earth metals such as Be, Mg, Ca, Sr, Ba and Ra. It is known that these substances have antinutrimental activity, although its mode of action is not well known. Findings suggest that have a role of enzyme inhibition, since they form complexes with protein and human hinder the assimilation of this macronutrient (Jean, 1998). The tannins have little relevance in the human diet and are mainly found in coffee, tea and some fruit (Cervera, 2001).

There is a general consensus among dieticians that diet plays a vital role in the support system of the body. Proper diet provides the strength and nutrition that individuals need to prevent disease; reading up on organic food information will help to build up immunity. Organic production of food includes cultural, biological, and mechanical practices that foster cycling of resources, promoting ecological balance and conserving biodiversity. Comparison studies of health in populations that habitually consume organically- or conventionally-produced foods clearly indicate the potential health benefits of organic foods. In order to be better supported in the future, more research of better quality is necessary than that which is currently available (Williams, 2002).

4   Materials and Methods

4.1   Sample Preparation

The *Opuntia ficus indica*, var. redonda, were from the experimental field of Universidad Nacional Autonoma de Mexico, located on "Los Lores" farm, in Silao, Guanajuato Mexico were harvested during the summer of 2009 from July to August. The environmental conditions were: an average temperature of 18.4° C and the pluvial precipitation was about 600 mm per year. Each sample was made up of 4 kg of nopal pads which were collected from several plants in the same sampling areas, but were at different maturity stages. In order to know the age of cladodes, new nopal pads were marked and dated as they were sprouting. This was the first day of ten different dates the pads were harvested. The others include day 40, 50, 60, 70, 80, 90, 100, 115, 125, and 135, respectively. The samples were transported to the laboratory and the pads were classified and separated into ten groups according to their age, this being 40, 50, 60, 70, 80, 90, 100, 115, 125, and 135 days, respectively, as has already been mentioned. All samples were analyzed in triplicate.

4.2   Washed and Dry Vacuum Process

The thorns of nopal pads were removed manually then washed with distilled water and disinfected using commercial 10% sodium hypochlorite solution in order to eliminate microorganisms. These samples were sectioned into small slices (3 mm) in order to facilitate the drying process. The prickly pads were then dried using a vacuum system for 12 hours at 10^{-2} Torr, and 45 °C, Vacuum is often employed as a process for removing bulk and absorbed water (or other solvents) from a product. Combined with heat, vacuum can be an effective method for drying. High degrees of dryness can be attained at relatively low temperatures. This allows for fast and effective drying of temperature sensitive products. Lower moisture content can be achieved when using vacuum and heat than can be achieved with heat only. Additionally, drying under a vacuum can prevent oxidation of sensitive product that cannot be dried in the presence of air. Vacuum drying systems can also recover the solvent that is removed from the product, if required. Often the part to be dried is placed into a vacuum drying chamber. However, if the part can withstand, and is designed for vacuum, the inside of the part can be evacuated and dried without the use of a vacuum chamber. Finally, the pads were pulverized in order to obtain a powder using a hammer mill (Pulvex 200, Mexico) equipped with a 0.5 mm screen. These dry vacuum powdered samples were used to determine mineral content by utilizing atomic absorption.

4.3   Chemical Approximate Analysis

The moisture content of the resulting nopal flour was determined by desiccation at 40 °C for 24 h, according to the 934.01 method as described in the Association of Official Analytical Chemists techniques (AOAC, 2000). The chemical analyses of the prickly pads were carried for ten groups at different maturity stages. This included protein, carbohydrates, fat, non organic components (ash) and humidity. Analyses were done in triplicate according to the AOAC techniques (AOAC, 2000). The evaluation of the flours was performed using specific methods for different components. Explanations of these tests follow.

Mineral ash content was evaluated with the 942.05 method (AOAC, 2000), using 2 g samples, determined at 550 °C for 24 h in order to remove organic material. The samples were placed in shallow, relatively broad ashing dishes that had been ignited. The samples were then cooled in desiccator, and weighed once they reached room temperature.

Nitrogen (N) concentration was ascertained by applying the Kjeldahl method 2001.11 (AOAC, 2000), using a 0.5 g sample.

The carbohydrate free nitrogen extract, was determined by calculating the differences in 100 g of all the components using AOAC official method 986.25 1986 (AOAC, 2000). Crude fiber was determined according to the 991.42 and 993.19 AOAC methods. Fat was analyzed by petroleum ether extraction using a Soxhlet apparatus according to the 920.39 AOAC methods (AOAC, 2000).

4.4   Determination of Tannins Content

The content of tannins in the nopal powders was measure by colorimetric method using vanillin as reactive chromospheres and catechin as tannin pattern (Jean, 1998). A 0.500 g of sample in assay tubes was extracted with 5 ml of hydrochloric acid in methanol for 20 min at room temperature with constant agitation After centrifugation for 10 min, 5 ml of vanillin-HCl (2% vanillin and 1% HCl) reagent was added to 1 ml aliquots and the colour developed after 20 min at room temperature was read at 500 nm., using white as a solution prepared by mixing 1 ml of the sample and 5 ml of hydrochloric acid: methanol. Correction for interference light natural pigments in the sample was achieved by subjecting the extract to the conditions of the reaction, but without vanillin reagent. A standard curve was prepared using catechin after correcting for blank and tannin concentration was expressed in g/100 g. The content of tannins obtained through a calibration curve using catechin as standard. The analysis was performed in triplicate.

4.5   Atomic Absorption Spectroscopy (AAS)

The Ca, Mg, K, and Na contents were determined using the dry-ashing procedure 968.08 (AOAC, 2000). The Ca, Mg, K, Na ions concentrations were measured with a double beam atomic absorption spectrometer, a Analyst 300 Perkin Elmer, USA. The organic components were previously eliminated at 550 °C for 24 h.

4.6   Mass Spectrometry ICP-MS

The mineral elements lithium (Li), vanadium (V), phosphorus (P), manganese (Mn) iron (Fe), cobalt (Co), arsenic (As), zinc (Zn), selenium (Se), cadmium (Cd), and thallium (Tl) of prickly pads powder were quantified by means of mass spectrometry ICP-MS following the Environmental Protection Agency Guidelines (EPA, 1995). The tests were carried out following the method of AOAC (984.27) (AOAC, 2000) using a Thermo Jarrel Ash, Model IRIS/ ICP ICP Spectrophotometer. The IRIS Optical Emission Spectrometer is inductively coupled argon plasma, optical emission spectrometers which uses Echelle optics and a unique charge injection device, solid state detector in order to provide complete and continuous wavelength coverage over the typical analytical wavelength range. The IRIS is equipped with Radial Plasma for the widest range of applications. The unit includes ICP, chiller, power supply, and autosampler, computer with software loaded with no software media, service and operation manual.

4.7   Statistical Analysis

Data, based on three replicates were subjected to analysis of variance. Standard deviation of each individual nutrient regarding maturity stage mean was computed and variations between maturation stages were evaluated by using Tukey test at a 5% level of probability (P = 0.05). All statistical data was calculated using stat graphics.

5   Results and Discussion

5.1   Chemical Proximal Analysis

Prickly pads powders present a large decrement in humidity in relation to the fresh prickly pads which is inherent to the vacuum drying process (Table 1); this procedure prevents the proliferation of microorganisms to render the pads edible (Geankoplis, 2006).

Prickly pads age (days)	Prickly pads weight (g)	Moisture (g)	Ash (g)	Fat (g)	Crude Fiber (g)	Protein (g)	Carbohydrates (g)
40	100	5.03cd	17.65a	2.16e	11.00a	7.07b	42.94a
50	150	8.81e	19.59b	2.37 f	13.26b	8.99e	53.04b
60	200	5.43d	20.64c	2.38 f	16.14c	8.39d	53.01b
70	250	4.85bcd	21.09d	1.62bc	19.03d	8.92e	55.53d
80	300	4.36ab	21.64e	1.53ab	18.73d	7.25b	53.53bc
90	350	4.81bc	21.92f	1.50ab	19.12d	7.78c	55.15cd
100	400	4.08a	22.80g	1.42a	20.11de	8.29d	56.73d
115	450	4.58abc	22.91h	1.72c	21.48e	8.48d	59.20e

Table 1: Chemical composition of dehydrated prickly pads on 100 g of sample (*Opuntia ficus indica*). Results for each component *versus* age followed with the same letter in the column were not different significantly (P < 0.05).

The fat content of the powders decreased as a function of age and not direct relationship related to age-days was observed (R^2= 0.3319 (Table 1). The decreases noticed were perhaps due to physiological changes or climatic conditions such as precipitation or irrigation where the plants were grown (AOAC, 2000). For protein, no related changes were observed (Table 1), which was low for all studied ages and similar to those of other vegetables (Lee *et al.*, 2005). Findings suggest that physical conditions such as water availability, temperature, and light/dark periods are primarily implicated in protein synthesis. Several studies demonstrated that protein synthesis increasing as a cellular protection when the soil is too acid or saline (Aguilar & Peña, 2006, Drennan & Nobel 2000, Nobel & Israel, 1994).

Carbohydrate content of old prickly pads showed significant increases from 42.94 mg/g at day 40 to 60.77 mg/g at day 135. Furthermore, they also showed a direct relationship (R^2=0.5446) pertaining to age. As with all vegetables, carbohydrates are the main component in prickly pads (Stintzing & Carle, 2005).

The ash content of minerals Ca and Fe were increased from 40 to 135 days old samples, whereas P, Mn and Zn not showed age related changes. The lineal regression analysis showed a positive relationship (R^2=0.7158) in regard to prickly pads age. The Ca and Fe content increased from 40 to 135 days samples (Figure 1 A and B, Table 2).

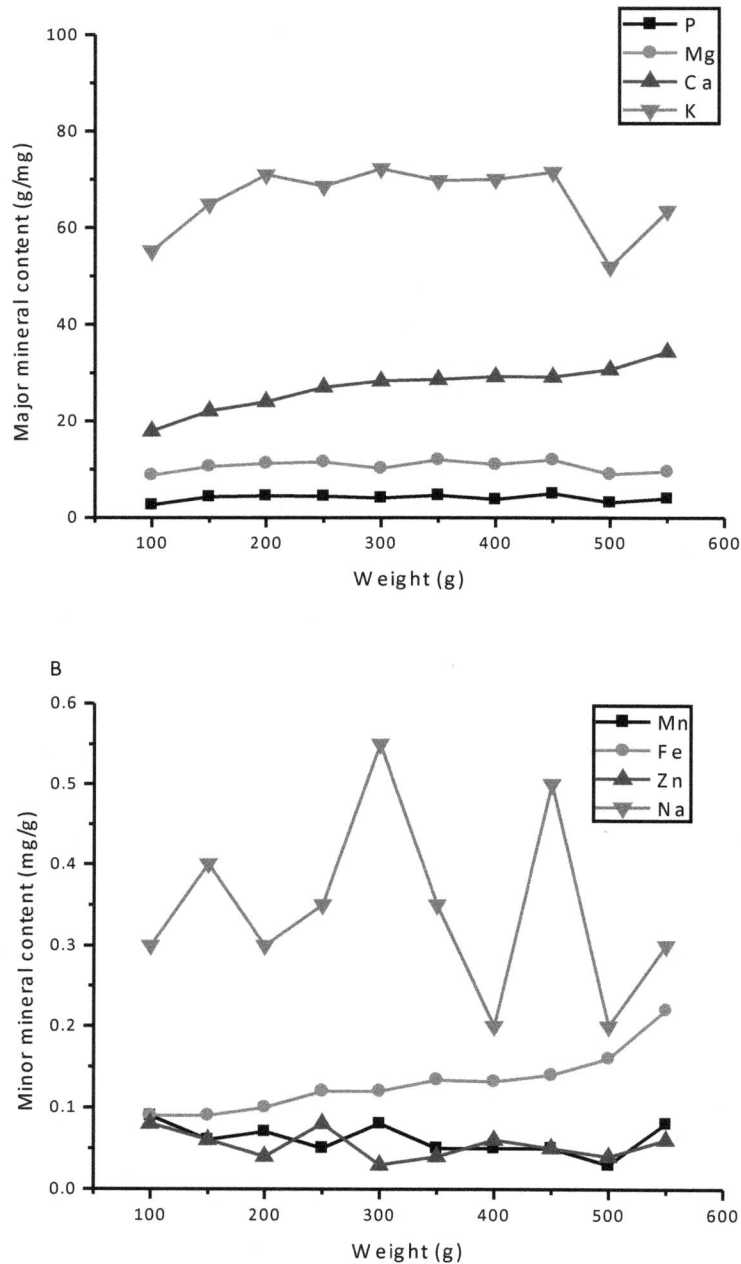

Figure 1: Major mineral content (A) and minor mineral content (B), of prickly pads at different maturational stage (Weight). Values are mean from triplicates samples.

Mineral	Maturity stage (age-days) (mg/g)									
	40	50	60	70	80	90	100	115	125	135
Phosphorus	2.59a	4.26b	4.48b	4.39 b	4.06b	4.60b	3.77abc	5.00c	3.15a	3.94
Manganese	0.09	0.06 a	0.07a	0.05 a	0.08	0.05a	0.05a	0.05a	0.03a	0.08a
Iron	0.09a	0.09 a	0.10a	0.12 b	0.12b	0.134b	0.132bc	0.14c	0.16	0.22
Zinc	0.08	0.06	0.04	0.08	0.03	0.04	0.06	0.05	0.04	0.06
Magnesium	8.80a	10.60 e	11.20f	11.5 g	10.2d	12.00h	11.00f	11.95h	8.95b	9.55c
Calcium	17.95	22.10a	24.00a	27.00 b	28.35bc	28.65bc	29.20bc	29.15c	30.70c	34.40
Potassium	55.20a	64.75bc	70.90d	68.50bcd	72.20 d	69.70cd	69.95d	71.45d	51.80a	63.35b
Sodium	0.30	0.40	0.30	0.35	0.55	0.35	0.20	0.50	0.20	0.30

Table 2: Mineral composition of prickly pads powder at different maturational stage age-days. Results for each mineral *versus* age followed with the same letter in the horizontal line were not different statistically significant (P < 0.05). Note that the values marked with de same letter in horizontal way do not showed differences according to age.

The vanadium, cobalt and selenium showed minimal changes in relation to age with maximal content at 80, 90, and 100 age-days. For the lithium, arsenic, cadmium and thallium content, the data revealed minimal content without important changes associated with ages. These findings suggest that the prickly pads powders might be a complement to daily diet due to their essential micro minerals content (Tables 2 and 3). Further suggesting that some elements of ash chemical composition depend on different factors, such as pH, water availability, soil texture and composition where the nopal grow. These results are in line with previous studies which reported that prickly pads contain the main minerals in carbonates, chlorides, sulfates and phosphates (Frati et al., 1991, Granados & Castañeda, 1997).

Mineral	Maturity stage (age-days) (mg/100g)									
	40	50	60	70	80	90	100	115	125	135
Lithium	0.80	0.23	1.0	1.4	0.99	0.07	0.55	0.18	0.19	0.29
Vanadium	0.33a	1.43b	1.61b	1.66b	2.27b	2.19b	2.07ab	0.68a	0.94	0.79a
Cobalt	0.16a	0.13ab	0.15abc	0.14bde	0.18c	0.12d	0.10de	0.15de	0.11e	0.21
Arsenic	0.14	0.05	0.04	0.00	0.007	0.00	0.04	0.002	0.00	0.00
Selenium	0.38	0.14	0.13	0.001	0.05	0.13	0.09	0.005	0.00	0.01
Cadmium	0.05	0.00	0.03	0.08	0.00	0.01	0.00	0.00	0.00	0.06
Thallium	0.07	0.06a	0.06a	0.06a	0.06a	0.06a	0.06a	0.07a	0.82	0.06

Table 3: Minor mineral composition, of prickly pads powder at different maturational stage, age-days. Results for each mineral *versus* age followed with the same letter in the arrow were not different statistically significant (P < 0.05).

5.2   Tannin content

The content of tannins in the prickly pads, modified depending on their stage of maturation, as shown in Figure 2, with statistically significant (p < 0.05) differences between the samples. The behavior of the antinutrimental factor in the prickly pads remained undefined, i.e. not maintained a relationship with the maturation state of the prickly pads, as noted in the case of minerals.

In general terms was detected a higher content of tannins in the prickly pads at 500-550 g of weight. In this regard, has established that a high concentration of this antinutrimental component in food can give them an astringent taste, clot alkaloids and albumins, in addition to being a chelating agent and sequestrate heavy metals (Otero & Hidalgo, 2004). With regard to content of tannins is observed increase as it increases the age, what suggest that samples of the old prickly pad, being at this age when can play their antinutrient action. In contrast, old prickly pads have the advantage for implement antioxidant action.

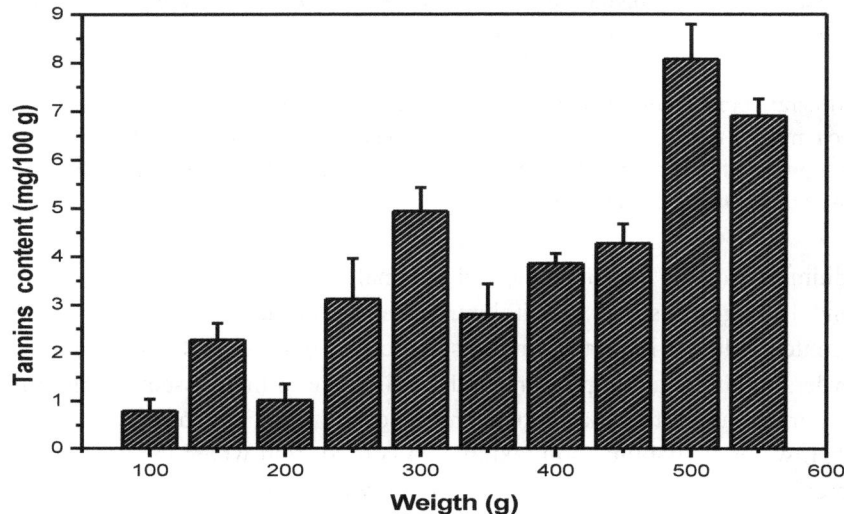

Figure 2: Tannins content of prickly pads (mg/100 g dry sample), at different developmental stages.

5   Perspectives and Conclusions

The crude fiber showed a positive relationship related to the age, however, the soluble dietary fiber tended to have negative relationship, suggesting than older nopal is better source of insoluble. Several researchers have observed decrements in the LDL-cholesterol and triglycerides when individual dietary intakes were supplemented with prickly pads at 40-50 age-days (Jieun et al., 2011; Junyong et al., 2012; Reid et al., 1995; Sáenz, 1997). The data showed different fiber and mineral content along life cycle of prickly pads, each maturity stages can also be used for distinct purposes (Hernández-Pérez et al., 2005, Lee et al., 2005, Reid et al., 1995). In addition, antioxidant properties are due to the phenols and flavonoids composition in *Opuntia spp* (Feugang et al., 2006, Gallegos-Infante et al., 2009, Guevara-Figueroa, 2010, Medina-Torres et al., 2011, Palumbo et al., 2003).

Because nutritional deficiencies associated to degenerative disease are currently widespread in many poor areas of the world, attention should be focused on inexpensive solutions. Nopal powders can be an economic alternative when used as dietary supplement in all seasons, without the need fresh nopal. The dried products represent certain advantages for transport and preservation for prolonged periods in optimal conditions to ensure maximum nutritional quality and availability (Rodríguez-Félix & Cantwell,

1988). Functional and organic foods that have secondary benefit for health are preferred for human consumption instead off other classic cultivated foods regarding their chemical treatment; often organic foods are preferred for human consumption instead off other classic cultivated foods regarding their chemical treatment (OMS, 2005, Williams, 2002). Prickly pads are good option between food recommendations for people with diabetes and health care providers aware of beneficial nutrition interventions. For achieve nutrition-related goals requires a coordinated team effort that includes the persons with diabetes and involves them in the decision-making process. While the long-term goal of diabetes research must remain the cure and the prevention of the disease and reasonable near-term goals might include amelioration of the symptoms or prevention of complications. Prickly pads can ameliorate the diabetes damage mainly for their soluble fiber content at younger maturity stages. In is well known that surplus calories in the daily diet induce pathological alterations leading to insulin resistance. For this reason the food intake in terms of habit, the individual must be emphasized ingest nutrients discrete so the follow adequate dietary patterns (Mozaffarian & Ludwig, 2010). These directions can then be followed by public health experts, legislators and the food industry in order to ensure correct labeling and information to the consumer. Only extensive multinational studies will be capable of unraveling their relevance and the underlying molecular interactions, not only between the genes themselves but with environmental factors such as diet and healthy life style (Korner *et al*, 2008). Directions for ameliorate or prevent diseases can be followed by health experts, legislators, and the food managers in order to ensure correct food combination. Only extensive multidisciplinary studies will be capable of give the lines for the adequate pattern of feeding, and together with a good life style based on the diet and exercise.

Acknowledgements

This project was partially supported by the National Council of Science and Technology of Mexico (CONACyT), Grant 91211. The authors want to thank MS Aracelí Aguilera Barreiro, and Carolina Muñoz Torres for their technical support.

References

Aguilar, B.G., & Peña, V.C.B. (2006). *Alteraciones fisiológicas provocadas por sequía en nopal (Opuntia ficus-indica). Revista Fitotecnia Mexicana. 29: 231-237.*

Andrade-Cetto, A. & Wiedenfeld, H. (2011). *Anti-hyperglycemic effect of Opuntia streptacantha Lem. Journal of Ethnopharmacology. 133: 940-943.*

Association of Official Analytical Chemists (AOAC). *Official methods of analysis, 17th edn. (2000). Gaithersburg, Maryland, USA.*

Bailey, C.C. (2002). *Diabetes. Indian Journal of Experimental Biology. 37: 190-192.*

Bennet, C. (2004). *Distribution of carbohydrate, protein, fat metabolism for diabetes. Journal of Diabetic Association of India. 4: 256-259.*

Betancourt-Domínguez, M.A., Hernández-Pérez, T., García-Saucedo, P., Cruz-Hernández, A. & Paredes-López, O. (2006). *Physico-chemical changes in cladodes (nopalitos) from cultivated and wild cacti (Opuntia spp.). Plant Foods for Human Nutrition.61: 115-119.*

Chauhan S.P., Sheth N.R., Jivani N.P., Rathod IS, Shah PI. (2010). *Biological actions of Opuntia species. Systematic Reviews in Pharmacy. 1: 146-151.*

Cameron-Smith, D., Collier, G.R., & Odea, K. (1994). *Effect of soluble dietary fibre on the viscosity of gastrointestinal content and the acute glycaemic response in the rat. British Journal of Nutrition. 71: 563-571.*

Cervera, P. (2001). *Alimentación y dietoterapia. Cap. 5. In: Antinutrientes. Mc Graw Hill Interamericana. España: 89-92.*

Drennan, P.M., & Nobel, P.S. (2000). *Responses of CAM species to increasing tmospheric CO_2 concentrations. Plant, Cell and Environment. 23: 767-81.*

Eastwood, M.A. & Morris E.R. (1992). *Physical properties of dietary fibre that influence physiological function: Amodel for polymers along the intestinal tract. The American Journal of Clinical Nutrition. 55: 436-442.*

Easwaran, P., Galibois, I., Destosiers, T. Guevin, N. Lavigne C. & H. Jacques, (1994). *Effect of dietary fibre mixtures on glucose and lipid metabolism and on mineral absorption in the rat. Annals of Nutrition and Metabolism. 38: 203-211.*

Environmental Protection Agency (EPA). (1995). *A guide to the biosolids risk assessments for the EPA part 503 rule. Washington: Office of Water. USA.*

Feugang, J.M., Konarski, P., Zou, D., Stintzing, F.C., & Zou, C. (2006). *Nutritional and medicinal use of cactus pear (Opuntia spp) cladodes and fruits. Frontiers in Bioscience. 11: 2574-2589.*

Franz, M.J., Bantle, .JP., Beebe, C.A., Brunzell, J.D., Chiasson, J.L., Garg, A., Holzmeister, LA, Hoogwerf, B., Mayer-Davis, E., Mooradian, A.D., Purnell, J.Q., & Wheeler, M. (2002). *Evidence-based nutrition principles and recommendations for the treatment and prevention of diabetes and related complications. Diabetes Care. 25: 148-198.*

Frati, M.A.C., Xilotl, D.N.,Altamirano, P., Ariza, R., & López, L.R. (1991). *The effect of two sequential doses of estreptacantha upon glycemia. Archivos de Investigación Médica (Mexico). 22: 333-336.*

Galibois, I. I. Desrosiers, T.T., Guévin, N.N., Lavigne, C. C. & Jacques, H. H. (1994). *Effects of dietary fibre mixtures on glucose and lipid metabolism and on mineral absorption in the rat. Annals of Nutrition and Metabolism 38: 203-211.*

Gallaher, C.M., Lee, S., & Prosky, L. (1995). *International survey on dietary fibre definition, analysis and reference materials. Journal of AOAC International. 78: 22.*

Gallegos-Infante, J.A., Rocha-Guzman, N.E., González-Laredo, R.F., Reynoso-Camacho, R.; Medina-Torres, L., & Cervantes-Cardozo, V. (2009). *Effect of air flow rate on the polyphenols content and antioxidant capacity of convective dried cactus pear cladodes (Opuntia ficus indica). International Journal of Food Science and Nutrition. 60: 80-87.*

Geankoplis, C.J. (2006). *Procesos de transporte y operaciones unitarias. (4th ed.) México: Continental.*

Gebremariam, T., Melaku, S., Yami, A. (2006). *Effect of different levels of cactus (Opuntia ficus-indica) inclusion on feed intake, digestibility and body weight gain in tef (Eragrostis tef) straw-based feeding of sheep. Animal Feed Science and Technology. 131: 42-51.*

Granados, S.D., & Castañeda, P.A.D. (1997). *El nopal historia, fisiología, genética e importancia. México. Trillas.*

Guevara-Figueroa, T., Jiménez-Islas, H., Reyes-Escogido, M.L., Mortensen, A.G., Laursen, B.B., Lin, L-W., De León-Rodríguez, A., Fomsgaard, I.S., & Barba de la Rosa, A.P. (2010). *Proximate composition, phenolic acids, and flavonoids characterization of commercial and wild nopal (Opuntia spp.). Journal of Food Composition and Analysis. 23: 525-532.*

Hernández-Pérez, T., Carrillo López, A., Guevara-Lara, F., Cruz-Hernández, A., & Paredes-López, O. (2005). *Biochemical and nutritional characterization of three prickly pear species with different ripening behavior. Plant Foods for Human Nutrition. 60: 195-200.*

Hill, J.O., & Prentice, A.M. (1995). *Sugar and body weight regulation. The American Journal of Clinical Nutrition. 62: 264S-273S.*

Institute of Medicine. (2002). Dietary reference intakes: energy, carbohydrate, fiber, fat, fatty acids, cholesterol, protein, and amino acids. Washington, DC, National Academies Press.

Jackson, K.G., Taylor, G.R.J. Clohessy A.M., & Williams, C.M. (1999). The effect of the daily intake of inulin on fasting lipid, insulin and glucose concentrations in middle-aged men and women. British Journal of Nutrition. 82: 23-30.

Jean A. (1998). Análisis nutrimental de los alimentos. Edit. Acribia, Zaragoza España.

Jieun P., Sahng-Wook H. & Yong-Suk S. (2011). Effects of Cheonnyuncho (Opuntia humifusa) seeds treatment on the mass, quality, and the turnover of bone in ovariectomized rats. Food Science and Biotechnology. 20: 1517-1524.

Johnson, I.T., & Gee, J.M. (1986). Effect of gelforming gums on the intestinal unstirred layer and sugar transport in vitro. Gut. 22: 398-403.

Junyong, K., Jinho P., Seong H.C., Shoji, I., & Youngju S. (2012). Opuntia humifusa supplementation increased bone density by regulating parathyroid hormone and osteocalcin in male growing rats. International Journal of Molecular Sciences. 13: 6747–6756.

Kavishankar, G.B., Lakshmidevi, N., Mahadeva Murthy, S., Prakash, H.S. & Niranjana S.R. (2011). Diabetes and medicinal plants-A review. International Journal of Pharmaceutical and Biomedical Science 2: 65-80.

Korner, A., Kiess, W., Stumvoll, M., & Kovacs, P. (2008). Polygenic contribution to obesity: genome-wide strategies reveal new targets. Front Hormone Research. 36: 12-36.

Lafrance, L., Rabasa, R., Poisson, D., Ducros F., & Chiassion, J.L. (1998). Effects of different glycemic index food and dietary fiber intake on glycemic control in Type I diabetic patients on intensive insulin therapy. Diabetic Medicine. 15: 972-978.

Luo, C., Zhang W., Sheng, C., Zheng, C., Yao, J., & Miao, Z. (2010). chemical composition and antidiabetic activity of Opuntia Milpa Alta extracts. Chemistry and Biodiversity. 7: 2869-2878.

Lopez, J.L. Jr. (2007). Use of opuntia cactus as a hypoglycemic agent in managing type 2 diabetes mellitus among Mexican American patients. Nutrition Bytes. 12: 1-6.

Lee, Y-C., Pyo, Y-H., Ahn, C-K., & Kim, S-H. (2005). Food functionality of Opuntia ficus-indica var. Cultivated in Jeju Island. Journal of Food Science and Nutrition. 10: 103-110.

Le Houérou, H.N. (1996). The role of cacti (Opuntia spp.) in erosion control, land reclamation, rehabilitation and agricultural development in the Mediterranean Basin. Journal of Arid Environments. 33: 135-159.

Lusi, S., Trowell, H., & Burkitt, D. (1986). Physiological role of dietary fibre: a ten year review. Journal of Dentistry for Children. 53: 444-447.

Manuel-y-Keenoy, B., & Perez-Gallardo, L. (2012). Metabolic impact of the amount and type of dietary carbohydrates on the risk of obesity and diabetes. The Open Nutrition Journal. l6: 21-34.

Medina-Torres, L, Vernon-Carter, EJ., Gallegos-Infante, J.A., Rocha-Guzman, N.E., Herrara-Valencia, E.E. Calderas, F & Jimenez-Alvarado, R (2011). Study of the Antioxidant Properties of Extracts Obtained from Nopal Cactus (Opuntia ficus-indica) Cladodes After Convective Drying. Journal of the Science of Food and Agriculture. 91: 1001-1005.

Moharib, S.A. (2000). Studies on intestinal enzyme activity and nutritive values of dietary fibres in rats. Bulletin of Faculty of Agriculture, University of Cairo. 51: 431-446.

Moller, D.E. (2001). New drug targets for type 2 diabetes and the metabolic syndrome. Nature. 414: 821-827.

Moreno Álvarez, M. J., García Pantaleón, D. Camacho, D. B., Medina Martínez C. & Muñoz Ojeda, N. (2008). Bromatological evaluation of tune Opuntia elatior Miller (Cactaceae). Revista de la Facultad de Agronomía (LUZ). 25: 68-80.

Musabayane CT. (2012). The effects of medicinal plants on renal function and blood pressure in diabetes mellitus. Cardiovascular Journal of Africa. 23: 462-468.

Mozaffarian, D., & Ludwig, D.S. (2010) Dietary guidelines in the 21st Century-a time for food. Journal of the American Medical Association. 304: 681-682.

Nobel, P.S., Israel AA. (1994). Cladode development, environmental responses of CO2 uptake, and productivity for Opuntia ficus-indica under elevated CO2. Journal of Experimental Botany. 45: 295-303.

OMS. (2005). Departamento de inocuidad de los alimentos. Organización mundial de la salud. Biotecnología moderna de los alimentos, salud y desarrollo humano: estudio basado en evidencias.

Otero, M.J., Hidalgo, L.G. (2004). Taninos condensados en especies forrajeras de clima templado: efectos sobre la productividad de rumiantes afectados por parasitosis gastrointestinales (una revisión). Livestock Research for Rural Development Vol. 16, Art. #13.

Palumbo, B., Efthimiou, Y., Stamatopoulos, J., Oguogho, A., Budinsky, A., Palumbo, R., & Sinziger, H. (2003). Prickly pear induces upregulation of liver LDL binding in familial heterozygous hypercholesterolemia. Nuclear Medicine Review. 6: 35-39.

Periago, M.J., Ros, G., López, G., Martínez, M.C., & Rincón, F. (1993). The dietary fiber components and their physiological effects. Revista Española de Ciencia y Tecnología de Alimentos. 33: 229-246.

Piga, A. (2004). Cactus pear, a fruit of nutraceutical and functional importance. J Profess Assoc Cactus Dev. 9-22.

Prasad, N.N., Khanu, M.F. Siddalingaswamy, M., & Santaram, K. (1995). Proximate composition and dietary fiber content of various food/rations processed to suit the Indian palate. Food Chemistry. 52: 371-378.

Reid, I.R., Ames, R.W., Evans, M.C., Gamble, G.D., & Sharpe, S.J. (1995). Long-term effects of calcium supplementation on bone loss and fractures in postmenopausal women a randomized controlled trial. American Journal of Medicine. 98: 331-335.

Rodriguez-Felix, A., & Cantwell, M. (1988). Developmental changes in composition and quality of prickly pear cactus cladodes (nopalitos). Plant Foods for Human Nutrition. 38: 83-93.

Rodríguez-García, M.E., De Lira, C., Hernández-Becerra, E., Cornejo-Villegas, M.A., Palacios-Fonseca, A.J., Rojas-Molina, I., Reynoso, R., Quintero, L.C., Del real, A., Zepeda, T.A. (2007). Physicochemical characterization of prickly pads (Opuntia ficus indica) and dry vacuum prickly pads powders as a function of the maturation. Plant Foods for Human Nutrition. 62: 107-112.

Sáenz, C. (2000). Processing technologies: an alternative for cactus pear (Opuntia spp.) fruits and cladodes. Journal of Arid Environments. 46: 209-225.

Sáenz, H.C. (1997). Cladodes: a source of dietary fiber. Journal of the Professional Association for Cactus Development. 117-123.

Saris, W.H. (2003). Sugars, energy metabolism, and body weight control. The American Journal of Clinical Nutrition. 78: 850S-857S.

Stintzing, F.C, & Carle, R. (2005). Cactus stems (Opuntia spp.): A review on their chemistry, technology, and uses. Mol Nutr Food Res. 49, 175-194.

Stintzing, F.C.; Schieber, A., & Carle, R. (2001). Phytochemical and nutritional significance of cactus pear. Eur Food Res Technol. 212: 396-407.

Williams, C.M. (2002) Nutritional quality of organic food: shades of grey or shades of green? Proc Nutr Soc. 61, 19-24.

World Health Organization. (1998). Obesity: preventing and managing the global epidemic. Report No.: 98.1.1998. Geneva.

Zhao, L. Y., Lan, Q. J., Huang, Z. C., Ouyang, L. J., & Zeng, F. H. (2011). Effect of a newly identified component of Opuntia dillenii polysaccharides. Phytomedicine. 18: 661-668.

Diabetics' Awareness of Oral Disorders Associated with Diabetes Mellitus

Aziza Eldarrat

City of London Dental School, London, UK

1   Introduction

Diabetes mellitus is made up of a group of metabolic disorders characterized by inappropriate blood hyperglycaemia, due to failure of the pancreatic beta cells to produce insulin and/or inability of the body to use the insulin produced because of insulin resistance in the body cells. Diabetes mellitus is a growing problem worldwide, it affects five percent of the world's population and the number of cases is doubling every generation (King *et al.*, 1998).

The medical professionals have been aware of diabetes mellitus and have studied it for many years, but have made little progress in halting its spread. In fact, the prevalence of diabetes mellitus has been increasing worldwide at such a rate that recently the World Health Organization (WHO) declared the disease an epidemic. Worldwide, the number of estimated cases of diabetes mellitus has increased from 30 million in 1985 to 135 million in 1995 (Smyth & Heron, 2006). Furthermore, WHO reported that by the year 2030 the number of estimated cases of diabetes mellitus is projected to increase to 366 millions. In most of the world, this increase is directly attributed to a genetic predisposition to the disease and also to lifestyle changes that modern development has brought on, such as a high-sugar diet, physical inactivity, obesity, as well as other aetiological factors.

2   Global Prevalence of Diabetes Mellitus

The estimated number of the global prevalence of diabetes mellitus in the year 2000 and the projections for year 2030, as reported by the WHO Global Burden of Disease Study, in the Middle Eastern, United States of America, Canada, European, Asian and African countries are shown in Figures 1, 2, 3 and 4, respectively. Worldwide, the number of people with diabetes mellitus is expected to double between 2000 and 2030 in most of the countries shown in the Figures (1-4). The greatest increase in the number of people with diabetes by 2030 among the Middle Eastern countries will be in Egypt, as seen in Figure 1 in close proximity to 7 million diabetic cases. In the Asian countries the estimated number will be massive, about 80 million diabetic cases, in India (Figure 3) and approximately 5 million diabetic cases in Nigeria among the African countries (Figure 4). This terrifying increase in the estimated number of people with diabetes mellitus by year 2030 in these countries (Egypt, India and Nigeria) could be attributed to the increase in population growth, aging, prevalence of obesity and physical inactivity.

2.1   Global Prevalence of Diabetes Mellitus by Population Age in Developed and Developing Countries

The global prevalence of diabetes mellitus by population age in year 2000 and 2030 for the developed countries is increasing in certain age groups. It has been shown that by the year 2030 it is projected that there will be a remarkable increase in the estimated number of diabetic cases in the age group 65 years and above, reaching 58 million cases from 26 million cases in the year 2000. There is also a projected increase in the estimated number of diabetic cases from 24 to 32 million cases in the age group 45-64 years by the year 2030. However, it is projected that the estimated cases for the age group 20-44 years will remain the same (5 million cases) without a noticeable change by 2030. Whereas, in the developing countries the estimated diabetic cases for the same age group (20-44 years) are projected to increase from 30 million cases in the year 2000 to 55 million cases in the year 2030. There will also be a terrifying in-

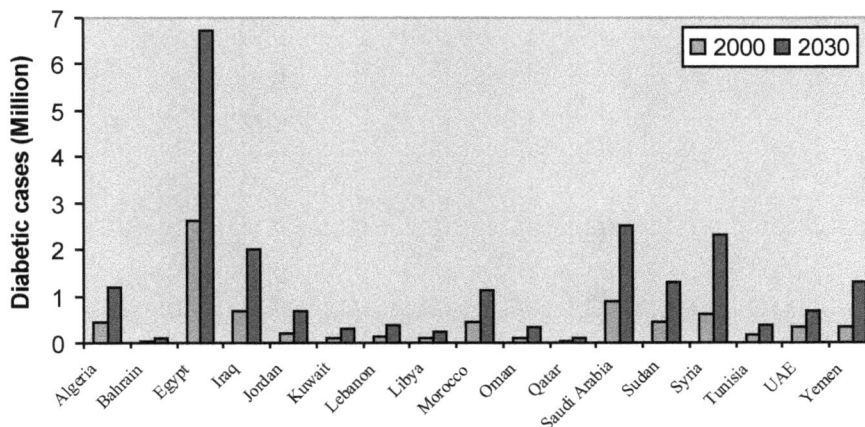

Figure 1: Prevalence of diabetes mellitus in the Middle Eastern countries. Adapted with permission from: http://www.who.int/diabetes/facts/world_figures/en/index.html

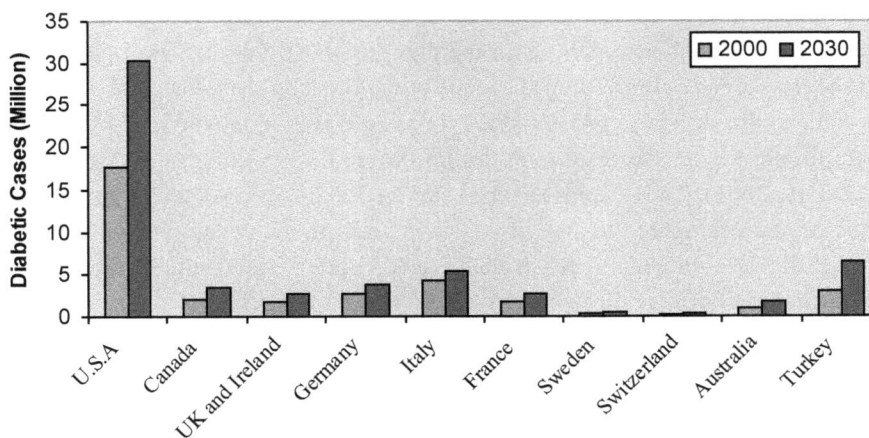

Figure 2: Prevalence of diabetes mellitus in the U.S.A., Canada and some European countries. Adapted with permission from: http://www.who.int/diabetes/facts/world_figures/en/index.html

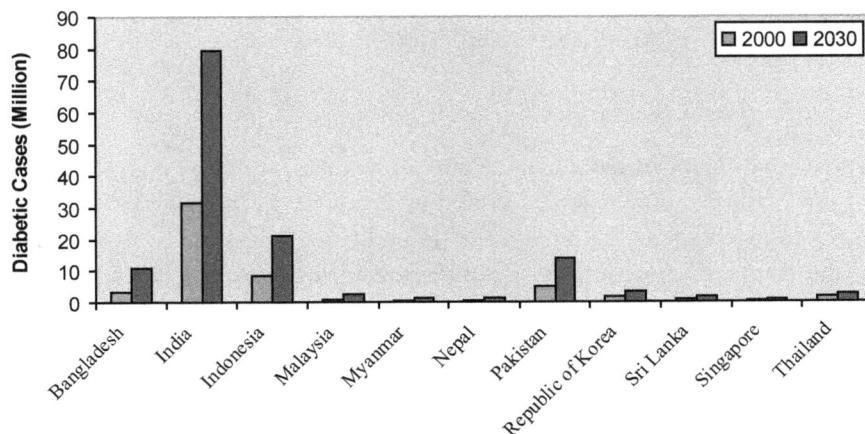

Figure 3: Prevalence of diabetes mellitus in some Asian countries. Adapted with permission from: http://www.who.int/diabetes/facts/world_figures/en/index.html

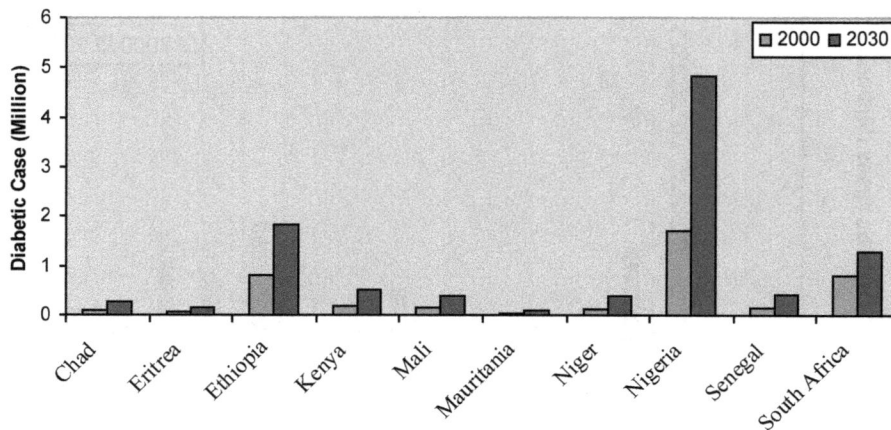

Figure 4: Prevalence of diabetes mellitus in some African countries. Adapted with permission from: http://www.who.int/diabetes/facts/world_figures/en/index.html

crease in the prevalence of diabetes mellitus in the age groups 45-60 years and 60-above years as compared to that of the developed countries for the same age groups by the year 2030. The estimated number of people with diabetes for age group 45-64 years, in the developing countries, is dramatically increased from 60 to 145 million cases and from 28 to 82 million cases for the age group 65 years and above by the year 2030 (Wild *et al.*, 2004). The decrease in the estimated diabetic cases for years 2000 and 2030 in the age group 65-above years compared to age group 45-64 years in the developing countries can be attributed to the failure of diabetic patients to reach that age (65-above years) due to serious diabetes mellitus complications. Cardiovascular disease (coronary artery disease) as result of diabetes complications is increasing the number of deaths among people with diabetes in these developing countries, as well as increased prevalence and associated consequences of other complications of diabetes mellitus (Wild *et al.*, 2004). The reported evidence suggests that the current and future increase of the global prevalence of diabetes mellitus in both developed and developing countries creates morbidity and mortality for millions of people worldwide (Mealey, 2000).

3   Pathophysiology of Diabetes Mellitus

3.1   Mechanism of Action of Insulin

Insulin is a hormone that regulates carbohydrate and fat metabolism in the body. Presence of glucose in the bloodstream stimulates the production of insulin by beta-cells in the Islets of Langerhans of the pancreas. Insulin binds to receptors on the target cells (in particular muscle cells, liver cells and adipose tissue) facilitating the uptake of glucose from the bloodstream into the cells. This leads to lowered blood glucose levels because glucose leaves the bloodstream and enters the cells to be utilized for energy, which acts as a negative feedback cycle causing a decrease in the production of insulin. Therefore, an increase in blood glucose level (hyperglycaemia) will result from decreased insulin production or in cases of peripheral resistance to insulin. On the other hand, an increase in insulin production will cause decrease in blood glucose level (hypoglycaemia). Insulin is the only hormone in the body that lowers blood glucose levels while, other hormones such as glucagons, growth hormone, thyroid hormone, catecholamines (epinephrine) and glucocorticoids all increase blood glucose levels.

3.2   Pathophysiology of Type 1 Diabetes Mellitus

The cause of type 1 diabetes mellitus is an autoimmune destruction of pancreatic beta-cells in the Islets of Langerhans of the pancreas resulting in an absolute insulin deficiency. Hence, the term insulin-dependent diabetes mellitus is used because the pancreatic beta-cells no longer produce insulin making the body dependant on exogenously administered insulin. The actual reason behind the autoimmune beta-cell destruction is unknown but one theory suggests that an environmental factor such as a viral infection is the cause of this destruction (Mandrup-Poulsen, 1998). Genetics do also play a role in increasing the risk of this autoimmune condition.

3.3   Pathophysiology of Type 2 Diabetes Mellitus

There is a strong genetic influence in acquiring Type 2 diabetes mellitus, however, it is also affected by acquired factors such as obesity, advancing age and inactive lifestyle (Mandrup-Poulsen, 1998). In type 2 diabetes mellitus the beta-cells in the Islets of Langerhans of the pancreas do produce insulin, but the tissues do not utilize it because the target cells have increased resistance to insulin. This leads to persistent hyperglycemia. Glucose accumulates in the bloodstream increasing the demand for insulin production by the beta-cells, and eventually the beta-cells can no longer cope with this increased demand and undergo apoptosis.

4   Classification of Diabetes Mellitus

The American Diabetes Association characterized diabetes mellitus into two major forms of diabetes, Type 1 and Type 2. Type 1 previously termed insulin-dependent diabetes mellitus (IDDM) or juvenile-onset diabetes and Type 2 termed as non-insulin-dependent diabetes mellitus (NIDDM) or adult-onset diabetes. Type 1 is characterized by defects in insulin secretion, and subdivided further into Type A (immune related) and Type B (idiopathic), and Type 2 is mainly characterized by insulin resistance (The Expert Committee on the Diagnosis and Classification of Diabetes Mellitus, 1998).

In addition to the mentioned causes, diabetes mellitus can also be brought about by pregnancy, certain drugs, or it could occur as a result of some autoimmune diseases, genetic disorders or as a result of infection (Manfredi et al., 2004). All types of diabetes mellitus are characterized by hyperglycaemia or elevated plasma glucose level.

Type 1 affects mostly children and young adults but it can occur at any age, while type 2 commonly occurs in adults after the age of forty, but it also affects young adults due to the increase in childhood obesity (Delong & Burkhart, 2008).

4.1   Pre-diabetes Mellitus Stage

An active stage of progressive beta cell deterioration and insulin resistance is typical of pre-diabetes stage. It manifests before the development of impaired glucose tolerance and clinical diabetes. The level of blood glucose is higher than normal level but not high enough for a diagnosis of diabetes. The pre-diabetes stage usually takes years to develop into clinical diabetes mellitus. As reported by the American

Diabetes Association, about 57 million Americans are at the pre-diabetes stage in the United States of America.

4.2   Plasma Glucose Levels Associated with Pre-diabetes and Diabetes Mellitus Stages

As recommended by the Expert Committee on the Diagnosis and Classification of Diabetes Mellitus (1998), the primary methods to diagnose diabetes mellitus and monitor blood glucose levels by fasting plasma glucose test or oral glucose tolerance test or combination of both tests. In addition to the relevant classical clinical symptoms of diabetes include polyuria, polydypsia, chronic fatigue, and unexplained weight loss. Currently, glycosylated haemoglobin test is used to investigate and confirm plasma glucose level over past weeks to months.

Pre-diabetes stage is diagnosed when the fasting plasma glucose (FPG) levels reach 100-125 mg dl^{-1} along with a corresponding impaired oral glucose tolerance test (OGTT) at a level of 140-199 mg dl^{-1} as seen in Table 1. Clinical diabetes is diagnosed when the FPG equals or above 126 mg dl^{-1} and the OGTT equals or above 200 mg dl^{-1} (The Expert Committee on the Diagnosis and Classification of Diabetes Mellitus 1998).

Plasma glucose test	Normal	Pre-diabetes	Diabetes mellitus
Fasting plasma glucose (FPG)	< 100 mg/dl	100 -125 mg/dl	≥126 mg/dl
Oral glucose tolerance test (OGTT)	< 140 mg/dl	140 -199 mg/dl	≥200 mg/dl

Table 1: Plasma glucose levels associated with normal, pre-diabetes and diabetes mellitus stages

4.3   Glycosylated Haemoglobin Test

The glycosylated haemoglobin (HbAlc) test is currently considered to be the best measure and the gold standard for assessing glycaemic control. The estimation of HbAlc level provides an accurate and objective measure of glycaemic control over past weeks to months (Hirsch & Parkin, 2005). The HbAlc test measures the amount of glucose that is bound to haemoglobin molecule. In normal conditions, red blood cells do not contain any glucose when they are formed. As the red blood cells move through the circulatory system, glucose molecules become attached to the haemoglobin molecules within red blood cells in an irreversible process known as glycosylation. The HbAlc test is based on the glycosylation process and measures the amount of glucose that is bound to molecules of haemoglobin A1c (Delong & Burkhart, 2008). The higher the level of glucose in the blood, the more glucose molecules become attached to the haemoglobin within the red blood cells. The amount of glucose that is bound to the haemoglobin molecule reflects the average level of glucose that the cell has been exposed to over time (60 to 80 days). HbA1c test is used to determine if the patient has had glycaemic control over the past 3 months or not (Allen *et al.*, 2008). Table 2 lists the guidelines for evaluating the results of the HbAlc test using the HbAlc glycaemic index. People with diabetes mellitus are considered under good control with HbAlc glycaemic index of less than 7%, moderate control 7-10% and poor control >10% (Delong & Burkhart, 2008).

The HbA1c glycaemic index	
Normal	<6%
Good control	<7%
Moderate control	7-10 %
Poor control	>10%

Table 2: The HbA1c Glycaemic Index

4.4   Relationship between Glycaemic Control and Diabetes Complications

Several studies showed a significant association between diabetes mellitus complications and glycaemic control scores. It has been shown that diabetics suffering from various types of oral infections such as periodontal disease and mouth mucosal soreness also exhibited poor glycaemic control scores. A recent study showed a significant association ($p<0.05$) between pain experience due to oral infections and glycaemic control scores among diabetic participants (Eldarrat, 2011a). As observed in the study, diabetic participants who indicated they always experienced pain due to oral infections over the last three months had poor glycaemic control (HbA1c >10%), while diabetic participants who indicated they occasionally experienced such pain had a moderate level of glycaemic control (HbA1c ≤8%), and those who never experienced pain had good glycaemic control (HbA1c <7%). Moreover, another study showed a significant association ($p<0.05$) between dentate status of diabetics and their glycaemic control scores. It was found in the study the higher proportion of diabetic participants in the dentate group had lower glycaemic control scores (Allen *et al.*, 2008). Furthermore, other investigators have shown a direct relationship between glycaemic control scores and the incidence of microvascular complications among people with diabetes (Hirsch & Parkin, 2005)

5   Complications of Diabetes Mellitus

Diabetic patients should be alerted that poor glycaemic control has negative consequences on their general health and health-related quality of life. When diabetic patients do not carefully control their blood glucose levels, their risk for serious systemic and oral complications will be much higher than diabetic patients with good control of their blood glucose levels.

5.1   Pathophysiology of Diabetes Mellitus Complications

The serious complications of diabetes mellitus mostly arise as a result of macrovascular and microvascular complications (Steinberg, 1997; Steffes, 1997; Klein, 1997). The macrovascular complications include increased thickness of arterial walls, increased lipid deposition, atheroma formation and development of micro-thrombi. The increased arterial wall thickness results from growth factor-induced stimulation of smooth-muscle cell proliferation. The rise of growth factors in diabetic individuals is due to the oxidation of circulating low-density lipoprotein (LDL) which increases the oxidant stress within the vascular system (Brunzell and Chait, 1997). This leads to chemotaxis of monocytes and macrophages in blood vessel walls, where oxidised LDL causes alterations in cellular adhesion and increased production of cytokines and growth factors.

The microvascular complications arise from changes in endothelial basement membrane, due to proliferation of endothelial cells and changes in their function, which result in vascular permeability alterations. Another factor that causes diabetes mellitus complications is the formation of advanced glycation endproducts (AGE's) which accumulate in the body plasma and tissues. The AGE's are formed as a result of the metabolic dysregulation which lead to non-enzymatic glycation and oxidation of proteins, lipids and nucleic acids. The AGE's binding to specific cellular receptors on the surface of monocytes and macrophages, rendering them hyper-responsive upon stimulation. This also leads to increased production of pro-inflammatory cytokines and growth factors which contribute to the chronic inflammatory processes of atherosclerotic lesions formation, altered wound healing and increased tissue destruction in response to antigens (Southerland *et al.*, 2006; Nishimura *et al.*, 2007).

5.2 Systemic Complications

Persistent hyperglycaemia in uncontrolled diabetic cases has repeatedly been reported to be associated with serious complications of diabetes mellitus, and these complications are responsible for the high rate of morbidity and mortality seen in the diabetic population (Mealey, 2000). The complications that result from persistent hyperglycaemia and lack of glycaemic control can be both chronic and acute complications.

The most common chronic complications are the macrovascular diseases (macroangiopathy), which include coronary artery, peripheral vascular and cerebrovascular diseases. The microvascular (microangiopathy) complications manifest as retinopathy, nephropathy, among other diseases. List of the systemic complications of diabetes mellitus due to long-standing persistent hyperglycaemia is shown in Table 3. The most common acute complications are diabetic ketoacidosis, hyperosmolar hyperglycaemia as well as other acute infections (Manfredi *et al.*, 2004; Skamagas *et al.*, 2008).

5.3 Oral Complications

In terms of diabetes mellitus oral consequences, the disease manifests itself in several ways. When diabetes mellitus is left uncontrolled for an extended period, it negatively affects the flow of salivary glands and results in xerostomia. It also causes sialosis, taste impairment, dental caries, periodontal disease, fungal infections, lichen planus, geographical tongue and fissured tongue (Sheppard, 1942; Russotto, 1981; Murrah, 1985; Lamey *et al.*, 1992; Greenspan, 1996; Manfredi *et al.*, 2004; Burt, 2005; Siudikiene *et al.*, 2008). List of oral complications of diabetes mellitus is show in Table 3.

5.3.1 Xerostomia (Dry Mouth)

In xerostomia or dry mouth, the salivary flow is reduced to such an extent that the oral cavity loses the beneficial properties of saliva. Saliva plays a vital role in the mouth as it helps in talking, chewing, tasting, swallowing and digesting food. One of the most common consequences of xerostomia is diffused pain in the mouth "burning mouth syndrome" due to dry mucosal surfaces irritation, especially in patients wearing dentures (Manfredi *et al.*, 2004). In addition, saliva controls the bacteria in the mouth, so lack of saliva would increase the risk of oral infections. When saliva secretion is not enough to wash and cleanse the oral cavity, oral biofilm and debris accumulate at a faster rate than in normal situation, this could be a factor in the increasing risk for dental caries (Rees, 1994; Finney *et al.*, 1997). Moreover, saliva has a role in the sense of taste, impaired saliva production in patients with diabetes mellitus could account for the impairment of taste observed in some diabetic patients (Hardy *et al.*, 1981). When the antimicrobial actions are negated in presence of high blood and saliva glucose levels, the growth and adhesion of yeast and Candida organisms is promoted (Knight & Fletcher, 1971; Odds *et al.*, 1978; Samaranayake *et al.*, 1984). The clinical manifestations of xerostomia are listed in table 4.

Systemic Complications of Diabetes Mellitus	Oral Complications of Diabetes Mellitus
1. Vascular system 　a. Macrovascular complications 　　• Accelerated atherosclerosis 　　• Coronary artery disease 　　• Myocardial disease 　　• Ischaemic heart disease 　　• Cerebrovascular (stroke) disease 　　• Peripheral vascular disease 　　• Gangrene of feet 　b. Microvascular complications 　　• Retinopathy (vision changes, blindness) 　　• Nephropathy (renal failure) 2. Nervous system 　• Peripheral sensory neuropathy (paraesthesia, anesthesia, reduced motor function) 　• Autonomic neuropathy (abnormal pupillary reflexes, cardiac autonomic disturbance, postural hypotension, impotence) 3. Muscular system 　• Myopathy (weakness & exercise intolerance) 4. Alterations in wound healing	• Xerostomia (mouth dryness) • Periodontal disease • Dental caries • Sialosis • Taste impairment • Fungal infections • Oral lichen planus • Geographical and fissured tongue • Sever TMJ dysfunction

Table 3: List of the serious systemic and oral complications of diabetes mellitus

Clinical manifestations of xerostomia
• Dry mouth
• Thick saliva
• The feeling of not being able to swallow or talk properly due to sticky saliva
• Rough, dry, red tongue
• Dry feeling in the throat as well as the mouth
• Burning sensation in the mouth
• Sensitivity to salty or spicy foods
• Bad breath
• Mouth sores
• Cracked lips
• Difficulty wearing dentures
• Unusual thirst

Table 4: The clinical manifestations of xerostomia

5.3.2   Periodontal Diseases

Gingivitis and periodontitis are the most common periodontal diseases affecting diabetics. Periodontitis is a chronic inflammatory disease, affecting 5-15 % of the diabetic and non-diabetic populations (Burt, 2005). However, the prevalence of periodontitis is higher in individuals with diabetes (17%) than in individuals without diabetes (9%) (Soskoline & Klinger, 2001). Furthermore, diabetic patients with uncontrolled blood glucose levels have been shown to be three times more susceptible to develop periodontitis than those with normal blood glucose levels (Li CL, et al., 2002). It has also been shown that diabetic smokers at a higher risk of developing severe periodontitis than non-smoking diabetics (Skamagas et al., 2008).

The main causative factors for periodontal disease are poor oral hygiene and bacterial biofilms composed of anaerobic gram-negative microorganisms. Diabetes mellitus has been described as the risk factor for initiation and progression of periodontal disease (Albandar, 2002). The greater risk of periodontal disease progression was associated with type 2 diabetes mellitus and it can be considered a risk factor for periodontitis (Nilo et al., 2009). It has been suggested that diabetes mellitus alters bacteria-host interactions by prolonging the inflammatory response and dysregulating cytokine production (Naguib et al, 2004; Graves et al, 2005).

Periodontal disease is considered a risk factor for diabetes and its serious complications, such as vascular disease, neuropathy, and retinopathy. Several researchers have advanced the notion that there is a bidirectional relationship between periodontitis and diabetes mellitus (Bartolucci & Parkes, 1981; Ureles, 1983). They have suggested that not only does uncontrolled diabetes increase the patients' susceptibility for developing periodontitis, but also severe periodontitis increases the risk for microvascular and macrovascular complications in diabetic patients (Thorstensson et al., 1995; the American Academy of Periodontology, 1999; Lalla & D'Ambrosio, 2001). The prevalence of diabetes mellitus in individuals with periodontitis is double that of individuals without periodontitis (Tsai et al., 2002).

Diabetes mellitus causes oral complications by pathological changes in oral microflora, phagocytic activity of the polymorphonuclear leucocytes and connective tissue. When this occur, the patient's ability to fight off infection is impaired, which increases the possibility of developing periodontitis (Manfredi et al., 2004). Compared to non-diabetic patients, it has been shown by several investigators that diabetes mellitus may modulate periodontal tissue destruction by reducing the polymorphonuclear leukocyte function, chemotaxis, adherence, and phagocytosis (Manouchehr-Pour et al, 1981; McMullen et al, 1981). Moreover, other investigators reported that accumulation of advanced glycation end products in the periodontium, as a result of protein glycation due hyperglycaemia, stimulate monocytes to the site and interact with receptors on the cell surface of monocytes. The interaction between advanced glycation end products and monocyte receptors induces a change in monocyte phenotype, upregulating the cell and significantly increasing the production of pro-inflammatory cytokines, such as prostaglandin E2, interleukin (IL)-1β, IL-6 and tumor necrosis factor (TNF)-α (Salvi et al, 1998; Rachon et al, 2003). This may be a mechanism by which increased tissue loss may occur in people with diabetes mellitus. Diabetes mellitus-related changes associated with the development and progression of periodontal disease, due to impaired polymorphonuclear leukocyte function, collagen production and bone formation. These changes brought by the disease resulted in decreased host response, ability to maintain periodontal tissues and periodontal bone levels. While increased collagenase production and presence of advanced glycation end products led to increased periodontal tissue destruction and decreased healing/repair processes. Additionally, pathological changes in small blood vessels (microangiopathy) reduce blood flow to the periodontium and compromise the transfer of nutrients necessary to maintain tissue health (Delong &Burkhart, 2008).

Clinical studies provided evidence to support the fact that periodontal infections have an adverse effect on glycaemic control and may increase the risk for diabetes complications.

Investigators showed that treatment of periodontal infections in diabetic patients helps them in establishing and maintaining good glycaemic control and acts to delay the onset or development of the oral complications of diabetes (Taylor & Borgnakke, 2008). Moreover, two consecutive recent studies reported that the glycaemic control of sixty participants with type 2 diabetes mellitus and had moderate to severe periodontal disease was significantly improved after receiving effective non-surgical periodontal treatment consisted of scaling and root planning over a period of 6 months (Koromantzos et al., 2011; Koromantzos et al., 2012). Other investigators assessed the effect of periodontal therapy on glycaemic control for fifty-two diabetic patients, aged 55-80 years, with uncontrolled type 2 diabetes mellitus (HbA1c, 7.5-11.0%) and had severe periodontitis. In the study, the diabetic group received non-surgical periodontal treatment combined with systemic doxycycline l00mg per day for 14 days. They found that periodontal treatment significantly improved periodontal status of the diabetic group (P<0.05), and decreased the level of fasting plasma glucose (Promsudthi et al., 2005). Taking into consideration the aforementioned bidirectional relationship between periodontal diseases and diabetes mellitus, the prevention and treatment of periodontal diseases through proper oral hygiene and regular dental check-ups are of paramount importance for diabetic patients.

5.3.3   Dental Caries

Diabetics with elevated HbA1c levels exhibit higher levels of glucose in their saliva which combines with oral biofilm to form an acid, causing the salivary pH to drop. Salivary pH of >5 is critical for enamel demineralization and initiating the decay process. Siudikiene et al., (2008) have shown that in diabetic children, a high concentration of salivary glucose and albumin, as well as high oral biofilm scores were the single most important factors in diabetic children tooth caries. The investigators imply poor glycaemic control as a reason behind caries in children with diabetes mellitus. Similarly, patients with well-controlled blood glucose levels tend to have reduced caries rates (American Academy of Periodontology, 2000). On the other hand, another study revealed no response on the prevalence of caries among people with diabetes mellitus type 2 (Collin et al, 1998). It has been suggested that the increase in liability to caries among people with diabetes mellitus may be due to an increase in glucose concentration in saliva and gingival crevicular fluid, but it is also more likely that diabetic patients neglect oral hygiene due to gingival inflammation.

5.3.4   Sialosis

Sialosis is asymptomatic non-inflammatory, non-neoplastic enlargement of salivary glands. The enlargement of salivary glands is as a result of the fatty infiltration of interstitium and enlargement of acinar cells. Sialosis may increase the risk for calculus formation and obstruction of salivary ducts. It commonly affects parotid glands but submandibular glands can be affected (Donath and Seifert, 1975). It has been reported that 10- 25% of people with diabetes mellitus may develop sialosis as a complication of longstanding diabetes mellitus (Murrah, 1985; Lamey et al., 1992). While other investigators reported only 3% of type 1 diabetic patients may develop sialosis (Guggenheimer et al., 2000).

5.3.5 Taste Impairment

People with diabetes mellitus lose the sweet taste of food, this sweet taste impairment is usually ignored, and as result undiagnosed diabetics may crave more sweet food causing further aggravation of their hyperglycaemia (Lamey *et al*, 1992). Diabetic patients with polydypsia and hyperglycaemia favour sugary drinks. The changes in taste sensation may indicate taste receptors abnormities among diabetic patients (Hardy *etal*, 1981).

5.3.6 Fungal Infections

Diabetic individuals with uncontrolled diabetes are at increased risk of fungal infections (Lamey *et al*,1992; Lalla and D'Ambrosio, 2001). Among candida species isolated from the oral cavity of diabetic patients;*Candida albicans* is the most prevalent (Willis *et al*, 1999) and *Candida dubliniensis*, (Willis *et al*,2000; Manfredi *et al*, 2002). Oral candidosis is more dangerous to those with diabetes mellitus than to those without. Reports express a correlation between fungal infections and diabetes mellitus (Ueta *et al*, 1993; Guggenheimer *et al*, 2000b).

5.3.7 Oral Lichen Planus

Lichen planus often appears as white oral lesion and it can be seen intra-orally as striated network, bullous or erosive lesions. Studies have reported a low prevalence of oral lichen planus in people with diabetes mellitus. The prevalence reported by several investigators was 0.17% (Borghelli *et al*, 1993), 4% (Van Dis and Parks, 1995) and 3.65% (Petrou-Amerikanou *et al*, 1998). Erosive form of oral lichen planus has a higher prevalence than other forms in diabetic patients (Lundstrom, 1983; Bagan-Sebastian *et al*,1992). These studies suggested that there is no strong relationship between oral lichen planus and diabetes mellitus. Scully and el Kom (1985) suggested a relationship between oral lichen planus, diabetes mellitus and hypertension, and the lesion most likely reflects lichenoid reactions associated with sulphonlyureas and/or antihypertensive drug therapy, rather than lichen planus.

5.3.8 Geographic and Fissured Tongue

Geographic tongue is also known as benign migratory glossitis. Geographic tongue is characterized by inflammation patches affecting the dorsum of the tongue. Geographic and fissured tongue, may affect around 8% of the people with diabetes mellitus (Wysocki and Daley, 1987; Guggenheimer *et al*, 2000), and a higher prevalence of fissuring of the tongue has been reported in type 1 diabetes mellitus patients as a result of longstanding complication of diabetes mellitus (Guggenheimer *et al*, 2000). Even though, an association between geographic tongue and diabetes mellitus has been suggested by some investigators (Wysocki and Daley, 1987), such an association has not been reported by others (Guggenheimer *et al*, 2000).

5.3.9 Temporomandibular Joint Dysfunction

Temporomandibular joint dysfunction is a diversity of conditions that affect temporomandibular joints, jaw muscles and nerves, associated with chronic facial pain. It has been reported that peripheral diabetic neuropathy, as a consequence of longstanding diabetes mellitus, may be a risk factor for severe temporomandibular joint dysfunction (Collin *et al*, 2000).

6   Diabetic Patients' Awareness and Attitude towards Their Oral

6.1   Diabetics' Awareness of Diabetes Mellitus Disease

The prevalence of diabetes worldwide has been increasing epidemically. It is estimated by WHO that 366 million people are expected to suffer from diabetes mellitus by 2030. The recent rise in diabetes is not a genetic shift only but also an environmental shift as a result of lifestyle habits. The prevalence of type 2 diabetes is higher than type 1 diabetes. The majority of people with diabetes have type 2 diabetes (90-95%), unfortunately, most of these people are unaware that they have diabetes mellitus (Delong & Burkhart, 2008). However, some diabetics know that they have the disease but do not know which type of diabetes they have although they are under diabetes medications. The disease may stay "silent" and the majority of people with diabetes mellitus do not realize they have diabetes mellitus until serious complications occur. Eldarrat (2011a) found among diabetic participants, 71% had type 2 diabetes, 18% of the participants suffered from type 1 and 11% did not know which type of diabetes they had. Similarly, another study showed that more than half of the diabetic participants (58%) had type 2 diabetes, 26% had type 1, and 16% did not know what type of diabetes they had (Eldarrat, 2011b). Other investigators found 27% of diabetic participants had type 1 diabetes, 66% type 2 and 7% did not know what type of diabetes they had (Allen *et al.*, 2008).

6.2   Diabetics' Awareness of Their Increased Risk for Complications

Reported evidence clearly confirms that people with diabetes have more knowledge about their increased risk for systemic complications associated with diabetes than they do for oral complications. Several recent studies reported that diabetic patients are much less informed of their risk for oral diseases in comparison with their knowledge of their increased risk for systemic diseases (Bowyer *et al.*, 2011; Eldarrat 2011a; Eldarrat 2011b; Allen *et al.*, 2008). Bowyer *et al.*, (2011) found the people with diabetes have poor awareness of oral care and health complications associated with diabetes mellitus. Likewise, Eldarrat (2011a) assessed the awareness of two hundred diabetic patients for their increased risk for systemic and oral diseases, and found the percentage of diabetic participants' awareness of their increased risk for eye disease 90%, heart disease 83%, kidney disease 83%, periodontal disease 66%, oral fungal infection 47%, and dental caries 44%. Another study showed that the percentage of diabetic participants who were aware of their increased risk for eye disease was 85%, heart disease 75%, kidney diseases 90%, periodontal disease 60%, dental caries 54% and oral fungal infections 42% Eldarrat (2011b). Similar findings were reported by other researchers, who assessed the knowledge of one hundred and one diabetic patients of their risk for periodontal disease, their attitude towards oral health and their oral health-related quality of life. Those researchers found that 98% of the diabetic participants were aware of their increased risk for eye disease, 84% for heart disease, 94% for kidney disease and 33% for periodontal disease (Allen *et al.*, 2008). Furthermore, in the same study, the diabetic participants with HbA1c levels >9%, which represents poor glycaemic control and at the highest risk for periodontal disease, 62% of these diabetic participants were unaware of their risk for periodontal disease (Allen *et al.*, 2008).

6.3   Diabetics' Awareness of Their Increased Risk for Dry Mouth

The knowledge of diabetic patients of their increased risk for oral diseases such as periodontal disease, tooth caries and fungal infections as a result of dry mouth is inadequate. More than 70% of the diabetic participants were suffering from dry mouth and, of these, 60% were unaware of the serious consequences of dry mouth on their oral health (Eldarrat, 2011b). It is well known that a significant reduction of salivary flow leading to dry mouth, and it is the most common oral manifestation of diabetes mellitus. It is of paramount importance to inform and make diabetics aware of the beneficial properties of saliva. Saliva's function of washing and cleansing the oral cavity is known to prevent the accumulation of oral biofilm and debris. The accumulation of oral biofilm could be a contributing factor to increase the risk for periodontal disease and dental caries in diabetics (Rees, 1994; Finney *et al.*, 1997). In addition, saliva has antimicrobial actions, when these actions are impaired, in presence of high blood and saliva glucose concentrations, the risk Candida organisms' growth is increased (Manfredi *et al.,* 2004). Therefore, diabetics should be informed and educated about the importance of keeping the oral cavity moist by stimulating salivary flow and frequent water drinking.

6.4   Diabetics' Awareness of Periodontal Disease

Serious periodontal disease not only can cause tooth loss, but can also cause changes in the shape of bone and gingival tissues. The gingival tissues become uneven, and dentures may not fit well. Diabetics often have sore gums from dentures. If chewing with dentures is painful, individuals with diabetes might choose foods that are easier to chew but not right for their diet and overall health. Eating the unhealthy foods can disturb blood sugar level (Allen *et al.*, 2008). It has been shown that the common knowledge of people with diabetes of periodontal disease signs is bleeding during brushing. It has been found that the majority of diabetics were aware that bleeding during brushing (70%), swollen and red-colored gingival (63%), and soreness of gingival (19%) are the signs of periodontal disease (Eldarrat, 2011b). Evidence is emerging to confirm the bidirectional relationship between diabetes mellitus and periodontal disease. Periodontal disease is one of the chronic infections which affect glycaemic control and associated with increased risk for diabetes complications. Awareness of diabetic patients and their physicians of the role of periodontal disease in glycaemic control of diabetics is important to maintain good oral health, glycaemic control and possibly delay the onset or progression of diabetic complications.

6.5   Diabetics' Awareness of the Influence of Oral Health on Overall Health

The influence of oral health on overall health of people with diabetes has been confirmed by several investigators. Many studies in the literature have highlighted the effect of periodontitis on diabetes mellitus. As reported by the previous studies that severe periodontitis may increase patients' susceptibility to develop diabetes and raise their risk for diabetes serious complications (Thorstensson *et al.*, 1995; the American Academy of Periodontology, 1999; Lalla & D'Ambrosio, 2001). Several investigators reported that periodontitis may initiate and /or accelerate insulin resistance in the body by enhancing the systemic immune response activation, initiated by cytokines (Salvi *et al.*, 2008; Mealey and Rose, 2008). A parallel relationship has been suggested between the severity of periodontitis and blood cytokine (TNF–a) levels, which is closely linked to insulin resistance (Engebretson *et al.*, 2004). The predominance of gram-negative anaerobic bacteria in periodontal infection may serve as a chronic source of systemic bacteremia and locally produced inflammatory mediators like Tumour Necrosis Factor (TNF-a), Interleukins (IL1 & IL6) and Prostaglandin (PGE2) by monocyte cells. These mediators have been shown to have effects on glucose and lipid metabolism and to antagonize insulin action in the body (Ling *et al.*, 1995). Furthermore, several clinical studies using non-surgical periodontal therapy reported a beneficial effect of periodontal therapy on glycaemic control of people with diabetes mellitus (Grossi *et al.*, 1997; Rodrigues *et al.*, 2003; Kiran *et al.*, 2005). Poorer glycaemic control has been shown to be associated with increased levels of cytokines, in the gingival crevicular fluid in individuals with type 2 diabetes mellitus and periodontitis (Engebretson *et al.*, 2004). Moreover, a significant association was shown between dentate status of diabetics and their glycaemic control scores, as a higher proportion of diabetic patients in the dentate group were found to have lower glycaemic control scores (Allen *et al.*, 2008). Another study reported that the majority of the edentulous diabetic participants (66%) did not have dentures and ate selected soft foods which were easy to chew and swallow (Eldarrat 2011b). Thus, edentulous people with diabetes are deprived of the benefits of eating healthy food. This has negative consequences on their glycaemic control, general health and health-related quality of life. Therefore, awareness of people with or without diabetes mellitus of the associations between oral health and overall health is the first crucial step to prevent and control the disease.

6.6   Diabetics' Attitude towards Their Oral Hygiene

Maintaining proper oral hygiene through oral self-care is also lacking in diabetic patients. A recent study assessed diabetic patients' attitude toward using a toothbrush and dental floss as part of their oral self-care, indicated that 19% of the diabetic respondents did not use a brush on a daily basis, 31% brushed twice a day, and a significantly higher number of respondents (50%) brushed once a day. In addition, a significant proportion (66%) never used dental floss to clean between their teeth, 11% reported using dental floss once a day, and 23% did not use it on daily basis (Eldarrat, 2011b). Similar results were reported by several investigators who found that of 299 participants only 29% brushed their teeth on a twice-daily basis (Bakhshandeh et al., 2008). Bowyer et al., (2011) found a significant number of respondents (67.2%) brushed their teeth at least twice a day, whereas only 15.3% used dental floss on daily basis. Other investigators found that diabetic women reported brushing their teeth more frequently than diabetic men and the differences in plaque and calculus indices were significantly lower in diabetic women than those of diabetic men (Karikoski *et al.*, 2001).

6.7   Diabetics' Attitude towards Their Regular Dental Check-ups

In fact, regular dental check-up visits are essential and may help in the detection of diabetic cases, in particular those who are unaware of the disease. Dental professionals are frequently the first to identify and refer patients with diabetes mellitus because of the oral findings from routine oral examinations. Investigators have reported that good oral condition is strongly associated with frequent dental visits (Karikoski *et al.*, 2001). The same investigators showed a significant association only between frequent dental visits and reduced amount of calculus, when they assessed the effects of oral self-care on periodontal health among adults with diabetes (Karikoski *et al.*, 2001). Even though, regular dental check-up visits are important to keep good oral health for diabetic patients, several investigators clearly showed that diabetic participants' attitude towards their oral health by keeping regular dental check-ups is poor. A study showed that about 40% of the diabetic participants had not visited a dental clinic for one year, and the main reason to visit a dental clinic was to receive treatment for pain and/or discomfort (Eldarrat, 2011b).

Moreover, in various surveys, investigators showed that the percentages of diabetic patients who kept regular dental check-ups were 37% (Kelly *et al.*, 1998), 47% (Allen *et al.*, 2008), 59% (Bakhshandeh *etal.*, 2008), 14% (Eldarrat, 2011b) and 79.8% (Bowyer *et al.*, 2011).

6.8   Diabetics' Attitude towards Keeping Their Teeth

A study assessed the response and decision made by diabetic patients about whether they would wish to save a loose tooth. 24% of diabetic participants would prefer extraction for a loose posterior tooth and

16% of an anterior tooth without consent. Diabetic participant response towards dentist consent before extraction of a loose anterior tooth was favored by 70%. Time and cost factors were less likely to influence the consent for extraction of either anterior or posterior tooth (Eldarrat, 2011b).

6.9   Diabetics' Sources of Awareness

Sources of knowledge and awareness of people with diabetes mellitus for their increased risk of oral diseases were found inadequate and receiving limited advice from healthcare professionals. Bowyer and co-investigators reported that 69% of diabetic respondents had never received any oral health advice related to their diabetes. The authors concluded that many adults with diabetes have poor awareness of oral care and health complications associated with diabetes. Training and advice for both healthcare professionals and patients concerning the importance of good oral health in patients with diabetes are needed (Bowyer *et al.*, 2011). Other studies showed that the source of information for diabetic patients regarding their increased risk for oral diseases mainly came from a dentist, and other sources such as television programs, the internet, magazines, and friends (Eldarrat 2011a & Eldarrat 2011b). In fact, it is the dentist's role to be a part of the healthcare team in order to help reduce the incidence and adverse impact of diabetes mellitus on oral health (Ali and Kunzel, 2011).

7   Conclusion

The dramatic increase of the global prevalence of diabetes among adults and children is attributed to a genetic shift and an environmental shift as a result of modern lifestyle habits such as unhealthy diet, obesity, physical inactivity. Despite the worldwide recognition of the dangers of diabetes mellitus, diabetic patients' awareness of and attitudes toward their increased risk for oral diseases has not been fully addressed. Diabetic patients are much less informed of their risk for dental diseases in comparison with their knowledge of their increased risk for systemic diseases. Thus, it is necessary for dental professionals and related government agencies to promote awareness of the relationship between diabetes mellitus and oral heath in order to prevent harmful complications. Education programmes to increase public awareness as a first step to prevent the disease and long-term complications. Health professionals in both the dental and medical fields and as well as the nutritionists need to take the responsibility to develop programs to educate the public about diabetes mellitus and the serious oral and systemic complications of the disease.

Acknowledgements

The author wishes to express her gratitude to the World Health Organization (WHO) for giving the permission to use the published data for regional and global prevalence of diabetes mellitus.

References

Albandar, J.M. (2002). Global risk factors and risk indicators for periodontal diseases. Periodontology, 29, 77-106.

Allen, E.M., Ziada, H.M., O'Halloran, D., Clerehugh, V., & Allen, P.F. (2008). Attitudes, awareness and oral health-related quality of life in patients with diabetes. Journal of Oral Rehabilitation, 35(3), 218-223.

Ali, D. & Kunzel, C. (2011). Diabetes mellitus: update and relevance for dentistry. Dentistry Today, 30(12), 45-50.

American Diabetes Association. (2005). Position statement: Standards of medical care in diabetes. Diabetes Care, 27, 524-536.

American Academy of Periodontology, Research, Science and Therapy Committee (2000). Position paper: Diabetes and periodontal diseases. Journal of Periodontology, 71, 664–678.

Bagan-Sebastian J.V., Milian-Masanet, M.A., Penarrocha-Diago, M. et al (1992). A clinical study of 205 patients with oral lichen planus. Journal of Oral Maxillofacial Surgery 50, 116-118.

Bakhshandeh, S., Murtomaa, H., Vehkalahti, M.M., Mofid, R., & Suomalainen, K. (2008). Oral self-care and use of dental services among adults with diabetes mellitus. Oral Health Preventive Dentistry 2008, 6(4), 279-286.

Bartolucci, E.G. & Parkes, R.B. (1981). Accelerated periodontal breakdown in uncontrolled diabetes: Pathogenesis and treatment. Oral Surgery Oral Medicine Oral Pathology, 52, 387-390.

Borghelli, R.F., Pettinari, I.L., Chuchurru, J.A. et al (1993). Oral lichen planus in patients with diabetes. An epidemiologic study. Oral Surgery Oral Medicine Oral Pathology 75, 498-500.

Bowyer, V., Sutcliffe, P., Ireland, R., Lindenmeyer, A., Gadsby, R., Graveney, M., Sturt, J., Dale, J. (2011). Oral health awareness in adult patients with diabetes: a questionnaire study. British Dental Journal, 23, 211(6):E12.

Brunzell, J.D. and Chait, A. (1997). Diabetic dyslipidemia: pathology and treatment. In: Porte D, Sherwin RS, editors. Diabetes mellitus. 5th ed. Stamford (CT): Appleton & Lange.

Burt B.A. (2005). Position paper: epidemiology of periodontal diseases. Journal of Periodontology 76, 1406-1419.

Centers for Disease Control and Prevention (2005). Dental visits among dentate adults with diabetes-United States, 1999 and 2004. MMWR Morb Mortal Wkly Rep, 54(46), 1181-1183.

Collin, H.L., Uusitupa M., Niskanen L. et al (1998). Caries in patients with non-insulin-dependent diabetes mellitus. Oral Surgery Oral Medicin Oral Pathology Oral Radiology Endodontics, 85, 680-685.

Delong, L. & Burkhart, N. (2008). Endocrine disorders. In General and oral pathology pp 147-178, philadelphia: lippincott Williams & Wilkins.

Donath K., Seifert G. (1975). Ultrastructural studies of the parotid glands in sialadenosis. Virchows Arch A Pathololgy Anatomy Histology 365, 119-135.

Eldarrat, A. (2011a). Awareness and attitude of diabetic patients towards their increased risk for oral diseases. Oral Health and Preventive Dentistry, 9 (3), 235-241.

Eldarrat, A. (2011b). Diabetic Patients: Their Knowledge and Perception of Oral Health. Libyan Journal of Medicine, 6, 5691-5696.

Engebretson SP, Hey-Hadavi J, Ehrhardt FJ, Hsu D, Celenti RS, Grbic JT, et al. (2004). Gingival crevicular fluid levels of interlukin-1beta and glycemic control in patients with chronic periodontitis and type 2 diabetes. J Periodontol. 75, 1203-1208.

Finney, L.S., Finney, M.O., & Gonzalez-Campoy, J.M. (1997). What the mouth has to say about diabetes. Careful examinations can avert serious complications. Post graduation Medicine, 102, 117-126.

Graves, D.T., Naguib, G., Lu, H., Leone, C., Hsue, H., & Krall, E. (2005). Inflammation is more persistent in type 1 diabetic mice. Journal of Dental Research, 84, 324-328.

Greenspan, D. (1996). Xerostomia: diagnosis and management. Oncology, 10, 7-11.

Grossi SG, Skrepcinski FB, DeCaro T et al. (1997). Treatment of periodontal disease in diabetics reduces glycated hemoglobin. J Periodontol, 68, 713-19.

Guggenheimer J, Moore PA, Rossie K et al (2000). Insulin-dependent diabetes mellitus and oral soft tissue pathologies. I. Prevalence and characteristics of non-candidal lesions. Oral Surgery Oral Medicine Oral Pathology Oral Radiology Endodontics 89, 563-569.

Hardy, S.L., Brennand, C.P., & Wyse, B.W. (1981). Taste thresholds of individuals with diabetes mellitus and of control subjects. Journal American of Diet Association, 79, 286-289.

Hirsch, I.B. & Parkin, C.G. (2005). Is A1c the best measure of glycaemic control? USEndocr-Rev.at:http//www.touchbriefing.com/cdps/cditem.cfm/nid=1479 &cid=5.

Karikoski, A., Ilanne-Parikka, P. & Murtomaa, H. (2001). Oral self-care and periodontal health indicators among adults with diabetes in Finland. Acta Odontology Scand 59, 390-395.

Kelly, M., Steele, J., Nuttall, N., Bradnock, G., Morris, J., & Nunn, J. (1998). Adult dental health survey: oral health in the United Kingdom. London: TSO, 2000.

King, H. (1998). Global burden of diabetes, 1995-2025: prevalence, numerical estimates, and projections. Diabetes Care, 21, 1414.

Kiran M, ArpakN, Unsal E, Erdoan MF (2005). The effect of improved periodontal health on metabolic control in 1ype 2 diabetes mellitus. J CIin PeriodontoI , 32, 266-272.

Klein R. (1997). Retinopathy and other ocular complications in diabetes. In: Porte D, Sherwin RS, editors. Diabetes mellitus. 5th ed. Stamford (CT): Appleton & Lange.

Knight, L. & Fletcher, J. (1971). Growth of Candida albicans in saliva: stimulation by glucose associated with antibiotics, corticosteroids, and diabetes mellitus. Journal of Infectious Disease, 123, 371-377.

Koromantzos, P.A., Makrilakis, K., Dereka, X., Katsilambros, N., Vrotsos, I.A., Madianos, P.N. (2011). A randomized, controlled trial on the effect of non-surgical periodontal therapy in patients with type 2 diabetes. Part I: effect on periodontal status and glycaemic control. Journal of Clinical Periodontology, 38(2), 142-147.

Koromantzos, P.A., Makrilakis, K., Dereka, X., Offenbacher, S., Katsilambros, N., Vrotsos, I.A., Madianos, P.N. (2012). Effect of non-surgical periodontal therapy on C-reactive protein, oxidative stress, and matrix metalloproteinase (MMP)-9 and MMP-2 levels in patients with type 2 diabetes: a randomized controlled study. Journal of Periodontology, 83(1), 3-10.

Lalla, R.V. & D'Ambrosio, J.A. (2001). Dental management considerations for the patient with diabetes mellitus. Journal American of Dental Association, 132, 1425-1432.

Lamey, P.J., Darwazeh, A.M., & Frier, B.M. (1992). Oral disorders associated with diabetes mellitus. Diabetes Medicine, 9, 410-416.

Li, C.L., Tsai, S.T., & Chou, P. (2002). Comparison of metabolic risk profiles between subjects with fasting and 2-hour plasma glucose impairment: The Kinmen Study. Journal Clinical Epidemiology, 55(1), 19-24.

Ling PR, Istfan NW, Colon E, Bistrian BR. (1995). Differential effects of interleukin-1 receptor antagonist in cytokine- and endotoxin-treated rats. Am J Physiol. 268, E255-E261.

Lundstrom, I.M. (1983). Incidence of diabetes mellitus in patients with oral lichen planus. International Journal of Oral Surgery 12, 147-152.

Mandrup-Poulsen, T. (1998). Recent advances — diabetes. British Medical Journal 316, 1221-1225.

Manfredi, M., McCullough, M.J., Al Karaawi, Z.M., et al (2002). The isolation, identification and molecular analysis of Candida spp. isolated from the oral cavities of patients with diabetes mellitus. Oral Microbiology Immunology 17, 181-185.

Manfredi, M., McCullough, M.J., Vescovi, P., Al-Kaarawi, Z.M., & Porter, S.R. (2004). Update on diabetes mellitus and related oral diseases. Oral Diseases, 10, 187-200.

Manouchehr-Pour, M., Spagnuolo, P.J., Rodman, H.M. & Biss-ada, N.F. (1981). Impaired neutrophil chemotaxis in diabetic patients with severe periodontitis. Journal Dental Research, 60, 729-730.

McMullen,J.A., Van Dyke, T.E., Horoszewicz, H.U., & Genco, R.J. (1981). Neutrophil chemotaxis in individuals with advanced periodontal disease and a genetic predisposition to diabetes mellitus. Journal of Periodontology, 52, 167-173.

Mealey, B.L. (2000). Diabetes mellitus. In: Rose, L.F., Genco, R.J, Mealey, B.L, Cohen ,D.W, editors. Periodontal medicine. Toronto, Canada: BC Decker Inc.

Mealey BL, Rose LF. (2008). Diabetes mellitus and inflammatory periodontal disease. Current Opinion Endocrinology Diabetes and Obesity.15, 135-41.

Murrah, V.A. (1985). Diabetes mellitus and associated oral manifestations: a review. Journal of Oral Pathology, 14, 271-281.

Naguib, G., Al-Mashat, H., Desta, T., & Graves, D.T. (2004). Diabetes prolongs the inflammatory response to a bacterial stimulus through cytokine dysregulation. Journal of Investi Dermatology, 123, 87-92.

Nilo, G.M.C., Mario, V.V., Carmelo, S. & Aubrey, S. (2009). The Relationship Between Diabetes Mellitus and Destructive Periodontal Disease: A Meta-Analysis. Oral Health Preventative Dentistry, 7, 107-127.

Nishimura, F., Iwamoto, Y., Soga, Y. (2007). The periodontal host response with diabetes. Periodontololgy 2000, 43, 245–253.

Odds, F.C., Evans, E.G., Taylor, M.A, & Wales, J.K. (1978). Prevalence of pathogenic yeasts and humoral antibodies to Candida in diabetic patients. Journal of Clinical Pathology, 31, 840-844.

Petrou-Amerikanou, C., Markopoulos, A.K., Belazi, M. et al (1998). Prevalence of oral lichen planus in diabetes mellitus according to the type of diabetes. Oral Diseases 4, 37-40.

Promsudthi, A., Pimapansri, S., Deerochanawong, C. & Kanchanavasita, W. (2005). The effect of periodontal therapy on uncontrolled type 2 diabetes mellitus in older subjects. Oral Diseases, 11, 293-298.

Rachon, D., Mysliwska, J., Suchecka-Rachon, K., Sem-etkowska-Jurkiewicz ,B., Zorena, K., Lysiak-Szydlowska, W. (2003). Serum interleukin-6 levels and bone mineral density at the femoral neck in post-menopausal women with type 1 diabetes. Diabetes Medicine, 20, 475-480.

Rees, T.D. (1994). The diabetic dental patient. Dental Clinical North America, 38, 447-463.

Rodrigues, D.C., Taba, M.J., Novaes, A.B, Souza, S.L., Grisi, M.F. (2003). Effect of non-surgical periodontal therapy on glycemic control in patients with type 2 diabetes mellitus. Journal of Periodontology, 74(9), 1361-1367.

Russotto, S.B. (1981). Asymptomatic parotid gland enlargement in diabetes mellitus. Oral Surgery Oral Medicine Oral Pathology, 52, 594-598.

Salvi, G.E., Beck, J.D., Offenbacher, S. (1998). PGE2, IL-1 beta, and TNF-alpha responses in diabetics as modifiers of periodontal disease expression. Annual of Periodontology, 3, 40-50.

Salvi, G.E., Carollo-Bittel, B., Lang, N.P. (2008). Effects of diabetes mellitus on periodontal and peri-implant conditions. Update on association and risks. Journal of Clinical Periodontology, 35(S-8), 398-409.

Samaranayake, L.P., Hughes, A., & MacFarlane, T.W. (1984). The proteolytic potential of Candida albicans in human saliva supplemented with glucose. Journal of Medical Microbiology, 17, 13–22.

Scully, C. and el Kom, M. (1985). Lichen planus: review and update on pathogenesis. Journal of Oral Pathololgy 14, 431-458.

Sheppard, I.M. (1942). Oral manifestation of diabetes mellitus: a study of one hundred cases. Journal of American Dental Association, 29, 1188-1192.

Siudikiene, J., Machiulskiene, V., Nyvad, B., Tenovuo, J., & Nedzelskiene, I. (2008). Dental caries increments and related factors in children with type 1 diabetes mellitus. Caries Research, 42(5), 354-362.

Skamagas, M., Breen, T.L., & LeRoith, D. (2008). Update on diabetes mellitus: prevention, treatment, and association with oral diseases. Oral Disease, 14(2), 105-114.

Smyth, S. & Heron, A. (2006). Diabetes and obesity: the twin epidemics. Nature Medicine, 12(1), 75-80.

Soskoline, W. & Klinger, A. (2001). The relationship between periodontal disease and diabetes: An overview. Annuals of Periodontology, 6, 91–98.

Southerland, J.H., Taylor, G.W., Moss, K., Beck, J.D., Offenbacher, S. (2006). Commonality in chronic inflammatory diseases: periodontitis, diabetes, and coronary artery disease. Periodontology 2000 40, 130–143.

Steffes, M.W. (1997). Pathophysiology of renal complications. In: Porte D, Sherwin RS, editors. Diabetes mellitus. 5th ed. Stamford (CT): Appleton & Lange.

Steinberg, D. (1997). Diabetes and atherosclerosis. In: Porte D, Sherwin RS, editors. Diabetes mellitus. 5th ed. Stamford (CT): Appleton & Lange.

Taylor, G.W. & Borgnakke, W.S. (2008). Periodontal disease: associations with diabetes, glycemic control and complications. Review. Oral Diseases, 14(3), 191-203.

The American Academy of Periodontology (1999). Diabetes and periodontal diseases. Journal of Periodontology, 70, 935-949.

The Expert Committee on the Diagnosis and Classification of Diabetes Mellitus (1998). Diabetes Care, 21, 5-19.

Thorstensson, H., Dahlen, G., & Hugoson, A. (1995). Some suspected periodonto-pathogens and serum antibody response in adult long-duration insulin-dependent diabetics. Journal Clinical Periodontology, 22, 449-458.

Tsai, C., Hayes, C., & Taylor, G. (2002). Glycemic control of type 2 diabetes and severe periodontal diseases in the US adult population. Community Dental Oral Epidemiology, 30(3), 182–192.

Ureles, S.D. (1983). Case report: a patient with severe periodontitis in conjunction with adult-onset diabetes. Compendium Continue Education of Dentistry, 4, 522-528.

Van Dis, M.L. and Parks, E.T. (1995). Prevalence of oral lichen planus in patients with diabetes mellitus. Oral Surgery Oral Medicine Oral Pathology Oral Radialogy Endodontics 79, 696-700.

Willis, A.M., Coulter, W.A., Fulton, C.R., et al (1999). Oral candidal carriage and infection in insulin-treated diabetic patients. Diabet Med 16, 675-679.

Willis, A.M., Coulter, W.A., Hayes, J.R., et al (2000). Factors affecting the adhesion of Candida albicans to epithelial cells of insulin-using diabetes mellitus patients. J Med Microbiol 49, 291-293.

World Health Organization, Country and regional data on diabetes / Prevalence of diabetes worldwide. Available from URL: [http://www.who.int/diabetes/facts/world_figures/en/index.html].

Wysocki, G.P., Daley, T.D. (1987). Benign migratory glossitis in patients with juvenile diabetes. Oral Surgery Oral Medicine Oral Pathology 63, 68-70.

Retropharyngeal Abscess in Diabetics: A Challenge

Olushola Abdulrahman Afolabi
Department of Ear, Nose and Throat
University of Ilorin, Nigeria

Joseph Olusesan Fadare
Department of Medical Pharmacology and Therapeutics
Obafemi Awolowo University, Nigeria

Stephen A Ogah
Department of Ear, Nose and Throat
University of Ilorin Teaching Hospital, Nigeria

Ezekiel O.Oyewole
Department of Anaesthesia
Federal Medical Center, Nigeria

1   Introduction

A retropharyngeal abscess (RPA) is one of the potentially serious deep space neck infections. It is an infection with abscess collection in the retropharyngeal space. It is due to suppuration of retropharyngeal lymph nodes within the retropharyngeal spaces of the neck (Afolabi *et al.* 2011). It is found to affect all age groups from neonates to elderly (Basel Al-Sabah *et al.* 2004, Ganglani 1996). Most publications reported a higher incidence among males than in females this seems to be a common consensus in the literature as it has been observed that males tends to respond to medical treatment better than the females (Basel Al-Sabah *et al.* 2004, Craig & Schunk 2003).

It is the most common deep neck infection in children (Afolabi *et al.* 2011, Ganglani 1996), but the literature is scanty, and most of the publications are case reports or small series with few retrospective and prospective study(Afolabi *et al.* 2011, Basel Al-Sabah 2004). Knowledge of the retropharyngeal space and its relationship to the other compartments is important in understanding the presentation, treatment, and complications of deep neck infections (Basel Al-Sabah *et al.* 2004). An abscess in this location is an immediate life-threatening emergency with the potential for airway compromise in all age groups. If the abscess compresses the larynx and upper trachea or ruptures due to pressure effect the symptoms of upper airway obstruction may develop either following the compression or aspiration of the purulent material (Afolabi *et al.* 2011). The invasion of contiguous structure, sepsis and other catastrophic complications may also result from this pathology (Choi *et al.* 1997). RPA can be of traumatic or non- traumatic origin. The traumatic is usually due to injury to the pharyngeal mucosa which may be from foreign body such as fish bone (Afolabi *et al.* 2011), or laryngeal mask (Eoin *et al.* 2009), animal bones, office pin, or any other material that breaches the mucosa into the submucous layer of the pharynx this can occur in all age group with the highest morbidity in the extreme of ages. The non-traumatic RPA is largely a disease of younger children, as a result of developmental aspects of the neck lymphatic system. Studies have shown that over 95% of the cases occurred in children under the age of 6. However, it is rather uncommon in adult, except in adult with diabetes, it may develop spontaneously especially in undocumented injury to the throat in patients with poorly controlled diabetics and those who are debilitated and the elderly (Okeowo 2004;, Cowan & Hibbert 1997;, Craig & Schunk 2003). Several studies have shown that diabetes mellitus is indeed a predisposing factor for deep neck infections and that the infections are also very severe leading to death in many instances (Mazita *et al.*, 2006; Glynn *et al.*, 2007; Sapunar *et al.*, 2008). Delay in diagnosing this condition results in high morbidity and mortality (Craig & Schunk 2003;, Ganglani & Edward 1995).

2   Anatomy of the Retropharyngeal Space and Pathogenesis of Retropharyngeal Abscess

The anatomy of the deep neck spaces is highly complex and can make precise localization of infections in this region difficult. Diagnosis of deep neck infections is difficult because they often are covered by a substantial amount of unaffected superficial soft tissue. Deep neck infections many times are difficult to palpate and to visualize externally (Brito-Mutunayagam *et al.* 2007). The use of antibiotics in this current age has reduced the incidence of infections of the fascial spaces of the head and neck, but these infections continue to occur. Atypical presentations are not uncommon in diabetic patients and immunocompromised patients. Fascia envelops the muscles, vessels, and viscera of the neck. Fascia planes form where adjacent fascia condenses. Fascia spaces are potential spaces between these planes. The cervical fascia consists of two layers, the superficial or investing layer which is part of the deep cervical fascia (Figure 1 Axial slide of the neck). The superficial layer lies just below the skin, completely encircles the neck, and is continuous with fascia of the face and the superficial fascia of the muscles of the back. Within this layer lie the platysma muscles, external jugular vein, and lymph nodes. The deep fascia comprises three layers. The anterior layer envelops the trapezius, sternocleidomastoid, omohyoid, and strap muscles and the parotid and submandibular glands. The middle or visceral layer surrounds the pharynx, esophagus, larynx, trachea, and thyroid gland. The prevertebral layer covers the vertebral bodies and paraspinus muscles. Contributions from all three layers form the carotid sheath, which contains the vagus nerve, carotid artery, and internal jugular vein.

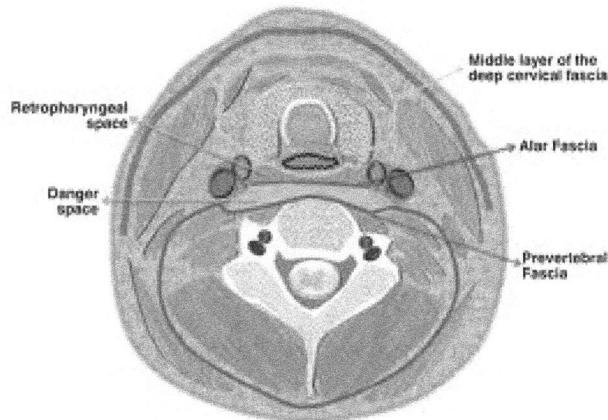

Figure 1: Section of the neck at about the level of the sixth cervical vertebra. Showing the arrangement of the fascia. Republished with permission from radiographics.rsna.org assessed on 24/12/2012.

Fascial spaces are potential avenues for the spread of infection. The spaces formed by fascia enveloping muscles offer some resistance of the spread of infection, whereas the spaces formed by fascia-enveloping viscera and vessels are associated with the most serious infections because they offer little resistance to this spread. The retropharyngeal space is located immediately posterior to the nasopharynx, oropharynx, hypopharynx, larynx and trachea (Cowan & Hibbert 1997;, Ganglani & Edward 1995). The visceral (that is, buccopharyngeal) fascia, which surrounds the pharynx, trachea, esophagus and thyroid, forms the anterior border of the retropharyngeal space. The retropharyngeal space is a potential space bounded anteriorly by pharyngeal muscle and its investing fascia, posteriorly by the alar layer of prevetebral fascia, superiorly by the skull base and inferiorly by the fusion of the anterior and posterior layers of fascia at the level of C7 it can also be said to lie between the visceral division of the middle layer of the deep cervical fascia around the pharyngeal constrictors and the alar division of the deep layer of deep cervical fascia posteriorly. It extends from the skull base to the tracheal bifurcation where the visceral and alar divisions fuse. It primarily contains retropharyngeal lymphatics (Gianoli *et al.*, 1991). Laterally, the space is bounded by the carotid sheaths and parapharyngeal spaces (Ganglani & Edward 1995). This potential space contains no important structures except lymph nodes which normally regress by the age of 3-4yrs (Milan & Cumming 1996) while some authors report it regresses by age of five years (Cmejrek *et al.* 2002). It extends superiorly to the base of the skull and inferiorly to the mediastinum at the level of the tracheal bifurcation. A midline raphae is present in this space making some infections appear unilateral. However without treatment infections can easily spread from one space to the adjacent space most especially the parapharyngeal space. The retropharyngeal space can become infected in three ways (Craig & Schunk 2003; Cowan & Hibbert 1997). Either infection spreads from a contiguous area affecting the retropharyngeal nodes or the space is inoculated directly secondary to a penetrating foreign body as we observed in our case in which a fish bone foreign body penetrated the retropharyngeal space as found intraoperatively. It may be through oropharyngeal injuries such as accidental lacerations, which are not uncommon in children who run and fall down after they have placed an object such as a toy, stick, pencil or toothbrush into their mouths (Craig & Schunk 2003; Wahbeh *et al.* 2002; Marom *et al.* 2007; Ologe & Afolabi 2007). There also are iatrogenic causes, which include instrumentation with laryngoscopy, endotracheal intubation, surgery, endoscopy, feeding tube placement and dental injection procedures (Marra & Hotaling 1996), which inoculate these organisms directly into the retropharyngeal space. Other common sources of infection in the retropharyngeal space are the nose, adenoids, nasopharynx, and sinuses. Infections of this space may drain into the prevertebral space and follow that space into the chest. Mediastinitis and empyema may ensue. Abscess in the space may push forward, occluding the airway at the level of the pharynx. It may appear as anterior displacement of one or both sides of the posterior pharyngeal wall because of involvement of lymph nodes, which are distributed lateral to the midline fascial raphe.

3   Bacteriology and Underlying Diseases

Various organism have been isolated from the retropharyngeal abscess however report from Taiwan in 2001 reported that the commonest pathogens were Streptococcus Viridans and Staphylococcus aureus, others were Klebsiella pneumoniae, Escherichia coli, Enterobacter spp., Prevotella spp., Salmonella spp. and Methicillin resistant staphylococcus aureus (MRSA) have been described (Tan *et al.,* 2001). Veillonella spp. and Morganella have also been isolated. Mixed infections were found in 46 percent of patients that was studied. It has been suggested that, at least in some paediatric patients, recent EBV infection may have an aetiological role in RPA formation (Tan *et al.*, 2001).

Another recent study conducted in Iran published in 2010 showed bacterial cultures for 40 cases of deep neck space retropharyngeal abscess and *Positive coagulase staph* was the most significant pathogen (31 out of 40, 77.5%), *Negative coagulase staph* was in second rank (7 cases, 17.5%) and then *β-hemolytic streptococcus* as well as *Entrobacter* (each one is 2.5%), *α-hemolytic streptococcus* (7.5%), *Klebsiella* and *Non hemolytic streptococcus* (each 5%) and finally *Pseudomonas* (2.5%). Forty five cases out of 147 ones (30.61%) had underlying diseases including diabetes (28 cases) (19%), immunodeficiency following the consumption of immunosuppressive medicines (10 cases) (6.8%), drug addiction (7 cases) (4.8%) (Hassan et al 2010). Klebsiella pneumonia has been consistently found in diabetic patients with deep neck abscesses; a retrospective study carried out in Singapore found that 41.2% of patients with deep neck abscesses had diabetes mellitus and 50% of their cultures were positive for Klebsiella pneumonia (Lee & Kanagalingam, 2011). Another retrospective study from Taiwan revealed Klebsiella pneumonia as the most common causative agent among diabetics while Streptococcus viridians was responsible in most non-diabetic patients (Huang *et al.*, 2005). Diabetes mellitus also predisposes to infections with not so common organisms; Citrobacter freundii and Streptococcus milleri have been isolated from diabetics with deep neck abscesses (Aderdour *et al.*, 2008; Hasegawa *et al.*, 2011). Penicillin-resistant *Staphylococcus pneumoniae* has been described as a causative organism in paediatric cases

(Parhiscar & Har-El 2001). Blastomycosis as a cause of RPA has also been described (Kobayashi 2002). Tuberculous abscesses are traditionally associated with cervical spine disease in adults, but have also been described in young children in the absence of neck disease (Hansen & Maani 2004).

4   Case Presentation

A 16-month-old Yoruba girl was referred from a peripheral hospital to the ear, nose and throat (ENT) unit of our hospital with a one-week history of fever, a six-day history of cough and a five-day history of neck swelling. Her fever was high grade with bouts of cough, and she had no history of contact with a person with chronic cough, no associated weight loss and no post-tussive vomiting. Her mother noticed neck swelling five days before presentation which was progressive and painful, with associated limited neck movement. The patient refused to eat, expectorated a thick tenacious secretion, and had episodes of irritability and excessive crying. The child had a previous history of left ear discharge which had resolved, and there was no history of hearing impairment or nasal symptoms. About three days prior to presentation, the child was noticed to be breathless, for which she was treated at a private hospital as a case of pneumonia and was placed on an antitussive and antibiotics. The patient's medical history and family and social history, as well as the review of systems, were not remarkable. An examination of the throat revealed poor oral hygiene; foul-smelling, thick, tenacious, straw colored secretion from the oral cavity and oropharynx; and a bulging posterior pharyngeal wall. The patient's neck showed a diffuse swelling which was tender. The ear, nose, chest and abdominal examinations were essentially normal. An assessment of retropharyngeal abscess was made to rule out parapharyngeal abscess as a differential diagnosis. Investigations revealed that the packed cell volume was 41%, and the electrolyte and urea examinations showed the following concentrations: sodium, 142 mM/L; potassium, 3.7 mM/L; urea 6.5 mM/L; and creatinine, 101 mM/L. Retroviral screening was done and was found to be negative for both HIV I and II.

X-rays of the soft neck tissue revealed widening of the prevertebral space containing areas of opacity and lucency extending from the base of the skull to the level of the seventh cervical spine (C7), which at the level of the second cervical vertebra (C2) was about 22 mm, with the laryngeal air column almost obliterated and anterior displacement of the airway and straightening of the cervical spine (Figure 2). There was lateral displacement of the trachea to the left from the anteroposterior view (Figure 3). The patient was resuscitated with intravenous fluid and antibiotics and was taken for examination under anesthesia and drainage of the abscess. The patient was placed in the anti-Trendelenburg position while under general anesthesia. Intubation was difficult but was finally achieved using a size 2.5 mm endotracheal tube inserted by an experienced anesthetist, and light packing with wet gauze was placed around the endotracheal tube. Anesthesia was induced with halothane in oxygen, and the trachea was secured with 1 mg/kg suxamethonium. Anesthesia was maintained with 66% nitrous oxide in oxygen and 0.5% to 1% halothane in oxygen, while muscle paralysis was induced with 0.1 mg/kg pancuronium. Analgesia was ensured with 2 µg/kg fentanyl. A Boyle-Davis mouth gag was introduced gently to expose the oral cavity and oropharynx, a cruciate incision was made using a size 11 surgical blade and a surgical probe was introduced to break down all loculi. About 30 to 40 mL of foul-smelling, purulent discharge was drained with the extrusion of a fish bone remnant from the abscess cavity. The culture revealed a growth of mixed organisms: Staphylococcus aureus, Klebsiella pneumoniae and anaerobic streptococci. Prior to extubation, residual neuromuscular block was antagonized with a combination of 0.04 mg/kg neostigmine and 0.02 mg/kg atropine. The patient was extubated but suddenly developed laryngeal spasm. Manual ventilation with a face mask was difficult as the patient's pulse oximetry was less than 80%. Anesthesia was deepened with halothane, and the patient's trachea was resecured with 1 mg/kg suxamethonium. The patient was ventilated manually with 100% oxygen in the improvised recovery room on account of poor respiratory function for about 8 to 10 hours, after which she was transferred to the postoperative ward, where her condition was satisfactory. The patient was maintained on intravenous antibiotics, analgesics and anti-inflammatory agents. The patient was discharged to home on the fifth day postoperatively.

5   Types of Retropharyngeal Abscess

5.1   Acute

This can be acute retropharyngeal or chronic retropharyngeal abscess. Acute Retropharyngeal space infections usually occur primarily as a sequela of upper respiratory tract infections that drain into the retropharyngeal lymph nodes. It may be a result of suppuration of retropharyngeal lymph nodes secondary to infection in the adenoids, nasopharynx, posterior nasal sinuses or nasal cavity (Afoabi et al., 2011; Cowan & Hibbert 1997; Ganglani & Edward 1995). In adults, it may result from foreign bodies or trauma from penetrating injury of posterior pharyngeal wall or cervical oesophagus. Rarely, pus from acute mastoiditis tracks along the undersurface of petrous bone to present as retropharyngeal abscess. The disease occurs primarily in young children. There is often a history of a recent upper respiratory tract infection. The acute is commoner in children although it also occurs in adults.

5.2   Chronic

The chronic retropharyngeal abscess is commoner in adults, It is tubercular in nature and it may arise from caries of cervical spine or tuberculous infection of retropharyngeal lymph nodes secondary to tuberculosis of deep cervical nodes. The former presents centrally behind the prevertebral fascia while the latter is limited to one side of midline as in true retropharyngeal abscess behind the buccopharyngeal fascia. Retropharyngeal tuberculous abscess is a rare presentation of the disease even in the presence of extensive pulmonary tuberculosis (Melchor et al., 1993). Sometimes, retropharyngeal tuberculous abscess causing stridor and threatening respiratory obstruction may be the only manifestation (Carroll et al., 1989). Tuberculous retropharyngeal abscess in adults is usually secondary to tuberculous involvement of cervical spine (Mathur & Bais 1997). The probable route of spread of tuberculosis to retropharyngeal space is via the lymphatic to a persistent retropharyngeal lymph node. Rarely, the abscess may be due to hemotogenous spread from pulmonary tuberculosis or tuberculosis elsewhere (Mayed & Hussam 2011). Tuberculous infection causes destruction, caseation, and necrosis of vertebrae or may present as an abscess. The abscess may remain close to the vertebra and present on the radiograph as pre vertebral or Para vertebral abscess or it may move distally along the tissue planes to present as cold abscess (Cowan & Hibbert 1997; Nussbaum et al., 1995). A delay in diagnosis and treatment can increase the risk of complications, including a spontaneous rupture of the abscess that can lead to trachea-bronchial aspiration or strider secondary to laryngeal edema. Early diagnosis is also essential in order to prevent the onset or progression of the neurological sequel of Pott's disease. (Parhiscar & Har-El 2001).

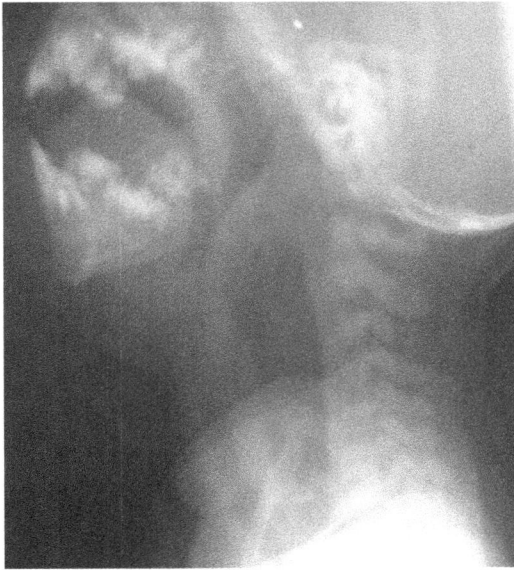

Figure 2: Lateral view X-ray showing the soft neck tissue revealing widening of the prevertebral space Containing areas of mixed opacity and lucency extending from the base of the skull to the level of the seventh cervical spine (C7), with the laryngeal air column almost obliterated, anterior displacement of the airway and straightening of the cervical spine.

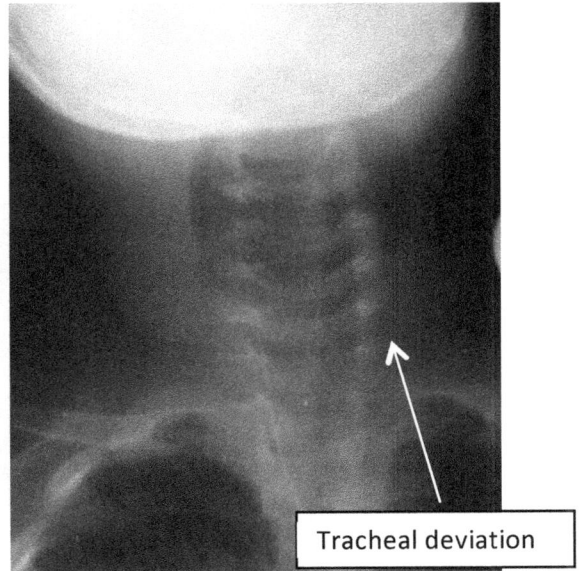

Figure 3: Anterio-Poterior view with deviation of the Tracheal to the left side of the patient

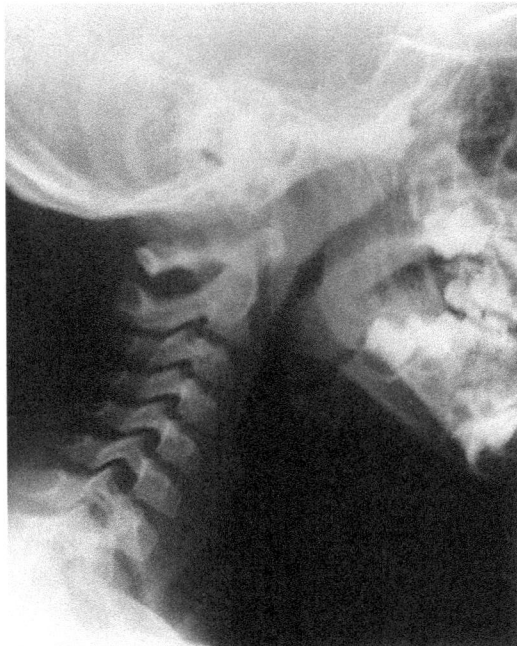

Figure 4: Lateral view showing post operative view with resolution of the retropharyngeal abscess.

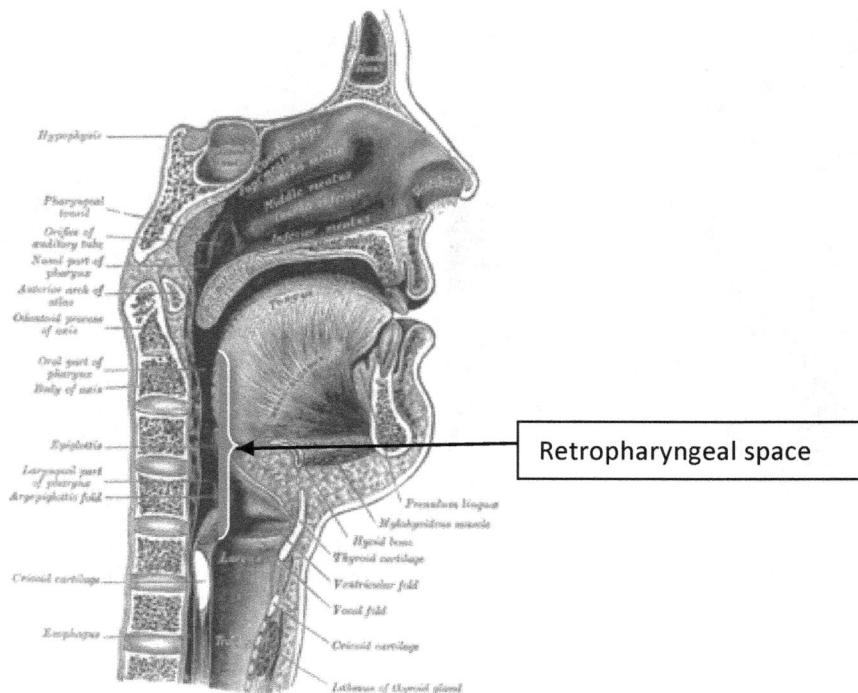

Figure 5: Sagittal section of Nose and Throat showing the retropharyngeal space. Republished with permission from translationdirectory.com assessed on 07/07/12 on google.com

6   Clinical Features

In children the symptoms include fever, sore throat, odynophagia, dysphagia, drooling, neck stiffness, muffled voice or hot potato speech in older patients, and difficulty in breathing (Afolabi *et al.*, 2011). Dysphagia and difficulty in breathing are prominent symptoms as the abscess obstructs the air and food passages, stridor and croupy cough may be present. Examination may reveal torticollis; limitation of neck movement; cervical tenderness; boggy, inflamed oropharyngeal mucosa; and a bulge or fluctuant swelling of the posterior pharyngeal wall either be central or to one side or both sides. Anteromedial displacement of the tonsil, and cervical edema or lymphadenopathy may also be observed. The classic presentation occurs in less than 10% of children (Mayed & Hussam 2011).

In adult, there may be few symptoms and little to find on examination. A history of previous tuberculous contact, pharyngeal trauma by fish or chicken bone, dental problems and intravenous drug abuse must be specifically sought. Also, history of symptoms suggestive of diabetes mellitus or family history of diabetes should be explored. Pain occurs at a relatively late stage and may be associated with fever. Neurological signs may develop due to cord compression. There may be bulging of the posterior pharyngeal wall on examination. There is usually nothing to feel in the neck unless the abscess is huge (Marcelle2008). Deficits of cranial nerves IX, X, and XII and Horner's syndrome may also be observed. The sites of spinal involvement with tuberculous spondylitis are paradoxical lesion, which is the most common site, central body lesion, anterior type in the anterior part of the vertebrae, appendicular type in the pedicle, lamina, transverse process and articular type in the posterior intervertebral joint (Tsui *et al.*, 2004).

The neurological deficit occurring with tuberculous spondylitis either due to cold abscess, granulation tissue, necrotic debris and sequestrae from bone or the inter-vertebral disc tissue, and occasionally vascular thrombo-sis of the spinal arteries (Mayed & Hussam 2011). Neck may show tuberculous lymph nodes in cases with caries of cervical spine.

7   Investigation

Lateral neck radiograph findings include air in the soft tissues, loss of the normal curvature of the cervical spine, and abnormal widening of the prevertebral soft tissue may be found as in the index case presented above which indicated the presence of a gas forming organism in the retropharyngeal space. In others it may just be a widened prevertebral space which is almost twice the size of the vertebral body of the individual involved. Occasionally radiologic interpretation of this area in children may be difficult because of difficulty in positioning, redundancy of normal soft tissue, and variation with inspiration and expiration. Computed tomographic scan with and without contrast can confirm the presence of an abscess and determine its extent in the neck spaces and other spaces involved. It will also demonstrate signs of infection and differentiate between cellulitis and abscess, the position, size, and extent of the abscess will be established, as well as its relationship to the great vessels. However a great deal of controversy exists regarding the utility of the computed tomographic (CT) scan, especially in young infants. Ring enhancement around an area of low attenuation on CT is not pathognomonic of an abscess. Even free air in the retropharyngeal area, which may be considered a sign of abscess, can be due to anaerobic infection, fistulous connection, or even a necrotic cavity of a neoplasm (Basel Al-Sabah *et al.*, 2004).

Chest radiograph is also done to ascertain there is no aspiration pneumonitis as this will increase the morbidity. Routine investigations should include urinalysis, random blood sugar, fasting blood sugar, haematocrit, WBC with differentials, serum electrolytes, urea and creatinine. Aderdour et al in a case report described a patient with retropharyngeal abscess who was found to have diabetes mellitus during routine laboratory work-up (Aderdour *et al.*, 2008).

8   Treatment

The treatment of any abscess is surgical drainage to let out the purulent content, if retropharyngeal abscess is present, surgical drainage is absolutely indicated. This is an emergency and the need to adjust or stop diabetic medication needs to be specifically addressed by the anaesthetist but generally tablets are not given on the morning of surgery and insulin given in either a reduced dosage subcutaneously with a covering intravenous infusion of 5 percent dextrose, or as a sliding scale as well as intra-operative monitoring of patient's vital signs, blood sugar as well as urine output. In a sliding scale the patient receives a constant dextrose infusion such as dextrose 4 percent with saline 0.18 percent (with potassium 20 mmol in 1000 mL bag) at 100 mL/h and an insulin infusion adjusted one to two hourly according to blood glucose (Adrian Pearce 2008). There is some evidence that tight control of glucose to a range of 4-6 mmol/L is beneficial (Adrian Pearce 2008).

Most abscesses can be drained intra-orally. To prevent aspiration, the patient is placed in the anti-Trendelenburg (head down), and the neck is extended. The procedure is usually done under general anaesthesia with an endotracheal intubation done by an experienced anaesthetist depending on the size of the abscess. If the abscess is huge with difficult intubation a prophylactic tracheostomy can be done under local anaesthesia and the balloon of the tracheostomy tube inflated to prevent the aspiration of purulent material. The patient will be in the anti-Trendelenburg position while under general anesthesia. If intubation was difficult a small size endotracheal tube can be usedas it is done in the case report above where a size 2.5 mm endotracheal tube was inserted by an experienced anesthetist, and light packing with wet gauze was placed around the endotracheal tube apart from inflation of the high volume low pressure balloon of the endotracheal tube. Anesthesia will be induced with halothane in oxygen, and the trachea will be secured with 1 mg/kg suxamethonium depending on the weight of the patient involved. Anesthesia will be maintained with 66% nitrous oxide in oxygen and 0.5% to 1% halothane in oxygen, while muscle paralysis will be induced with 0.1 mg/kg pancuronium. Ensure adequate analgesia with 2 µg/kg fentanyl where not available paracetamol, pentazocine, or diclofenac can be used. A right size Boyle-Davis mouth gag will be introduced gently to expose the oral cavity and oropharynx, while doing this care should be taken to avoid rupture of the abscess. A test aspirate will be done using a wide bore needle and syringe to take specimen for microscopy culture and sensitivity and also identify the point of maximum collection. A cruciate incision will be made using a size 11 surgical blade and a surgical probe will be introduced to break down all loculi and suctioned out. Prior to extubation, residual neuromuscular block will be antagonized with a combination of 0.04 mg/kg neostigmine and 0.02 mg/kg atropine to reverse the anesthesia. Prevention of laryngeal spasm can be achieved by extubating the patient using a no-touch technique when the patient is awake (Tsui *et al.*, 2004), as was done in the index case presented above or under deep anesthesia (possibly after a magnesium infusion) (Gulhas *et al.*, 2003), in the event that the awake extubation failed. Complications of laryngospasm can be prevented through application of a gentle jaw thrust, but if this fails, the depth of anesthesia can be increased with intermittent positive pressure ventilation on a ventilator. Larygeal spasm is an indication for admission into the intensive care unit in any age group.

In children, pharyngotonsillitis is the most common source, whereas odontogenic infections are the most common cause in adults. Infections may easily spread to and from this space. If an abscess is identified, drainage is required. Traditionally, the external, cervical approach had been used exclusively to drain these abscesses because it provides excellent exposure, but with the development of CT, many abscesses can be drained transorally. If the CT demonstrates that the abscess is medial to the great vessels, drainage of the abscess can be performed safely and effectively through a transoral approach. The transoral approach is technically easier to perform and is associated with less morbidity and shorter hospitalization generally for the patients however in the diabetic patients they usually have a longer duration of admission in view of the reduced immunity and hyperglycemic state that affects the body response to some of the drugs used (Estrada *et al.*, 2003). The external, cervical approach remains the approach of choice for abscesses that dissect along or are lateral to the great vessels. The incidence of surgical infection is increased in hyperglycemic diabetic patients in a number of different surgical populations. (Estrada *et al.*, 2003) Diabetic patients are also more susceptible to deep neck infections than the nondiabetic population. (Parhiscar & Har-El 2001; Chen *et al.*, 1998) Several aspects of immunity may deteriorate in short- or long-term hyperglycemia. Polymorphonuclear function is depressed particularly when acidosis is present (Joshi *et al.*, 1999). Furthermore, leukocyte adherence, chemotaxis, and phagocytosis may also be affected (Delamaire *et al.*, 1997; Gallacher *et al.*, 1995).

A chronic retropharyngeal abscess can be drained safely via a trans-oral route as described above or by an external route. (Marra & Hotaling, 1996). It is well accepted that if the spine is stable & there is no neurological deficit, or minimal neurological signs, anti tuberculosis drug therapy and conservative neck stabilization should be the initial treatment. If neurological signs are prominent on patient admission or develop later, or if there is cervical instability or significant degree of subluxation, then surgical debridement and stabilization are indicated (Joshi *et al.*, 1999; Delamaire *et al.*, 1997).

9   Differential Diagnosis

The differential diagnosis of lesions in the retropharyngeal spaces are: infected adenoidal hypertrophy, foreign body in the aerodigestive tract especially when they present with symptoms of upper airway obstruction and acute epiglottitis are the most important differential diagnosis in children (Lee et al 2001). In adult the differentials are nasopharyngeal carcinoma (Pak *et al.*, 1991), lipoma, malignant schwannoma, sarcoidosis, aberrant internal carotid artery, internal carotid artery pseudoaneurysm (Schmall & Stoll 2002), Forestiers disease, Kawasaki disease and haematoma following whiplash injury (Lee *et al.*, 2004). Appropriate preoperative imaging with CT or MRI and transoral diagnostic biopsy is, therefore, recommended (Anagnostara *et al.*, 2005).

10   Complications

Retropharyngeal abscess complication includes upper airway obstruction from the swelling, aspiration of the ruptured abscess leading to Aspiration pneumonitis, mediastinitis and empyema thoracis, other complications are pericardical effusion and jugular vein thrombosis, this complications are worsened by hyperglycemic state as seen in diabetic patients. The abscess may spread along the tissue plane predisposing to neck necrotizing fasciitis can cause dyspnea, delerium, mediastinitis, others are pericardial tamponade, DIC, neuropathy, diabetic ketoacidosis and neuropathy, overwhelming sepsis and death if blood sugar is uncontrolled in diabetics. It can also spread to involve vital neurovascular structure due to its anatomical relationship with the parapharyngeal space (Ganglani & Edward 1995). If the surgery is now done under general anaesthesia the patient also stand the risk associated with general anaesthesia and in diabetics there is associated problem of poor healing when sugar level is uncontrolled.

References

Aderdour L. Hassani R, Nejmi H, Elfakiri MM, Maliki O, Droussi H, Sassi A, Younous S, Samkaoui MA, Raji A (2008). Retropharyngeal abscess revealing diabetes: a case report]. Ann Endocrinol (Paris). 69:526-9.

Adrian Pearce. Preparation of the patient for surgery In Scott-Brown's Otolaryngology. Volume 1, 7th edition. Edited by: Kerr Michael Gleeson, George G Browning, Martin J Burton, Ray Clarke, John Hibbert, Nicholas S Jones, Valerie J Lund and Linda M Luxon (2008). Edward Arnold (Publishers) Ltd, An imprint of Hodder Education, a part of Hachette Livre UK, 338 Euston Road, London NW1 3BH. 38; 465-66.

Afolabi OA, Fadare JO, Oyewole EO, Ogah SA (2011). Fish bone foreign body presenting with acute fulminating retropharyngeal abscess in a resource challenged center: case report. J Med Case Reports. Apr 27;5(1):165.

Anagnostara T, Athanassopoulou T, Kailidou E, Markatos A, Eystathidis A, Papageorgiou S (2005). Traumatic retropharyngeal haematoma and prevertebral oedema induced by whiplash injury. Radiology. 1 1 : 1 45-9.

Basel Al-Sabah, Hashim Bin Salleen, Abdulrahman Hagr, Jeanne Choi-Rosen, John J. Manoukian and Ted L. Tewfik (2004) Retropharyngeal Abscess in Children: 10-Year Study The Journal of Otolaryngology, 33(6): 352-355.

Brito-Mutunayagam S, Y K Chew, K Sivakumar, N Prepageran (2007), Parapharyngeal and Retropharyngeal Abscess: Anatomical Complexity and Etiology. Med J Malaysia. 62(5): 413-415.

Carroll N., Bain RJ, Tseung MH. Edwards RH (1989). Tuber-culous Retropharyngeal Abscess producing respiratory obstruction, Thorax, 44 (7), 599.

Choi SS, Vezina LG, Grundfast KM (1997): Relative incidence and alternative approaches for surgical drainage of different types of deep neck abscesses in children. Arch Otolaryngol Head Neck Surg, 123:1271-1275.

Chen MK, Wen YS, Chang CC, Huang MT, Hsiao HC (1998): Predisposing factors of life-threatening deep neck infection: Logistic regression analysis of 214 cases. J Otolaryngol 27:141–4.

Cmejrek RC, Coticchia JM, Arnold JE (2002). Presentation, Diagnosis, and Management of Deep-Neck Abscesses in Infants. Arch Otolaryngology Head Neck Surg. 128: 1361-64.

Cowan DL, Hibbert J (1997): Acute and chronic infections of the pharynx and tonsils. In Scott-Brown's Otolaryngology. Volume 5. 6 edition. Edited by: Kerr AG, Hibbert J. Oxford Boston: Butterworth-Heinemann, Jordan hills, Oxford DX28DP;(4):5-6.

Craig FW, Schunk JE (2003): Retropharyngeal Abscess in Children: Clinical Presentation, Utility of Imaging, and Current Management. PEDIATRICS, 6(111):1394-1398.

Delamaire M, Maugendre D, Moreno M, Le Goff MC, Allannic H, Genetet B (1997): Impaired leucocyte functions in diabetic patients. Diabet Med 14:29–34.

Eoin D. Casey, Martin Donelly, Conan L. McCaul (2009), Severe Retropharyngeal Abscess after the Use of a Reinforced Laryngeal Mask with a Bosworth Introducer Anesthesiology, 110 (4): 943-945.

Estrada CA, Young JA, Nifong LW, Chitwood WR Jr: Outcomes and perioperative hyperglycemia in patients with or without diabetes mellitus undergoing coronary artery bypass grafting. Ann Thorac Surg 2003; 75:1392–9.

Gallacher SJ, Thomson G, Fraser WD, Fisher BM, Gemmell CG, MacCuish AC (1995): Neutrophil bactericidal function in diabetes mellitus: Evidence for association with blood glucose control. Diabet Med 12:916–20.

Gaglani MJ, Edwards MS (1995): Clinical indicators of childhood retropharyngeal abscess. Am J Emerg Med, 13:333-336.

Gaglani MJ, Moise AA, Demmler GJ (1996). Retropharyngeal abscess in the neonate. J Perinatol 16: 231–3.

Gianoli GJ, Espinola TE, Guarisco JL, Miller RH (1991): Retropharyngeal space infection: changing trends. Otolaryngol Head Neck Surg; 105(1): 92-100.

Glynn F, Skinner LJ, Riley N, Donnelly M (2007). Parapharyngeal abscess in an insulin dependent diabetic patient following an elective tonsillectomy. J Laryngol Otol.121:e16.

Gulhas N, Dumus M, Demirbilek S, Togal T, Ozturk E, Ersoy MO (2003): The use of magnesium to prevent laryngospasm after tonsillectomy and adenoidectomy: a preliminary study. Paediatr Anaesth, 13:43-47.

Hansen K, Maani C (2004). Blastomycosis presenting as a retropharyngea l abscess. Otolaryngology and Head and Neck 130 : 635-8.

Hassan Abshirini, Seyyed Mohammad Alavi, Hossein Rekabi, Faeze Hosseinnejad, Ali Ghazipour, Maliheh Yavari, Mitra Shabab (2010). Predisposing Factors for the Complications of Deep Neck Infection Iranian Journal of Otorhinolaryngology 22(60); 97-102.

Hasegawa J, Hidaka H, Tateda M, Kudo T, Sagai S, Miyazaki M, Katagiri K, Nakanome A, Ishida E, Ozawa D, Kobayashi T (2011). An analysis of clinical risk factors of deep neck infection. Auris Nasus Larynx.38:101-7.

Huang TT, Tseng FY, Liu TC, Hsu CJ, Chen YS (2005). Deep neck infection in diabetic patients: comparison of clinical picture and outcomes with nondiabetic patients. Otolaryngol Head Neck Surg.132:943-7.

Joshi N, Caputo GM, Weitekamp MR, Karchmer AW (1999): Infections in patients with diabetes mellitus. N Engl J Med 341:1906–12.

Kobayashi KI, Haruta T , Kubota M, Nishio T (2002).A case of retropharyngeal abscess caused by penicillin-resistant Stretococcus pneumoniae. Journal of Infection. 44 : 267-9.

Lee N N, Long G, Ngai S, Sa h r i r S, Parker A, Lamont AC (2004). Right internal carotid pseudoaneurysm mimicking an abscess in a child . Medical Journal of Malaysia. 59:685-7.

Lee SS, Schwa rtz RH, Bahadori RS (2001). Retropharyngeal abscess. Epiglottitis of the new millennium . Journal of Pediatrics. 138 : 435-7.

Lee YQ, Kanagalingam J (2011). Bacteriology of deep neck abscesses: a retrospective review of 96 consecutive cases. Singapore Med J. 52:351-5.

Marra S, Hotaling AJ (1996): Deep neck infections. Am J Otolaryngol, 17:287-298.

Marcelle Macnamara. Acute and chronic pharyngeal infection in Scott-Brown's Otorhinolaryngology, Head and Neck Surgery 7th edition Volume 2 Edited by Michael Gleeson, George G Browning, Martin J Burton, Ray Clarke, John Hibbert, Nicholas S Jones, Valerie J Lund, Linda M· Luxon and John C Watkinson (2008) published by Hodder Arnold in Great Britain 2008 by Hodder Arnold 152 (2): 2000-2002.

Marom T, Russo E, Ben-Yehuda Y, Roth Y (2007): Oropharyngeal injuries in children. Pediatr Emerg Care, 23:914-918.

Mathur N.N, Bais AS (1997), Tubercular Retropharyngeal Abscess in Early Childhood, Ind J Pediatr, 64 (6), 898.

Mayed. M. Radi and Hussam Makki (2011) Rare Presentation of a Common Disease (Tuberculous Retropharyngeal abscess) Biomedical Research 22 (1): 15-17.

Mazita A, Hazim MY, Megat Shiraz MA, Primuharsa Putra SH (2006). Neck abscess: five year retrospective review of Hospital University Kebangsaan Malaysia experience. Med J Malaysia. 61:151-6.

Melchor Diaz MA, Domingo Carrasco C., Monge Jodra R, Marino Espuelas J, Ontanon Martin M (1993), Tuberculous Retropharyngeal Abscess in an HIV Patient- Report of a Case, Acta Otorhinolaryngol Esp, 44(6), 467.

Millan SB, Cumming WA (1996). Supraglottic airway infections. Prim Care23:741–58.

Nussbaum E, Gaylan LR, Bergman TA et al (1995) .Spinal tuberculosis: a diagnostic and management challenge .J Neurosurgery. 83: 243-247.

Okeowo PA (2004): Pharynx-Infections (Tonsillitis, Quinsy, abscess) & TB. In Okeowo's Companion to Ear, Nose and Throat Diseases in the Tropics. Volume 3, 1st edition. Lagos, Nigeria: University of Lagos Press;109-114.

Ologe FE, Afolabi OA (2007): Penetrating pencil injury in the retromolar trigone: the need to play safe on playing ground. J Surg Surg Sci, 1:38-40.

Pak MW, Chan KL, Van Hassalt CA (1999). retropharyngeal abscess. A rare presentation of nasopharyngeal carcinoma. Journal of Laryngology and Otology.113 : 70-2.

Parhiscar A, Har-El G (2001): Deep neck abscess: A retrospective review of 210 cases. Ann Otol Rhinol Laryngol 110:1051–4.

Sapunar Z J, Cabello V A, Godoy R E (2008). Retropharyngeal phlegmon caused by a group B Streptococcus in a diabetic patient: report of one case]. Rev Med Chil.136: 351-5.

Schmal F, Stoll W (2002). Differential diagnosis and management of space occupying lesions. HND 50: 418-23.

Tan PT, Chang LY, Huang YC, Chiu CH, Wang CR, Lin TY (2001). Deep neck infection in children. *Journal of Microbiology, Immunology, and Infection.* 34: 287-92.

Tsui BC, Wagner A, Cave D, Elliot C, El-Hakim H, Malherbe S (2004): The incidence of laryngospasm with a "no touch" extubation technique after tonsillectomy and adenoidectomy. *Anesth Analg,* 98:327-329.

Wahbeh G, Wyllie R, Kay M (2002): Foreign body ingestion in infants and children: location, location, location. *Clin Pediatr (Phila),* 41:633-640.

Surgical Therapy of Erectile Dysfunction in Men with Diabetes Mellitus

Ahmad Al-enezi

Department of Surgery, Division of Urology
King Fahad Medical City Hospital, Riyadh, Saudi Arabia

Tariq Faisal Al-Shaiji

Department of Surgery, Division of Urology
Al-Amiri Teaching Hospital, Kuwait City, Kuwait

1   Introduction

Diabetes mellitus is a metabolic disorder characterized by defect in insulin secretion, insulin action or the combination of both. As a result, the amount of glucose in the blood increases while the tissue cells are starved of energy (Kumar *et al.*, 2004).

This uncontrolled hyperglycemia causes damage to both nerves and blood vessels, leading to serious myriad of complications such as ischemic heart disease, peripheral vascular disease and cerebral vascular disease which may ultimately result in death.

Sexual dysfunction including sexual drive, ejaculatory function and sexual satisfaction is undoubtedly one of the major health problems that impair the quality of life of diabetic patients at physical, psychological and social levels. Those have been well documented in the medical literature since 1978 (McCulloch *et al.*, 1980). Erectile dysfunction (ED) is defined as the inability to achieve and/or maintain sufficient erection satisfactory for sexual intercourse (NIH Consensus Conference, 1993). A fair number of males with Type 2 diabetes may complain of ED at some stage in their lives. ED also tends to occurs at a younger age group in the Type 1 diabetes mellitus (Klein *et al.*, 1996). There have been Substantial epidemiological studies which demonstrated that the odd ratio of developing ED in diabetics is 2–4 times more than the normal population (Lewis, 1996).

The treatment of ED compromises different modalities starting with first and second line measures which are minimally invasive in nature. Third line measures with surgical intervention are saved for patients' refractory to minimally invasive approaches. The aim of this chapter is to shed light on the pathophysiology of ED in DM followed by discussion of the surgical measures applied in this patient population with special emphasis on penile implants.

2   Pathophysiology of ED in DM

Erectile function in essence results from intricate psychological, neurological, hormonal and vascular interactions. Centrally, coordination of penile erection involves many cerebral and supraspinal transmitters and the details of which remain incompletely understood and by in large have been based upon experimental animal models. Currently many studies are investigating the role of centrally acting drugs for ED particularly patients that are refractory for phosphodiesterase type 5 (PDE-5) inhibitor drugs. Peripherally, erection is triggered either by tactile, visual, olfactory, or imaginary stimuli. The ultimate peripheral response is mediated by coordinated signals from the autonomic and somatic nervous systems to the smooth muscles of the corpora cavernosa in the penis and the striated muscles of the perineum. Blood flow to the penis is controlled by the autonomic erection center, the source of parasympathetic (S2–S4) and sympathetic (T12–L2) input to the pelvic plexus, as well as the cavernous nerves innervating the trabecular smooth muscle (Taub *et al.*, 1993).

The corpora cavernosa smooth muscles are two spongy cylinders which comprise the human penis. The penile muscles are highly specialized vascular structures which surrounds the penile urethra. In addition, the penile urethra traverses another spongy cylinder, the corpus spongiosum muscle at the glans of the penis. The vascular system within the penile tissues work in syncytium so that optimal erection occurs as a result of increased intracavernosal arterial inflow and reduced venous outflow. Those muscles become engorged during sexual activity. Neural stimulation is transmitted through the nervi erigentes, which release three important neurotransmitters: norepinephrine, acetylcholine and nitric oxide (NO).

Penile erection is predominantly mediated by parasympathetic neurotransmitters and NO and to a lesser extent by the other regulatory factors. For tumescence, intracavernosal oxygen and the enzyme NO synthase are both required essentially for the generation of nitric oxide. In turn, NO promotes the formation of cyclic GMP which causes smooth muscle relaxation and vasodilatation in the penile tissues. Sildenafil, Vardenafil and Tadalafil are drugs that act as (PDE-5) inhibitors and are widely used as first line treatment of patients with ED. The reverse is true during detumescence which occurs as a result of cyclic GMP metabolism via intracavernosal type 5 cyclic GMP phosphodiesterase. Norepinephrine pathways also play a lesser role in detumescence (Jeremy *et al.*, 1997).

In DM, the role of NO has a significant therapeutic implication. In fact, suboptimal and low levels of nitric oxide synthase have been found in diabetic patients in addition to testosterone deficiency. Testosterone deficiency results have been implicated in the pathophysiology of ED. Testosterone is critical for, nocturnal erections, libido and the maintenance of intracavernosal nitric oxide synthase activity (Mills *et al.*, 1992; Santen *et al.*, 1973). Hypogonadism has also been associated with ED and diabetes. According to Corona *et al.* (2004), Hypogonadism was demonstrated in 24.5% of men with diabetes and ED vs. 12.6% in those with ED. Testosterone supplementation in human diabetics with ED receiving pharmacological treatment has been advocated in the diabetics that did not respond to PDE5 inhibitors (Kalinchenko *et al.*, 2003).

On the other spectrum, the pathology of ED in DM is certainly multi-factorial and not solitary in nature. ED is more prevalent than retinopathy or nephropathy (Lehman *et al.*, 1983) in diabetic patients. According to a study by The Massachusetts Male Aging group, up to 75% of diabetic male patients have a predilection lifetime risk for developing ED (Feldman *et al.*, 1994; Metro *et al.*, 1999; Sarica *et al.*, 1994). Moreover, the age of onset of ED in diabetics occurs earlier in those who suffered from diabetes within 10 years from the onset in more than 50% of patients (Whitehead *et al.*, 1990). Interestingly, 12% of type 1 diabetic men had ED as the first diagnostic symptom (Koncz *et al.*, 1970). In the same vein, ED in diabetics could herald fatal cardiovascular disease (Gazzaruso *et al.*, 2004).

In the literature, the most common hypothesized mechanisms for developing ED in DM are as follows (Moore *et al.*, 2006):

1. The impairment of NO synthesis and the reduction of cGMP in diabetes (Costabile *et al.*, 2003).

2. The formation and accumulation of advanced glycation end-products (AGEs) in the corpus cavernosum leading to higher levels of oxygen free radicals and endothelia dysfunction (Cartledge *et al.*, 2001; Costabile *et al.*, 2003; Giuseppe *et al.*, 2006; Sullivan *et al.*, 1997).

3. Increased plasma serum and cavernosal levels of endothelin and the up regulation of endothelin-B receptor binding sites (Singh *et al.*, 2001; Takahashi *et al.*, 1990)

4. GTP-binding protein RhoA/Rho-kinase pathway and ET-1 induced vasoconstriction of the cavernosal smooth muscles (Park *et al.*, 2002; Wang *et al.*, 2002)

5. Autonomic, peripheral and central neuropathy (Agarwal *et al.*, 2003)

6. Deficiency in the cGMP-dependent protein kinase-1 (PKG-1) causing cavernosal smooth muscle relaxation (Chang *et al.*, 2004).

There have been several studies in the literature demonstrating a potential link between poor glycemic control and ED in diabetic patients. The increased levels of Hemoglobin (Hb)A1c has been associated with ED severity (Rhoden *et al.*, 2005a; 2005b). Nevertheless, here have been controversial results exist regarding the beneficial effects of intensive glycemic control on erectile function (Lu *et al.*, 2009).

The current evidence is scarce and many studies have failed to address whether ED would improve with intensive glycemic control. This is due to the fact that the vast majority was not specifically designed to test the hypothesis if intensive glycemic control would improve ED. Hence, this area remains a high priority for future research by utilizing objective questionnaires, large sample size and minimizing confounding factors.

3   Surgical Treatment of ED in DM

Surgical therapy for ED remains the gold standard surgical modality for patient's refractory to first and second line therapies. The surgical treatment with penile prosthesis was first described in the 1930s. Over the years significant developments were made to the prosthetic devices and materials leading to excellent functional and cosmetic results (Kim & Carso, 1993). On the other spectrum, penile arterial revascularization or venous surgery are other surgical treatment modalities for ED which tends to be effective only in a highly selected group of patients, mainly congenital or traumatic in nature and are being performed rarely.

3.1   Arterial Revascularization

Penile arterial bypass surgery was first described in the early 1970s (Michal et al., 1973; 1974), and has undergone many modifications since its early description. The risk factors in penile arterial insufficiency is strongly related to atherosclerosis such as is most frequently the result of general arteriosclerosis as hyperlipidemia, hypertension, cigarette smoking, and diabetes mellitus. The outcome of penile arterial revascularization in patients with such risk factors generally is unsatisfactory. According to the American Urological Association (AUA2005) guidelines, arterial reconstructive surgery could be offered as a treatment option only in healthy individuals with recently acquired ED secondary to a focal arterial occlusion and in the absence of any evidence of generalized vascular disease.

Several tests are available to confirm the diagnose such as Duplex ultrasonography of the penis with injection and stimulation test. In addition, selective penile or pudendal angiongram is essential prior to any surgical reconstruction.

Current surgical techniques for revascularization include anastomosis between the epigastric artery and the dorsal penile artery or the deep dorsal vein (Hauri et al., 1999; Virag et al., 1980). Young patients with arterial insufficiency due to pelvic trauma are generally ideal candidates for such procedures (Goldstein, 1988). Certain centers offer laparoscopic approach to minimize the morbidity and overall the long-term success is in the range of 34-80% spontaneous erections (Lund et al., 1995; Manning et al., 1988).

The commonest complications of the procedures are infection, bleeding, thrombosis of anastomosis and hyperemia in the glans of the penis.

3.2   Venous Surgery

Venogenic cause for ED is considered when sub-optimal erectile response to intracavernosal injection occurs despite a normal arterial response on duplex ultrasonography.

When venous leak is suspected in ED, cavernosometry and cavernosography can be used to delineate its location and the severity (Puyau et al., 1983; Rudnick et al., 1991; Wespes et al., 1986). Venous surgery should be contemplated only when cavernosography demonstrates visual evidence of penile venous leak.

Penile prostheses surgery tends to be more superior to venous surgery as venous surgical ligation has been associated with significant obliterations of arterial inflow in many cases. Hence penile venous surgery has been limited to patients under the age of 50. Venous surgery is relatively contraindicated in diabetics, and in patients refusing to quit smoking. Recognizable complications of venous surgery include numbness of the skin, shortening of penile length, penile curvature and hematoma formation.

The poor prognostic factors that affect the long term outcome and may also explain the high incidence of failure rate include increasing age, duration of ED, multiple leak sites, crural venous leak site, and the existence of arteriogenic insufficiency (Kim *et al.*, 1995; Motiwala *et al.*, 1993).

3.3   Prosthetic Surgery

Penile implants were first introduced to clinical practice almost 30 years ago (Scott *et al.*, 1974; Small *et al.*, 1975). It is estimated that one-third of patients with ED will not respond to contemporary medical treatments such as PDE-5 inhibitors and intracavernosal injection therapy. Moreover, half of the patients with ED have severe and irreversible damage; making those patients ideal candidates for penile prosthesis surgery (Moncada *et al.*, 2004).

Penile prosthesis is an irreversible surgery in the erectile corporal tissues which in essence means that any previous degree of normal physiological erections will be permanently lost. In other words, if there is an indication for the prosthesis to be removed such as infection or mechanical failure; complete ED will ensue.

There are three major classes of penile prosthesis which are semi-rigid, two-piece and three-piece inflatable implants. The semi-rigid prosthetic implants are technically easier to insert and have minimal mechanical failure rate. They are made of two cylinders. Their insertion is indicated in Patients with limited mentation or restricted manual dexterity. However, they are generally inferior to the inflatables; as the penis remains unable to achieve complete rigidity or flaccidity. The semirigids also have higher rate of prosthetic erosions. The two-piece inflatable prostheses have a pair of cylinders connected to a scrotal pump. The prosthesis cylinders are deflated by bending the middle part of the shaft of the penis. These two-piece is disadvantaged by less rigidity than the three-piece and less girth expansion. The two-piece also does not have better flaccidity than the three-piece upon deflation. The three-piece inflatable prosthesis is composed of a pair of cylinders which are implanted in the penis, a pump that is inserted in the scrotum and a reservoir that is placed in the extra peritoneal region of abdomen. The scrotal pump has a small button that allows inflatation and deflation of the cylinders.

3.3.1   Inflatable Three-Piece Penile Prosthesis Operation

The insertion of a three-piece penile prosthesis is considered the gold standard and provides the best option for patients due to its optimal rigidity and flaccidity as well as patient satisfaction. Hence in this part of the chapter, we have elected to focus on the surgical techniques and the management of pitfalls that are commonly encountered during the procedure.

Both large and small penises have been best served by the three-piece inflatable implants because semi-rigid and two-piece implants are difficult to conceal in such patients. Preoperative counseling of prospective patients is mandatory about the different methods available for treatment and explanation of how prosthesis works. Patients must be fully informed that any preexisting natural erection will be lost and that the procedure is irreversible. Another important fact that the patient must be aware of is that the length of the fully stretched flaccid penis preoperatively will be the maximal length obtained with a penile prosthesis.

3.3.2   Preoperative Preparations

Diabetic patients with better blood sugar control and HbA1C are less susceptible to infection than those with poorly controlled HbA1C (Bishop *et al*., 1992). On average, the presence of diabetes increases the infection rate in penile prosthesis from 3 to 8% (Wilson *et al*., 1998).

Active infection therefore anywhere in the body should be excluded, but especially in urine and skin. Patient should be encouraged to brush the genitalia with strong soaps for few days prior to the procedure. Preoperative antibiotics targeting gram-positive bacteria are recommended before skin incision. In addition, the following are vital:

- Shaving immediately before the procedure
- Alcohol-based skin preparation and a minimum of 10 minutes scrubbing should take place prior to the formal prepping and draping
- Draping for scrotal incision should be with extremity drape and self adhesive special drapes if possible
- Face masks, disposable gowns, and double-gloving are mandatory
- Traffic in and out of the operating room should be minimized and there must be laminar air flow if possible

3.3.3   Special Equipments

- Scott retractor, transverse penile strap, and hook retractors
- Small Deaver or similar retractors
- Brook's cavernosal dilators or Hegar dilators
- Rosello cavernotomes for cases of corporal fibrosis
- Furlow inserter with Keith needles
- DeBakey forceps and Metzenbaum scissors
- Long-blade nasal speculum
- Absorbable sutures for corporotomy, dartos fascia and skin closures

3.3.4   Surgical Steps

A Foley catheter is first inserted into the urethra and the bladder is emptied. A spigot is applied. A Scott retractor is then placed below the penis. A transverse skin incision is made at the penoscrotal junction. The incision can be modified to an inverted T-shape and extended when better corporal exposure is needed during difficult surgery, e.g., when there is corporal fibrosis (Figure 1). The dartos fascia is exposed and incised. Skin hooks are placed. The tunica albuginea of both corporas are exposed and the urethral catheter is palpated in the midline. This facilitates urethral exposure and minimizes its potential damage. A stab wound is made with a scalpel into each corpora and, using Metzenbaum scissors, a 2-cm vertical corporotomy is performed between two nonabsorbable 2-0 stay sutures (Figure 2).

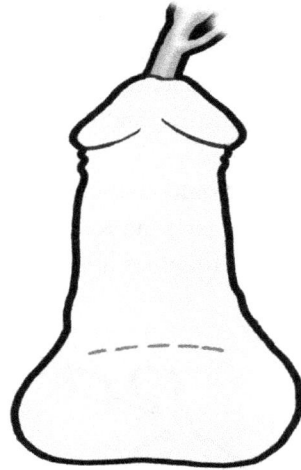

Figure 1: A Foley catheter is inserted to empty the bladder. A transverse skin incision is made at the penoscrotal junction. The incision can be modified to an inverted T-shape.

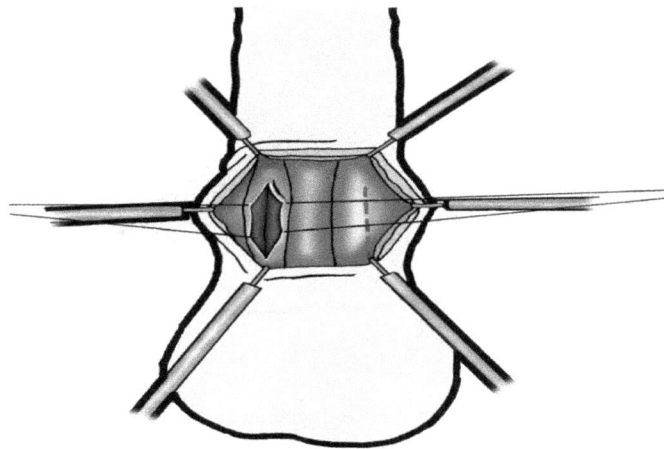

Figure 2: Skin hooks are in place. A stab wound is made into each corpora and a 2-cm vertical corporotomy is performed between two nonabsorbable 2-0 stay sutures.

Corporal dilatation is performed and directed laterally to avoid urethral injury. The corporal space is dilated with Brook's dilators or Hegar dilator from 10 mm up to 14 mm. proximally the dilator can be felt to hit on the ischiopubic ramus. An equal depth of the dilators should be achieved when performing proximal dilatation; this ensures that proximal perforation is highly unlikely. Both corporas are irrigated with antibiotic solution. Distally, the glans of the penis is palpated until maximal limit of dilatation is achieved by feeling the tip of the dilator bilaterally. At each side, a measurement is recorded proximally and distally each towards approximately mid-point of the corporotomy incision and, added together which determines the final length of the cylinder implant. There should be no more than 1 cm discrepancy between the two sides. Cycling of the connected corporal cylinders and pump is performed two or three times using sterile saline. This ensures the removal of any air bubble. The connecting tubes are gently clamped with rubber-shod clamps. The same preparatory steps are repeated for the reservoir.

The rear tip extenders of the cylinders are attached at this stage when needed. The proximal part of the corporal cylinder/rear tip extender is inserted first, and the back of a DeBakey forceps may be used to facilitate a gentle pushing into the corporal space.

The Furlow instrument is then inserted distally and laterally to avoid any 'crossover' into the contralateral corporal space. The Furlow is used to pass the Keith needle at the tip on each side to facilitate the distal placement of the cylinders. The corporotomies are closed using the 2-0 absorbable stay sutures (Figure 3).

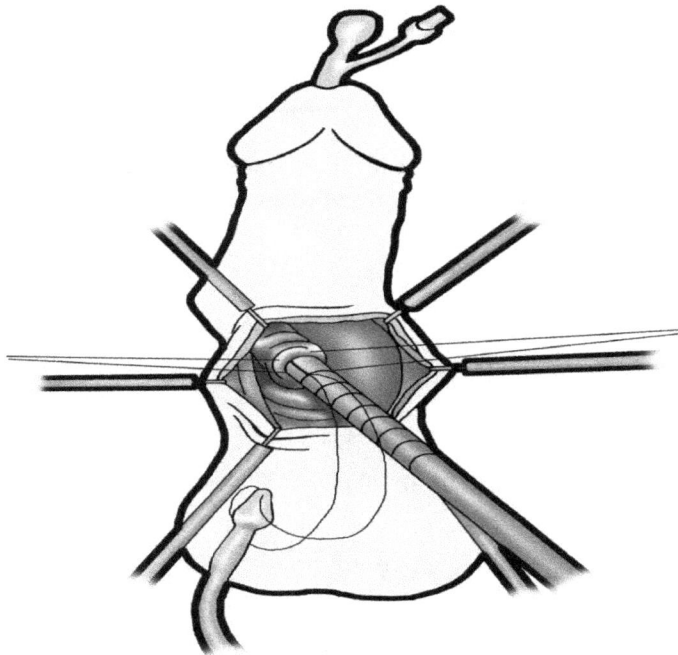

Figure 3: The Furlow is used to pass the Keith needle at the tip on each side to facilitate the distal placement of the cylinders.

A subdartos pouch is made for the pump in the middle of the scrotum or the hemiscrotum. A small incision is made through the dartos fascia and a long-blade nasal speculum or ring forceps is used to create the space. The pump is inserted into the subdartos pouch, ensuring that the deflation button llies anteriorly and inferiorly.

The tubing from the pump is preferably passed through separate stab incisions in the dartos fascia to emerge from the posterior aspect of the pouch. The opening of the top part of the pouch is closed with 2-0 nonabsorbable suture. Connection between the tubing of the pump and the cylinders is made. The reservoir tubing from the pump remains intact at this stage. A 50-ml syringe filled with normal saline is attached to the reservoir tubing. This allows testing of the prosthesis cylinders to ensure the function and quality of erection. In preparation for the reservoir placement, the spigot is removed from the Foley catheter and the bladder is fully drained. The size of the reservoir depends upon the surgeon's preference. However, a previous surgery on one side would make placement on the contralateral side preferable.

The external ring is identified using a small Deaver retractor and the index finger is used to palpate the spermatic cord, pushing it medially to protect it. A closed Metzenbaum scissors is then used to puncture the transversalis fascia. This permits access to the retropubic space. The index finger is inserted again to create a space. The retropubic location of the space is confirmed by feeling the back of the pubic bone, the symphysis pubis and the Foley balloon inside the bladder (Figure 4).

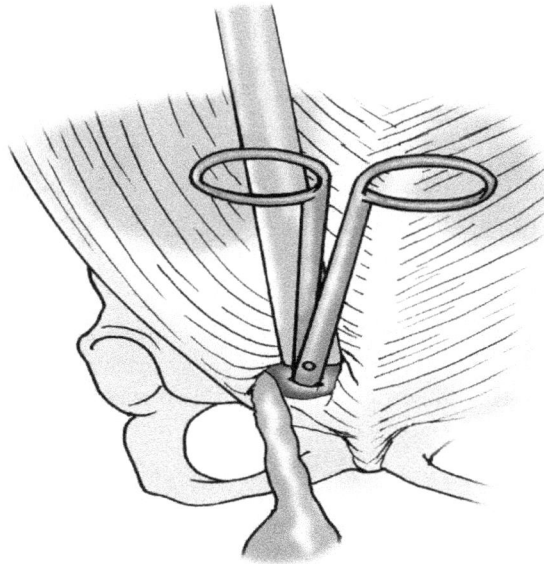

Figure 4: The external ring is identified using a small Deaver retractor. A closed Metzenbaum scissors is used to puncture the transversalis fascia allowing access to the retropubic space. The index finger is inserted again to create a space.

Through the same wound, a long-blade nasal speculum is inserted in the created transversalis fascia defect, the blades are pulled upward and lateral to gain access to this defect. The blades are gently spread apart, and the reservoir is inserted into the newly created retropubic space (Figure 5).

Alternatively, a Deaver can be placed to expose the space to permit placement of the reservoir. The reservoir is then filled with normal saline up to 5 mls above its manufactured capacity. With the tubing to the filling syringe left open, the syringe should spontaneously fill to 5 ml. If it fills more than this, the position of the reservoir space needs to be checked again to ensure that there is no pressure around the reservoir. Some reservoirs have lockout valves to prevent autoinflation. The correct position of the reservoir is confirmed again by palpation and it is ensured that the reservoir tubing is exiting through the transversalis fascia defect.

The final connection between the pump and the reservoir is completed and a last check is made of the connections between the three tubes. The rubber-shod clamps are removed and inflation and deflation of the prosthesis is carried out few times to make sure that it is functioning properly (Figure 6).

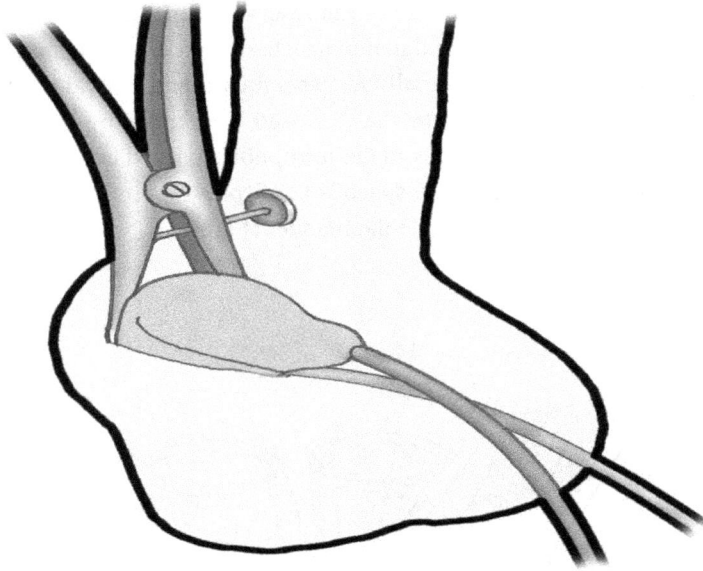

Figure 5: A long-blade nasal speculum is inserted in the created transversalis fascia defect. The blades are pulled upward and lateral to gain access to the defect. The blades are gently spread apart, and the reservoir is inserted into the newly created retropubic space.

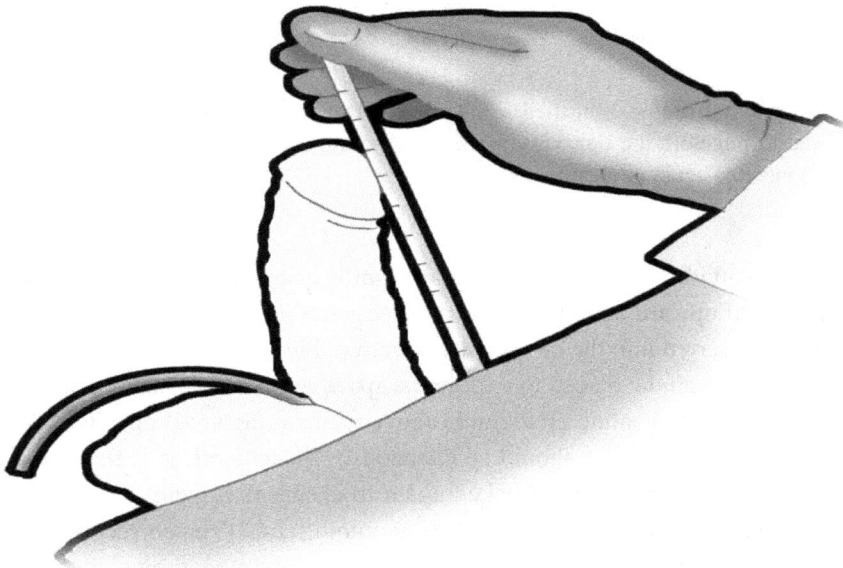

Figure 6: Once the final connection between the pump and the reservoir is completed and a last check is made of the connections between the three tubes, inflation and deflation of the prosthesis is carried out few times to make sure that it is functioning properly.

We prefer not to leave a drain routinely unless there is a particular concern, e.g., bleeding. If needed, a drain may be left *in situ* through a separate stab wound incision. The wound is then closed in two layers. The dartos fascia is closed with 2-0 absorbable suture and the skin is closed with 3-0 absorbable suture.

3.3.5 Post Operative Care

Antibiotics

Antibiotics are usually continued for 48 hours postoperatively. Some surgeons prefer to maintain antibiotics for a week after surgery and a longer period of time after revision surgery or in special circumstances, e.g., previous penile prosthesis infection.

Urinary catheter

The catheter facilitates identification of the urethra and the corpus spongiosum. It can be removed at the end of the procedure or retained for 24 hours after surgery.

Drain

Some surgeons prefer to use a drain to reduce the edema and to facilitate drainage of hematoma when it occurs. These drains are usually removed on postoperative day 1 or day 2 (Sadeghi-Nejad *et al.*, 2005).

Wound care

The penis is positioned over the suprapubic region pointing toward the umbilicus. The wound is covered with gauze and Mefix® tape is applied. The patient is reviewed in the outpatient clinic after 2 weeks to check the wound and to rule out autoinflation.

Pain

Pain following placement of a penile prosthesis is subjective and variable. It may be aggravated by preexisting conditions. For most patients, pain is no longer bothersome by 4–6 weeks.

Using the prosthesis

The cylinders are kept inflated for 24 hours and then partially deflated. This facilitates corporal hemostasis. At 4 weeks, the patient is advised to cycle the prosthesis. Patients are taught to operate the inflatable prosthesis at about 6 weeks. Other clinicians may prefer to leave the cylinders inflated for few weeks to allow creation of an adequate capsule, since keeping the prosthesis deflated after surgery for few weeks might results in prosthetic tip retraction under the glans and the creation of a capsule that is too short. A reasonable method is to leave the prosthesis partially (50%) inflated at the conclusion of the procedure; this will encourage proper modeling of the penis and also maintain good hemostasis.

3.3.6 Pitfalls and Specific Considerations

Infection

Despite the use of antibiotics and meticulous sterile environments and improved surgical techniques, infection rates remained relatively stable over decades till the introduction of antibiotic-coated implants. *Staphylococcus epidermidis*, *Staphylococcus aureus*, *Pseudomonas*, and *Candida albicans* are the most common skin-colonizing microorganisms implicated (Mulcahy *et al.*, 2008; Sausville *et al.*, 2009).

It has also been demonstrated that the incidence of infection is doubled (18.8%) in re-operation cases and in secondary implantation, uncontrolled diabetes, and paraplegia, as well as in the hands of inexperienced surgeons (Henry *et al.*, 2005; Lotan *et al.*, 2003). Overall, infection rates are generally 1.8%–10% for first-time prostheses and 7%–21% for replacements (Jarow *et al.*, 1996; Lane *et al.*, 2007).

Regardless of the microbiologic agent involved, it is advisable to remove the infected implant if the patient has not responded to antibiotic therapy. In such cases, all components of the infected implant should be removed to prevent a recurrence of infection. Also, the absence of clinical and microbiological evidence of infection must be ensured before embarking on any further surgery for penile prosthesis. It is essential to advise patients to use physiotherapy with a vacuum device in order to prevent excessive shrinkage of cavernosal tissue and consequent penile shortening.

An alternative to removal of all components and later reimplantation has been described by Mulcahy (Mulcahy *et al.*, 2003) who calls it the 'salvage or rescue' procedure. This involves removal of all prosthetic parts and irrigation of the wound with a series of antiseptic solutions, followed by replacement of the prosthesis during the same procedure. It is also demonstrated that the use of systemic antibiotics for 48–72 hours prior to the salvage improves the chances of success, with improvement or resolution of cellulitis suggesting that the chance of the salvage procedure succeeding would be higher. The advantage of the salvage procedure is that most of the length of the penis will be maintained. In addition, it is easier to place cylinders while the cavities in the corpora cavernosa are still open, rather than returning at a later date to create new cavities in the scar tissue.

Type of incision

The penoscrotal approach avoids possible injury to the dorsal sensory nerves, provides easier and more complete corporal exposure, and allows the pump to be anchored in the scrotal pouch. In a review by Montague and *Angermeier* (Montague *et al.*, 2000) for most primary penile prosthesis patients, the AMS Ultrex® prosthesis is recommended because it produces expansion in both girth and length of the penis. In primary patients with long penises and in men with Peyronie disease, the AMS 700CX® prosthesis is recommended. For secondary implants (penile prosthesis reimplantation), the urologist can still offer most of patients the AMS Ultrex® device. However, in men with previous urethral erosion or cylinder crossover complications, the recommendation is to use the AMS 700CX® prosthesis. When corporal dilation is limited because of cavernosal fibrosis, for instance after removal of an infected penile prosthesis, the smaller size AMS 700CXM® cylinders are a better option (Wilson *et al.*, 1994).

Cavernosal fibrosis

The multicomponent inflatable penile prosthesis has undergone sequential modifications that have afforded important functional advantages and have greatly reduced the potential for mechanical failure. This was made possible by the introduction of the Ultrex® cylinder, which consists of bi-directionally woven Dacron™ and Lycra™ layers situated between inner and outer layers of silicone. This allows expansion in girth from 12 mm to 18 mm, while resisting any possible aneurysmal bulge. However, oversizing and deformity maybe encountered.

Montague and Angermeier described a cylinder measurement technique that avoids the problem of oversizing that may occur particularly in the case of the length-expanding Ultrex® penile prosthesis, when cylinders that are too long can result in an S-shaped cylinder deformity. These types of deformities are sometimes difficult to diagnose. Wilson and Delk published an outstanding review describing the newer tools and techniques to enhance placement of an inflatable device in patients with severe fibrosis

(Montague *et al.*, 2000). This includes the use of specially designed cavernotomes for dilating fibrotic corpora, the use of downsized prosthetic cylinders, alternative procedures to fix cylinders in the face of perforation (as opposed to primary closure of the perforation), and replacing the original cylinders 1 year after the modified cylinders have served as tissue expanders. The cylinder sizing is of great importance (Wilson *et al.*, 1994).

Corporal sizing

A 2-cm corporotomy incision is used and the distal measurement is from the distal end of the corporotomy and the proximal measurement is from the proximal end of the corporotomy as outlined earlier within the surgical steps. The two measurements added together determine the total cylinder size. The aim is to insert a cylinder that extends to each end of the corpus cavernosum and lies comfortably inside the open corporotomy. With the cylinder completely filled with normal saline it will be possible to ascertain the final appearance. The use of a cylinder that does not match the length of the corpus cavernosum may result in the so called S-shaped cylinder deformity.

Difficult corporal closure

Straightforward corporotomy closure can be attained using horizontal mattress sutures or simple closure with absorbable stay sutures pre-placed on each side of the corporotomy before corporal dilatation. This prevents possible damage to the cylinders. When severe intracorporal fibrosis is encountered, corporal dilatation to accommodate the cylinder and subsequent closure over the prosthesis is usually challenging. Various materials have been utilized to cover the cylinders when primary closure of the tunica albuginea is not possible. These include synthetic graft, tunica vaginalis flaps, processed cadaveric dura mater, processed cadaveric skin, and processed cadaveric pericardium (Alter *et al.*, 1998; Fallon *et al.*, 1990; Herschorn *et al.*, 1995; Landman *et al.*, 1999; Reddy *et al.*, 1999; Smith *et al.*, 1998).

Corporal perforation and urethral injury

If corporal fibrosis is anticipated, wider transverse incisions or vertical penoscrotal incisions are the best approach for proximal exposure of the tunica albuginea. With careful dilation of the corpora cavernosa, the majority of the complications can be avoided.

If distal corporal perforation is identified during dilation (e.g., a distally placed dilator comes out the meatus or, when irrigating the distal corpora, the fluid emerges out of the meatus), the safest course of action is to terminate the procedure. An injured urethra should be repaired over a Foley catheter. Another procedure can be re-scheduled after 6 weeks. However, another option in cases of urethral perforation is urethral mobilization and suturing of the albugineal and urethral defect, followed by continuation with the procedure for prosthesis insertion. If the patient has a previous history of distal perforation or severe distal corporal fibrosis and previous urethral erosion, the urethra should be repaired through a circumcision incision. In addition, the patient should be warned about the possible need for temporary urinary diversion such as suprapubic catheter, vesicostomy, or perineal urethrostomy (Wang *et al.*, 2000).

The patient should receive broad-spectrum antibiotics for 3–4 weeks and a retrograde urethrogram should be performed before the catheter is removed. If distal perforation occurs during the dilatation of the second corpora cavernosum, the injury should be repaired and then either the cylinder can be inserted on the non-perforated side with concomitant urinary diversion or the procedure should be abandoned and both corpora irrigated with antibiotics. Proximal laceration of the urethra during scrotal exposure can be repaired, and insertion of the prosthesis may continue. Care must be taken to avoid contacting the suture lines when closing the urethral and albugineal defects before continuation with prosthesis implantation.

Correction for proximal perforation has also been attempted with the use of synthetic graft material to form a 'windsox;' however, this technique has been associated with significant postoperative graft infection (Carson & Noh, 2002).

For proximal perforation of the corporal body during implantation into scarred corporal tissues, a sling of nonabsorbable suture through the rear tip extender has been demonstrated to effectively keep the cylinder base out of the damaged tunica albuginea. When this sling is used most authorities advocate that the prosthesis should not be used for 3 months (Henry & Wilson, 2007); This minimizes trauma and early pressure on the prosthesis during the healing process.

Crossover

Crossovers are rarely complete, i.e., with the tip of both cylinders in one corporal body. The corporal septum tends to have windows, and the typical crossover is indicated by an over-and-back movement. Using the scrotal incision and placing the penis on stretch in the Scott retractor helps the surgeon to avoid this over-and-back movement. If crossover is suspected, both cylinders should be removed, and the corpora cavernosa should be re-dilated proximally and distally with a size 11 or 12 Hegar dilator in the opposite corpora. If the active dilator hits the opposite stationary Hegar, a crossover situation exists and needs to be managed accordingly. One of the techniques is to place the Hegar dilator on the side in which one of the cylinders resided as a reference point, whether proximal or distal. The surgeon then gently re-channels the crossover side, staying lateral and using the stationary Hegar as the reference point. The cylinder is inserted with the stationary Hegar in place. When the cylinder goes in correctly, the stationary Hegar is removed and the contralateral cylinder is inserted. It is not necessary to repair the crossover because the septum of the corpora is variable, has windows, and occasionally is filamentous.

Pump and reservoir problems

There are three reservoir sizes available with the AMS three-piece inflatable penile prostheses: 50 mls, 65 mls, and 100 mls The 50-mL reservoir is used for the CXM prosthesis. The 65-mL reservoir is used for the prosthesis and for the two smaller cylinder sizes of the Ultrex® prosthesis. The 100-mL reservoir is designated for the two largest cylinder sizes of the Ultrex® prosthesis. Correct placement of the reservoir into the retropubic space and a back pressure test are mandatory to prevent the problem of autoinflation of the prosthesis.

In special situations, the retroperitoneal space can be extremely fibrotic and the transversalis fascia thickened. This is often caused by previous surgery, such as cystectomy or renal transplantation, or it may be the result of radiation. The surgeon may elect to insert a two-piece inflatable device, make a separate incision for placement of the reservoir, or consider another location for reservoir placement. Paravesical or abdominal placement of the reservoir may be a better option in previously operated patients. The pump should be placed in a dependent and easily palpable scrotal position. Particular care should be taken to not dissect or tear small vessels in this region as a scrotal hematoma can easily develop.

When replacing the three-piece prosthesis for malfunction the best way to manage the reservoir of the original prosthesis is still a matter for debate. Removing a reservoir is far more difficult than its initial placement; a self-retaining long-blade nasal speculum may be used for removal of the reservoir utilizing an extended diathermy tip to cut down on the tubing, which is placed on gentle traction. Some surgeons leave the reservoir of the original three-piece device behind after removing the penile cylinders and the scrotal pump of the malfunctioning device. Rajpurkar *et al*. (2004) found that retained reservoirs are not susceptible to infection or erosion and can therefore be left behind.

Revision

Antiseptic washout and mechanical debridement of the bacterial biofilm within the corporal space are the mainstay techniques during revision prosthetic surgery. It is theoretically advisable to remove reservoirs at the time of revision surgery. Alternatively, new reservoirs may be placed in different locations if the surgeon decides to leave the old one behind because of the daunting task involved in removing some of them.

Peyronie disease

When penile curvature is present, whether due to Peyronie disease or other causes, CX prosthesis cylinders have more straightening properties than Ultrex® cylinders. The formercylinders are used in conjunction with 'modeling' of thepenis as described by Wilson and Delk (1994). Correcting the curvature deformity can be attained without the need for plaque incision or excision. It is necessary during modeling to initially clamp the cylinder input tubes to protect the pump from back-pressure flow. The prosthetic cylinders are inflated to high pressure, the input tube is clamped with rubber-shod clamps, and the penis is grasped with both hands and bent over the inflated cylinders at the region of maximum curvature. Bending is maintained for 90 seconds and then relaxed. It is worth noting that simple prosthesis insertion can produce complete straightening in up to 30% of patients. The rest of the patients may require additional procedures for residual curvatures (Ralph *et al.*, 2004; Pryor *et al.*, 2004).

A recent retrospective study by Garaffa *et al.* (2011) reported that modeling alone achieved more straightening on inflatable prosthesis (84%) than on a malleable prosthesis (54%) and procedures such as tunical plication or incision, with or without graft, can be used for any ventral curvature that persists after modeling.

In another study, Levine *et al.* (2010), reported a single center experience with IPP and straightening maneuvers as necessary in 90 men with medication-refractory ED and Peyronie disease. Additional intraoperative maneuvers used to straighten the penis following placement of the prosthesis included manual modeling, plaque incision and, if the defect created with incision was greater than 2 cm, an off-the-shelf human processed pericardial graft. In their study, IPP placement allowed reliable and satisfactory coitus for the great majority of men (91%). Mechanical failure was reported in 7%.

Patients with special conditions

For patients with complicated backgrounds such as kidney transplant or a neobladder, a simpler prosthesis should be contemplated than the three-piece inflatable penile prosthesis, for example, the two-piece or semi-rigid implant. Another solution is to place the reservoir outside the usual location (outlined above). In such cases, the surgeon makes a second incision and places the reservoir intra-abdominally or in the retroperitoneal space beneath the kidney. Three months after implantation, a tissue capsule would have formed around the reservoir and this will prevent increase in abdominal pressure from causing autoinflation.

Cold-glans syndrome

A common complaint after the insertion of a penile prosthesis is lack of glans engorgement after inflation. In the majority of patients this is due to inadequate sexual stimulation. In some patients, however, the glans is soft and cold despite proper sexual stimulation. Mulhall *et al.* (2004) found that most patients responded to sildenafil and reported higher satisfaction than with an implant alone. Lledo *et al.* (2011) have also reported similar results.

4   Future Research

There has been a tremendous enthusiasm in advancing further research ED in two main areas, first-line medical therapy and gene therapy. In medical therapy, the search for a drug which combines PDE5 inhibitory and NO-releasing properties aim to address the affect of multiple peripheral intracellular targets. On the other hand gene therapy for ED in diabetes and other conditions such as hypercholesterolaemia is still evolving as a therapeutic option.

Acknowledgement

We would like to express our special thanks to **Mr. Ibrahim El-Avvocato**, the artist behind the drawn figures.

References

Agarwal, S.K., Prakash, A., & Singh, N.P. (2003). *Erectile dysfunction in diabetes mellitus: Novel treatments. Interantion Journal of Diabetes Development Countries, 23, 94–98.*

Alter G.J., Greisman J., Werthman P.E., Seid A.S. & Joseph B.J. (1998). *Use of a prefabricated tunica vaginalis fascia flap to reconstruct the tunica albuginea after recurrent penile prosthesis extrusion. J Urol;159:128-32.*

Bishop, J.R., Moul J.W., Sehelnik, S.A., Pepas, D.S., Gormley, D.S. & McLeod, D.G. (1992). *Use of glycoslylated hemoglobin to identify diabetics at high risk for penile prosthesis infections. J Urol 1992; 147: 386–388.*

Carson, C.C. & Noh, C.H. (2002). *Distal penile prosthesis extrusion: Treatment with distal corporoplasty or gortex windsock reinforcement. Int J Impot Res 2002;14:81-4.*

Cartledge, J.J., Eardley, I. & Morrison, J.F. (2001). *Advanced glycation endproducts A review. Diabetologia, 44, 129–146.*

Chang, S., Hypolite, J.A., Velez, M., Changolkar, A., Wein, A.J., Chacko, S., & DiSanto, M. E. (2004). *Downregulation of cGMP- Dependent protein kinase-1 activity in the corpus cavernosum smooth muscle of diabetic rabbits. American Journal of Physiology Regulatory Integrative and Comparative Physiology, 287, R950–R960.*

Corona, G., Mannucci, E., Mansani, R., Petrone, L., Bartolini, M., Giommi, R., Forti, G. & Maggi, M. (2004). *Organic, relational and Psychological factors in erectile dysfunction in men with diabetes mellitus. Eur Urol 2004; 46:222–8.*

Costabile, R.A. (2003). *Optimizing treatment for diabetes mellitus induced erectile dysfunction. Journal of Urology, 170, S35–S39.*

Fallon B. (1990). *Cadaveric dura mater graft for correction of penile curvature in Peyronie disease. Urolog; 35:127-9.*

Feldman, H.A., Goldstein, I., Hatzichristou, D.G., Krane, R.J. & Mckinlay, J.B. (1994). *Impotence and its medical and psychosocial correlates: Results of the Massachusetts Male Aging Study. J Urol 1994;151:54–61.*

Garaffa, G., Minervini, A., Christopher, N.A., Minhas, S. & Ralph, D.J. (2011). *The management of residual curvature after penile prosthesis implantation in men with Peyronies disease. BJU Int 2011.*

Gazzaruso, C., Giordanetti, S., De Amici, E., Bertone, G., Falcone, C., Geroldi, D., Fratino, P., Solerte, S.B., Garzaniti, A. (2004). *Relationship between erectile dysfunction and silent myocardial ischemia in apparentl uncomplicated type 2 diabetic patients. Circulation; 110:22–6.*

Giuseppe, C., Ferdinando, F., Ciro, I., & Vincenzo, M. (2006). *Pharmacology of erectile dysfunction in man. Pharmacology & Therapeutics, 111, 400–423.*

Goldstein, I. (1988). Overview of types and results of vascular surgical procedures for impotence. Cardiovasc Intervent Radiol. 11(4): p 240-4.

Hauri, D. (1999). Penile revascularization surgery in erectile dysfunction. Andrologia, 1999. 31(Suppl 1): p. 65- 76.

Henry, G.D., Wilson, S.K., Delk, JR. 2nd, Carson, C.C., et al. (2005). Revision washout decreases penile prosthesis infection in revision surgery: A multicenter study. J Urol; 173:89-92.

Henry, G.D. & Wilson, S.K. (2007). Updates in inflatable penile prostheses. Urol Clin North Am; 34:535-47, vi.

Herschorn, S. & Ordorica, R.C. (1995). Penile prosthesis insertion with corporeal reconstruction with synthetic vascular graft material. J Urol; 154:80-4.

Jarow, J.P. (1996). Risk factors for penile prosthetic infection. J Urol 1996;156:402-4.

Jeremy, J.Y., Ballard, S.A., Naylor, A.M., Miller, M.A. & Angelini, G.D. (1997). Effects of sildenafil, a type-5 cGMP phosphodiesterase inhibitor, and papaverine on cyclic GMP and cyclic AMP levels in the rabbit corpus cavernosum in vitro. Br J Urol; 79(6):958.

Kalinchenko, S.Y., Kozlov, G.I., Gontcharov, N.P. & Katsiya, G.V. (2003). Oral testosterone undecanoate reverses erectile dysfunction associated with diabetes mellitus in patients failing on sildenafil. Aging Male. Jun; 6(2):94-9.

Kim, E.D. & McVary, K.T. (1995). Long-term results with penile vein ligation for venogenic impotence. J Urol; 153(3 Pt 1): p. 655-8.

Kim, J., & Carson, C.C. (1993). History of urologic prosthesis for impotence. Prob Urol; 7: p. 283-288.

Klein, R., Klein, B. E., Lee, K. E., Moss, S. E., & Cruickshanks, K. J. (1996). Prevalence of self-reported erectile dysfunction in people with long-term IDDM. Diabetes Care, 19, 135−14.

Koncz L, Balodimos MC. Impotence in diabetes mellitus. Med Times 1970;98:159–70.

Kumar, V., Cotran, R. S., & Robbins, S. L. (2004). Robbin's basic pathology (7th ed., pp. 641−655). Philadelphia: Saunders: An Imprint of Elsevier.

Landman, J. & Bar-Chama, N. (1999). Initial experience with processed human cadaveric allograft skin for reconstruction of the corpus cavernosum in repair of distal extrusion of a penile prosthesis. Urology 1999;53:1222-4.

Lane, B.R., Abouassaly, R., Angermeier, K.W., Montague, D.K. (2007). Threepiece inflatable penile prostheses can be safely implanted after radical prostatectomy through a transverse scrotal incision. Urology 2007;70:539-42.

Lehman, T.P. & Jacobs, J.A. (1983). Etiology of diabetic impotence. J Urol 1983;129:291–4.

Levine, L.A., Benson, J. & Hoover, C. (2010). Inflatable penile prosthesis placement in men with Peyronie's disease and drug-resistant erectile dysfunction: A single-center study. J Sex Med 2010;7:3775-83.

Lewis, R.W. (1996). Epidemiology of erectile dysfunction. Urologic Clinics of North America, 28, 209−216.

Lledo, E, Moncada, I., Jara, R., Carrera, P., Gonzalez-Chamorro, F., Llorente, A., Hernandez, C. (2011). Treatment with sildenafil of cold glans syndrome after hydraulic penile prosthesis implantation]. Actas Urol Esp Tech Case Report 2011; 3:76-83.

Lotan, Y., Roehrborn, C.G., McConnell, J.D., Hendin, B.N. (2003). Factors influencing the outcomes of penile prosthesis surgery at a teaching institution. Urol 2003;62:918-21.

Lu, C.C., Jiann, B.P., Sun, C.C., Lam, H.C., Chu, C.H., Lee, J.K. (2009). Association of glycemic control with risk of erectile dysfunction in men with type 2 diabetes. J Sex Med 2009; 6:1719–28.

Lund, G.O., Winfield, H.N. & Donovan, J.F. (1995). Laparoscopically assisted penile revascularization for vasculogenic impotence. J Urol, 1995. 153(6): p. 1923-6.

Manning, M., et al. (1998). Long-term followup and selection criteria for penile revascularization in erectile failure. J Urol, 1998. 160(5): p. 1680-4.

McCulloch, D.K., Campbell, I.W., Wu, F.C., Prescott, R.J., & Clarke, B.F. (1980). The prevalence of diabetic impotence. Diabetologia, 18, 279−283.

Metro, M.J., Broderick, G.A. (1999). Diabetes and vascular impotence: Does insulin dependence increase the relative severity? Int J Impot Res 1999;11:87–9.

Michal, V., et al. (1973). Direct arterial anastomosis on corpora cavernosa penis in the therapy of erective impotence. Rozhl Chir, 1973. 52(9): p. 587-90.

Michal, V., Kramar, R. & Pospichal, J. (1974). Femoro-pudendal by-pass internal iliac thromboendarterectomy and direct arterial anastomosis to the cavernous body in the treatment of erectile impotence. Bull Soc Int Chir, 1974. 33(4): p. 343-50.

Mills, T.M., Wiedmeier, V.T. & Stopper, V.S. (1992), Androgen maintenance of erectile function in the rat penis. Biol Reprod. 1992;46(3):342.

Moncada, I, Martinez-Salamanca, J.I., Allona, A., Hernandez, C. (2004). Current role of penile implants for erectile dysfunction. Curr Opin Urol 2004;14:375-80.

Montague, D.K. & Angermeier, K.W. (2000). Current status of penile prosthesis implantation. Curr Urol Rep 2000;1:291-6.

Moore, C.R., & Run, W. (2006). Pathophysiology and treatment of diabetic erectile dysfunction. Asian Journal of Andrology, 8(6), 675–684.

Motiwala, H.G., et al. (1993). Experience with penile venous surgery. Urol Int, 1993. 51(1): p. 9-14.

Mulcahy, J.J. (2003). Treatment alternatives for the infected penile implant. Int J Impot Res 2003;15 (Suppl 5):S147-9.

Mulcahy, J.J. (2008). Penile implant infections: Prevention and treatment. Curr Urol Rep 2008; 9:487-91.

Mulhall, J.P., Jahoda, A., Aviv, N., Valenzuela, R., Parker, M. (2004). The impact of sildenafil citrate on sexual satisfaction profiles in men with a penile prosthesis in situ. BJU Int 2004;93:97-9.

NIH Consensus Conference. Impotence. NIH Consensus Development Panel on Impotence. (1993). Jama, 270(1): p. 83-90.

Park, J.K., Lee, S.O., Kim, Y.G., Kim, S.H., Koh, G.Y., & Cho, K.W. (2002). Role of rho-kinase activity in angiotensin II-induced contraction of rabbit clitoral cavernosum smooth muscle. International Journal of Imporant Research, 14, 472–477.

Pryor, J., Akkus, E., Alter, G., Jordan, G., Lebret, T., et al. (2004). Peyronie's Disease. J Sex Med 2004;1:110-5.

Puyau, F.A. & Lewis, R.W. (1983). Corpus cavernosography. Pressure flow and radiography. Invest Radiol, 1983. 18(6): p. 517-22.

Rajpurkar, A., Bianco, F.F. Jr, Al-Omar, O., Terlecki, R., Dhabuwala, C. (2004). Fate of the retained reservoir after replacement of 3-piece penile prosthesis. J Urol 2004;172:664-6.

Ralph, D.J. & Minhas, S. (2004). The management of Peyronie's disease. BJU Int 2004;93:208-15.

Reddy, S.K., VandenBerg, T.L., Hellstrom, W.J. (1999). Use of cadaveric pericardium in the surgical therapy of Peyronie's disease. J Urol 1999;161:206.

Rhoden, E.L., Ribeiro, E.P., Riedner, C.E., Teloken, C., Souto, C.A. (2005a). Glycosylated haemoglobin levels and the severity of erectile function in diabetic men. BJU Int 2005;95:615–7.

Rhoden, E.L., Ribeiro, E.P., Teloken, C., Souto, C.A. (2005b). Diabetes mellitus is associated with subnormal serum levels of free testosterone in men. BJU Int 2005;96:867–70.

Rudnick, J., Bodecker R. & Weidner W. (1991). Significance of the intracavernosal pharmacological injection test, pharmacocavernosography, artificial erection and cavernosometry in the diagnosis of venous leakage. Urol Inl. 46(4): p. 338-43.

Sadeghi-Nejad, H., Ilbeigi, P., Wilson, S.K., Delk, J.R., et al. (2005). Multi-institutional outcome study on the efficacy of closed-suction drainage of the scrotum in three-piece inflatable penile prosthesis surgery. Int J Impot Res;17:535-8.

Santen, R.J. & Bardin, C.W. (1973). Episodic luteinizing hormone secretion in man. Pulse analysis, clinical interpretation, physiologic mechanisms. J Clin Invest. 1973;52(10):2617.

Sarica, K., Arikan, N., Serel, A., Arikan, Z., Aytac, S., et al. (1994). Multidisciplinary evaluation of diabetic impotence. EUrol 1994;26:314–8.

Sausville, J., Gupta, G., Forrest, G. & Chai T. (2009). Salmonella infection of a penile prosthesis. J Sex Med; 6:1487-90.

Scott, F.B., Bradley, W.E., Timm, G.W. (1974). Management of erectile impotence. Use of implantable inflatable prosthesis. Urology 1974;2:80-2.

Singh, R., Barden, A., Mori, T., & Beilin, L. (2001). Advanced glycation endproducts: A review. Diabetologia, 44, 129–146.

Small, M.P., Carrion, H.M., Gordon, J.A. (1975). Small Carrion penile prosthesis. New implant for management of impotence. Urology 1975;5:479-86.

Smith, C.P., Kraus, S.R., Boone, T.B. (1998). Management of impending penile prosthesis erosion with a polytetrafluoroethylene distal wind sock graft. J Urol 1998;160:2037-40.

Sullivan, M.E., Dashwood, M.R., Thompson, C.S., Muddle, J.R., Mikhailidis, D.P., & Morgan, R.J. (1997). Alterations in endotheli receptor sites in cavernosal tissue of diabetic rabbits: Potential relevance to the pathogenesis of erectile dysfunction. Journal of Urology, 158, 1966–1972.

Takahashi, K., Ghatei, M.A., Lam, H.C., O'Halloran, D.J., & Bloom, S.R. (1990). Elevated plasma endothelin in patients with diabetes mellitus. Diabetologia. 33(5):306-10,1990.

Taub, H., Melman, A., Christ, G.J. (1993). The relationship between contraction and relaxation in human corpus cavernosum smooth muscle. Urology 1993; 42: 698.

Virag, R., et al., (1980). Investigation and surgical treatment of vasculogenic impotency (author's transl)]. J Mal Vasc. 5(3): p. 205-9.

Wang, R. & Lewis, R.W. (2000). Reoperation for penile prosthesis implantation. In: Carson CC, editor. Current Clinical Urology Series on Urologic Prosthesis. Totowa, New Jersey: Humana Press Inc.; 2000. p. 231-47.

Wang, H., Eto, M., Steers, W.D., Somlyo, A.P., & Somlyo, A.V. (2002). RhoAmediated Ca2+ sensitization in erectile function. Journal of Biological Chemistry, 277, 30614−30621.

Wespes, E., et al., (1986). Pharmacocavernometry-cavernography in impotence. Br J Urol, 1986. 58(4): p. 429- 33.

Whitehead, E.D., Klyde, B.J. (1990). Diabetes-related impotence in the elderly. Clin Geriatr Med 1990;6:771– 95.

Wilson, S.K., Carson, C.C., Cleves, M.A., Delk, J.R. (1998). Quantifying risk of penile prosthesis infection with elevated glycosylated hemoglobin. J Urol 1998; 159: 1539,1540.

Wilson, S.K. & Delk, JR 2nd. (1994). A new treatment for Peyronie's disease: Modelling penis over an inflatable penile prosthesis. J Urol 1994;152:1121-3.

Infectious Gram-positive Bacteria Recovered From Diabetic Patients Under Dyalisis Treatments

Manuel Macía-Heras, Javier Donate-Correa, Gerardo Pulido-Reyes
Unidad de Investigación, Servicio de Nefrología
Hospital U. Ntra. Sra. de Candelaria, Spain

Sebastian Méndez-Álvarez
Unidad de Investigación, Servicio de Nefrología
Hospital U. Ntra. Sra. de Candelaria, Spain
Dpto. de Microbiología
Universidad de La Laguna, Spain

1   Introduction

Chronic kidney disease (CKD) has been recognized as a major health problem in the industrialized world. In fact, a great prevalence of earlier stages of CKD has been inferred (Eknoyan *et al.*, 2003). Based on data from the Third National Health and Nutrition Examination Survey, an awesome number of individuals in the United States have significantly decreased kidney function. There are even more individuals with manifestations of kidney damage (particularly albuminuria) without a significant decrease in kidney function. It is evident that most patients with CKD do not progress to End-Stage Renal Disease (ESRD; this term is the same as stage 5 CKD), but likely succumb to cardiovascular disease (CVD), which also is the leading cause of death for patients. In this setting the presence of infections and septicaemia has also contributed to an increase in morbidity and mortality. Stated otherwise, patients with CKD should have their disease detected and treated well before the onset of kidney failure and the need for dialysis or transplantation.

Existing epidemiological data suggest that infection in dialysis populations is associated with a marked increase in the use of health-care resources, as well as excess morbidity and mortality. For instance, patients undergoing peritoneal dialysis (PD) or hemodialysis (HD) have a notably increased risk of infection, particularly peritonitis in the former group and catheter-related bloodstream infection in the latter group. Moreover, infection in those patients on either form of dialysis is also associated with an increased risk of subsequent cardiovascular (CV) events; this increase in risk is only partially explained by underlying conditions, such as frailty. Thus, the presence of infection in a patient on dialysis has a substantial effect on CV mortality and morbidity, and should influence decisions regarding the use of therapies intended to minimize that risk.

2   Type 2 Diabetes as Leading Cause of CKD: Diabetic Nephropathy

The 21st century has the most diabetogenic environment in human history (Zimmet *et al.*, 2001; King *et al.*, 1998). Over the past 25 years, the prevalence of type 2 diabetes in the United States has almost doubled, with three to fivefold increase in India, Indonesia, China, Korea, and Thailand (Yoon *et al.*, 2006). In 2007, there were 246 million people with diabetes in the world, but by 2025, that number is estimated to reach 380 million. People with impaired glucose tolerance, a 'prediabetic state,' numbered 308 million in 2007, and this will increase to 418 million by 2025 (Sicree *et al.*, 2006). The increase in prevalence of diabetes will be greater in developing countries.

Diabetes is now the major cause of ESRD throughout the world in both developed and emerging nations (Reutens *et al.*, 2008). It is the primary diagnosis causing kidney disease in 20%–40% of people starting treatment for end-stage renal disease worldwide. In Australia, the number of new type 2 diabetes patients starting dialysis increased fivefold between 1993 and 2007 (ANZDATA Registry Report. 2008.). Between 1983 and 2005, there was a sevenfold increase in the number of new patients starting renal replacement therapy in Japan because of diabetes, accounting for 40% of all new-incidence patients (Yamagata *et al.*, 2008). In the United Kingdom Prospective Diabetes Study (UKPDS), the rates of progression of newly diagnosed type 2 diabetics between the different stages of diabetic nephropathy (normoalbuminuria, microalbuminuria, macroalbuminuria) and renal failure were 2%–3% per year (Adler *et al.*, 2003). Over a median of 15 years of follow-up for 4000 participants, almost 40% developed microalbuminuria, which represent the initial stage of kidney damage in patients suffering of diabetes (Retnakaran *et al.*, 2006). About 30% of the UKPDS (United Kingdom Prospective Diabetes Study) cohort developed renal impairment, of which almost 50% did not have preceding albuminuria (Retnakaran *et al.*, 2006). Reduced glomerular filtration rate and albuminuria caused by diabetic nephropathy are independent risk factors for CV events and death (Ninomiya *et al.*, 2009).

According to the WHO (World Health Organization), China and India will have about 130 million diabetics by 2025; they will consume about 40% of their countries healthcare budget in addition to reducing productivity and hindering economic growth. It was against this background that on December 21, 2006, the United Nations General Assembly unanimously passed Resolution 61/225 declaring diabetes an international public-health issue and identifying World Diabetes Day as a United Nations Day —only the second disease (after HIV/AIDS) to attain that status—. For the first time, governments have acknowledged that a noninfectious disease poses as serious a threat to world health as infectious diseases such as HIV/AIDS, tuberculosis, and malaria. The problems of diabetes are now seen as a major global public-health concern, especially in the developing world, which least can afford it. The first step to acting on diabetic kidney disease must encompass public-health campaigns aimed at preventing the development of type 2 diabetes. Medicare spending on the US ESRD program reached $26.8 billion in 2008. Furthermore, some 30% of the predicted US$1.1 trillion medical costs of dialysis worldwide during this decade will result from diabetic nephropathy (Lysaght 2002). Therefore, prevention of Diabetic Kidney Disease is important to improve health outcomes of persons with diabetes and to reduce the societal burden of chronic kidney disease (US Renal Data System, 2010).

3   Chronic Kidney Disease and Suceptibility to Infection

CKD and uremia milieu are associated with an increased susceptibility to infections and until recently the pathophysiology has been poorly understood. Infections remain a major cause of morbidity and mortality in patients with uremia and ESRD. Most of these infections are of bacterial origin and account for the majority of hospitalizations in this patient population. Infections were responsible for 12 to 22% of deaths among dialysis patients in the United States and Canada. Infections are the second most common cause of mortality in patients on dialysis, after coronary artery disease (US Renal Data System, 2006).

The presence of a substantial impairment of immunity in patients with uremia has been well documented (Descamps-Latscha *et al.*, 1994). Vascular access (VA) sites and PD catheters serve as ready portals of entry for pathogens. CKD and the subsequent need for maintenance HD can alter neutrophil function, reduce the ability for phagocytosis, depress natural killer cell activity, and can alter T and B cell function. These functional and quantitative abnormalities of cellular function account for the increased susceptibility to infection, and are independent of the cause of uremia. Various factors contribute to the altered cellular function in uremia. These include low albumin from malnutrition, metabolic acidosis, increased intracellular calcium, low molecular weight uremic toxins, and the presence of circulating inhibitors to chemotactic factors (Vanholder *et al*, 1996). Iron overload can impair immune function, enhances bacterial growth and virulence and thereby predisposes to an increased risk of infection in uremic patients (Sunder-Plassmann *et al*., 1999). Besides that, a decreased production of endogenous pyroxenes may cause a delay in recognition of infection (Lewis 1992). Skin test responses to standard antigens are impaired markedly in uremic patients. With the advent of dialysis for uremia, patients are subject to invasive procedures such as placement of intravenous catheters for temporary and permanent dialysis, what poses an increased risk of infections and for the same reasons dialysis patients are at increased risk of infections by resistant organisms.

In more recent years, convincing evidence has accumulated signaling that the immune system is chronically activated in clinically relevant uremic states (Foley 2007) (Table 1). As a result, many investigators believe that chronic activation with hypo-responsiveness may be the most accurate description of the immune dysfunction in clinical uremia. Some recent insights show several immune dysfunctions of advanced kidney disease. Thus one well-characterized observation in dialysis patients is that response rates to Hepatitis B vaccination are inexplicably low, and similar findings have been seen with other vaccines, such as tetanus or diphtheria; in contrast, vaccination responses to *Pneumococcus* are usually normal (Kohler *et al*., 1984). This hypo-responsiveness to hepatitis B vaccination seems to reflect impaired proliferation of T cells and decreased rates of production of T-cell growth factors, such as interleukin-2 (Girndt *et al*., 1993). Comparatively few antigens stimulate antibody production by B lymphocytes in complete independence of T cells; highly polymeric bacterial antigens, however, can elicit this response, among them the *Pneumococcus* vaccine. For most antigens, activation of helper T cells is required for both cellular and humoral immune responses. These findings suggest that defects in T-cell activation pathways may be an important component of the immune deficits of advanced CKD. Experimental studies suggest that the following may occur with uremia: defective co-stimulatory function of antigen-presenting cells, inflammatory activation of monocytes, and high levels of interleukin-12, leading to a reduced CD4þ/CD8þ T-lymphocyte ratio (Girndt *et al*., 1999). Finally, in HD patients the use of flow cytometry showed increased rates of apoptosis and smaller populations of naive and central memory T lymphocytes (Yoon *et al*., 2006).

Depressed neutrophil function.
Leukopenia secondary to complement activation.
Impaired phagocytosis.
Reduced natural killer cell activity.
Decreased T and B lymphocyte function.
Decreased T lymphocyte response to standar antigens.

Table 1: Host defense defects in uremia

4   Infections in Dialysis Modalities: Hemodialysis and Peritoneal Dialysis

Dialysis is a process by which waste products are removed from the body by diffusion from one fluid compartment to another across a semipermeable membrane. There are two different types of renal dialysis in common clinical usage: HD and DP. Both are acceptable modes of treatment of chronic renal disease. Over the past half century, the widespread use of dialysis to prolong life for people without kidney function has been a remarkable achievement (Himmelfarb *et al.*, 2010). As a result of its growth and evolution, the U.S. ESRD Program has often provided an early window into social, political, and economic developments in health care, and these changes have later been reflected throughout the U.S. health care system. Despite such successes, the use of dialysis in the treatment of ESRD is problematic in some respects. The number of patients treated, especially in the United States, has escalated and is far beyond early estimates. Aggregate dialysis-associated costs have increased accordingly, and morbidity and mortality among treated patients remain high despite considerable technical and scientific improvements. Our knowledge of which uremic toxins confer injury and of how they can be optimally removed during dialysis therapy remains incomplete. The limited numbers of clinical trials that have attempted to improve outcomes have had disappointing results, so well-designed and adequately powered clinical trials are needed. Ongoing studies are assessing whether longer or more frequent dialysis treatments, or both, can improve outcomes and whether these changes would be acceptable to most patients. However, substantive improvements for patients receiving dialysis will probably require major technological breakthroughs that will be predicated on an improved understanding of uremic toxins and uremic complications. Among these complications, infections represent the second leading cause in patient mortality and morbidity in the existing types of dialysis modalities.

The demographics of the dialysis population have changed dramatically over time. Less stringent selection of patients has led to treatment of an increasing proportion of elderly patients, patients with diabetes, and patients who are frail and have complex coexisting conditions (Moss 2001). The initiation of dialysis in patients with higher levels of residual kidney function has occurred concomitantly, particularly among patients older than 75 years of age. Among elderly nursing-home residents, the initiation of dialysis is associated with a substantial decline in functional status and high mortality. The factors driving these clinical practices, and their societal implications, are only beginning to be studied but may well lead to increased consideration of conservative management and palliative-care options for some patients (Murtagh *et al.*, 2007).

Dialysis patients have a strongly increased absolute risk and relative risk (RR) for morbidity and mortality from infectious diseases (Table 2). Infection accounts for 12 to 36% of the mortality in patients with ESRD and is second only to CVD as a cause of death (Nassar & Ayus, 2001) and septicemia is responsible for approximately three quarters of the infectious mortality. Infectious mortality is 1.66 times more frequent in PD than in HD. The annual mortality rate caused by sepsis is 100 to 300 times higher in patients with ESRD than in the general population (Laupland et al., 2004). A large cohort study reported that the increase in risk is not significantly altered by age, gender, or the presence of diabetes (Sarnak *et al.*, 2000). Other studies indicated that the risk for infection is linked to age, low Karnovsky index, type of VA, frequency of hospitalization, immunosuppressive therapy, use of a mistreatment heparin bolus, iron overload, and poor hygiene (Hoen *et al.*, 1998; Diskin *et al.*, 2007; Teehan *et al.*, 2004).

Malnutrition (Low albumin and low Karnovsky index).
Age.
Increased intracellular calcium.
Iron overload.
Low molecular weights toxins.
Decreased T lymphocyte response to standar antigens.
Invasive vascular and peritoneal procedures for dialisys access.
Poor hygiene

Table 2: Predisposing factors to infection in dialysis patients.

5   Hemodialysis

HD represents the most extended dialysis therapy worldwide. In this modality of dialysis blood is passed through an artificial kidney machine and the waste products diffuse across a man-made membrane into a bath solution known as dialysate, after which the cleansed blood is returned to the patient's body. In standard basis HD is accomplished usually in three- or four-hour sessions three times a week.

Infection as a cause of hospitalization for HD patients in the U.S. has increased in recent years. Between 1993 and 2006, hospitalization rates for infection rose 34%, and the rate of hospitalization for VA infections in HD patients more than doubled (US Renal Data System, 2008). The admission rate for pneumonia rose 7.3%, for bacteremia /septicemia 31%, and for cellulitis 20.3%. In 2006, there were 103 admissions per 1000 patient years with the diagnosis of bacteremia / septicemia and 129 per 1000 patient years with the diagnosis of VA-associated infection. Infection is reported as the second most common cause of death in HD patients (20.2% in 2006), after CVD (US Renal Data System, 2008). As previously referred patients on maintenance HD are strikingly vulnerable to infection for many reasons, including the immunodepressed state intrinsic to ESRD, the high prevalence of diabetes, exposure to other patients in the HD facility three times per week, frequent hospitalization, and the invasiveness of the HD procedure.

Many of the acute bacterial infections in HD patients are caused by *Staphylococcus aureus*, and are mainly related to temporary central venous catheters (CVCs). Also these infections can lead to sepsis and result in bacterial seeding/ infection of implants such as total hip/knee and cardiac valves. This is a serious complication that can result in significant additional morbidity and may require removal/ replacement of implants. Bacterial seeding/infection of compression spine fractures have also been reported resulting in long-term antibiotic therapy. Other infection-associated risks include pneumococcal pneumonia, which also remains common in the HD population. Pneumonia is one of many reasons that antibiotics are prescribed for HD patients which in turn increases the risk of developing colonization or infection with multidrug-resistant organisms (MDROs) such as methicillin-resistant *S. aureus* (MRSA).

6   Vascular Access and Infections

The necessity for vascular access in patients with renal failure can be temporary or permanent. The necessity for temporary access may vary from several hours (single dialysis) to months [if used to dialyze while waiting for an arteriovenous (AV) fistula to mature]. Temporary access is established by the percutaneous insertion of a catheter into a large vein (internal jugular, femoral, or, less desirably, subclavian). Construction of a permanent VA permits repeated angioaccess for months to years. An ideal permanent access delivers a flow adequate for the dialysis prescription, lasts a long time, and has a low complication rate. The autonomous AV fistula comes closest to satisfying these criteria because it has the best 5-year patency rate and during this period requires many fewer interventions than other access methods. Prosthetic accesses (AV grafts) are constructed by the insertion of a subcutaneous tube in a straight, curved, or loop configuration between an extremity artery and vein. Placement of a cuffed double-lumen silicone elastomer catheter (e.g., Perm-Cath device) or a pair of cuffed single-lumen catheters (e.g., Tesio catheter) into an internal jugular vein for permanent access is also done in selected circumstances. Although the autologous AV fistula is clearly the desired access for patients initiating HD, there is disproportionate use of AV grafts in the U. S. and an increasing dependence on cuffed indwelling central venous catheters. Guidelines developed by the National Kidney Foundation Dialysis Outcomes Quality Improvement initiative promote the increased construction of AV fistulas and earlier referral of patients to nephrologists, permitting early-access evaluation and early construction of an AV fistula or graft, thereby minimizing the use of venous catheter access. A second goal of the guidelines is to promote detection of access dysfunction prior to access thrombosis.

Infection is the leading cause of catheter loss and increases morbidity and mortality. Infection usually arises from the migration of the patient's own skin flora through the puncture site and onto the outer catheter surface, although it can also result from contamination of the catheter connectors, lumen contamination during dialysis, or from infused solutions. Catheters can also become colonized from more remote sites during bacteremia. Gram-positive bacteria (usually *Staphylococcus* species) are the most common culprits. In these setting access remains the Achilles heel of dialysis treatment, especially with regard to VA for HD due to its association with bacteremia, infections and sepsis that contributed to a great extent in the high rates of morbidity and mortality of HD patients. The incidence of VA-related bloodstream infection varies between medical facilities and can be influenced by the percentage of patients who receive dialysis via a central venous catheter (Marr *et al.*, 1998). As already mentioned several types of VA used in hemodialysis, listed in order of increasing risk of infection, are as follows: arteriovenous fistulas created from the patient's own blood vessels; arteriovenous grafts constructed from synthetic materials; tunneled CVCs; and non-tunneled CVCs (Marr *et al.*, 1998).

Several studies show that 48 to 89% of bacteremias in HD patients are related to a VA infection (Hoen *et al.*, 1998; Marr *et al.*, 1998; Nassar *et al.*, 2001). The type of VA is the most important predictor of the infection risk, with native fistulas being safer than grafts (RR 1.47), cuffed catheters (RR 8.49), and no cuffed catheters (RR 9.87) (Taylor *et al.*, 2002). Other studies reported a 10 to 30 times higher risk associated with noncuffed catheters than with native fistulas (Stevenson *et al.*, 2002). The incidence of bacteremia in HD patients varies from 7.6 to 14.4 episodes per 100 patient-years (Hoen *et al.*, 1998; Marr *et al.*, 1998). Although the type of VA has a major impact on the risk of bloodstream infections, it hardly affects the outcome of the subsequent infection (Inrig *et al.*, 2006). Major complications from VA related infections in dialysis are severe sepsis, metastatic mainly osteoarticular infections, and infective endocarditis. The risk for infective endocarditis in HD patients is 17.8 times higher than in the general population, mounting to 5.6 per 1000 patient-years (Abbott & Agodoa, 2002). Up to 57.9% of these episodes are caused by *S. aureus*, with an in-hospital mortality of approximately 50% (Kamalakannan *et al.*, 2007).

As previously mentioned Gram positive bacteria *S. aureus* is the most common microorganism implicated in vascular-access-related bloodstream infections, accounting for over half of HD catheter related infection (Nsouli *et al.*, 1979), followed by coagulase-negative staphylococci and has been associated with high morbi-mortality in these patients.

Of special interest is the control of MRSA. These species was first described in 1961 and has become a worldwide problem (Jevons, 1961), currently constituting the most commonly identified antibiotic resistant pathogen in many hospitals and contributing significantly to patient morbidity and mortality (Cosgrove *et al.*, 2003; Diekema *et al.*, 2004; Melzer *et al.*, 2003; Whitby *et al.*, 2003). Humans are the main natural reservoir of *S. aureus*. Although multiple body sites can be colonized by *S. aureus*, the rate of colonization is highest in the anterior nares (Wertheim *et al.*, 2005). In crosssectional population-based surveys, 10 to 50% of adults were colonized with *S. aureus* (Graham, 2006; von Eiff *et al.*, 2001). Longitudinal studies revealed three patterns of *S. aureus* nasal carriage (Wertheim *et al.*, 2005). Approximately 20% of healthy adults (range 12 to 30%) are persistent carriers and are colonized by a single strain over prolonged periods. Thirty percent (range 16 to 70%) are intermittent carriers that may harbor different strains in their nose over time. Fifty percent (range 16 to 69%) are persistent non carriers (von Eiff *et al.*, 2001). The large variation in the number of persistent and intermittent carriers between the available studies is the consequence of non-uniform definitions and methodological issues (Wertheim *et al.*, 2005). In addition to the anterior nares, *S. aureus* frequently colonizes the skin, the perineum, and the pharynx and, to a lesser extent, the gastrointestinal tract, the vagina, and the axillae *Staphylococci* can also survive for months on many types of surfaces and in environmental dust (Dancer *et al.*, 2008; Wertheim *et al.*, 2005). Airborne transmission is important in the maintenance of environmental reservoirs, but hands are the main vectors that transmit *S. aureus* from the environment to the nasal niche and from the nasal niche to several body sites, respectively. Although the presence of *S. aureus* in the nose elicits a subclinical immune response, this host response is ineffective to prevent further colonization once the germ has reached the anterior nares (Wertheim *et al.*, 2005). This may indicate that although the subclinical immune response provoked by nasal carriership is inadequate to prevent tissue invasion, it may decrease the devastating consequences of invasive *S. aureus* infection.

HD-patients as are patients with diabetes are at increased risk for intermittent or persistent carriership from the onset of dialysis (Wertheim *et al.*, 2005; Vandecasteele *et al.*, 2009). Importantly, incidence of invasive MRSA infection among dialysis patients is 100-fold higher than for the general population (Centers for Disease Control and Prevention (CDC), 2007). Moreover, *S. aureus* carriers who are on HD have a 1.8- to 4.7-fold increase of vascular VA infections and bacteremia compared with noncarriers (Wertheim *et al.*, 2005). The majority of dialysis patients carry the same strain on the hands and in the nose and also these strains are frequently the same as those recovered from subsequent infections (Ena *et al.* 1994). Similar to those in the general population (Wertheim *et al.*, 1994), the majority of *S. aureus* infections in HD patients therefore have to be considered autoinfections (Boelaert *et al.*, 2009). In summary, patients on dialysis have an increased rate of *S. aureus* nasal colonization which increases the risk of subsequent infection; eradication of nasal carriage would be beneficial (Golper *et al.*, 2000).Elimination of staphylococcal nasal carriage by topical nasal mupirocin application has been found to reduce the incidence of infection in patients on dialysis (Kluytmans *et al.*, 1997).

The Enterococci are the third group of microorganims responsible for bacteremia in HD patients. Particularly vancomycin-resistant enterococci (VRE) have emerged as an important nosocomial pathogen in these patients. A systematic literature review analysing the impact of vancomycin resistance on mortality by bacteremias showed that patients infected with VRE were more likely to die than those with vancomycin susceptible enterococci (Diaz-Granados *et al.*, 2005). Two species are especially important in enterococcal infections: *Enterococcus faecalis* and *Enterococcus faecium* although vancomycine resistance seems to be more extended in the last (Minnaganti *et al.*, 2001). Widespread and incorrect dosing of vancomycin in HD patients has probably led to the emergence of VRE.

Aerobic Gram-negative bacilli are responsible for the remainder HD infections. When these infective agents appear, inadequate disinfection of water treatment or distribution systems errors in dialyser reprocessing are usually involved. Among chronic hemodialysis patients, approximately 25% of blood stream infections are caused these bacteria (Marr *et al.*, 1998), and this percentage is increasing steadily.

7 Peritoneal Dialysis

In this type of dialysis therapy the waste products pass from the patient's body through the peritoneal membrane into the peritoneal (abdominal) cavity where the bath solution (dialysate) is introduced and removed periodically. Schematically there two standard modalities of PD: Continuous Ambulatory Peritoneal Dialysis (CAPD) and Automated PD (APD). CAPD represents a variation of PD that was developed as an alternative mode of dialysis for home dialysis patients, is a continuous dialysis process using the patient's peritoneal membrane as a dialyzer. The patient connects a two-liter plastic bag of dialysate to a surgically implanted indwelling catheter and allows the dialysate to pour into the peritoneal cavity. Four to six hours later, the patient drains the fluid out into the same bag and replaces the old bag with a new bag of fresh dialysate. This is done three to five times a day with the first exchange being made when the patient wakes up in the morning and the last exchange being made at bedtime. Because no machine is used, CAPD frees patients from the dietary restrictions associated with intermittent HD or intermittent PD. APD is a treatment modality that combines the advantages of the long-dwell, continuous steady state dialysis of CAPD, with the advantages of automation inherent in intermittent peritoneal dialysis. The major difference between APD and CAPD is that the solution exchanges, which are performed manually during the day by the patient on CAPD, are moved to nighttime with CCPD and are performed automatically with a peritoneal dialysis cycler. The long nighttime dwell of APD is moved to the daytime with CAPD. At night, the patient connects the catheter to the cycler system, which has several (two to four) five-liter containers of dialysate suspended. The cycler automatically empties the patient's peritoneal cavity of the all-day dwell. The cycler then cycles the nocturnal exchanges automatically while the patient sleeps; the number of nocturnal exchanges occurring at intervals of one to three hours (depending on the dialysis schedule) and the last exchange being instilled in the morning upon awakening. The patient then disconnects form the cycler and leaves the last two-liter inside the peritoneum to continue the daytime long-dwell dialysis.

The utilization of PD as an effective and feasible dialysis therapy CKD patients was extend world wide since the seventies and at present represent an attractive and first line dialysis option for patients with ESRD because it offers a very different lifestyle that enables people to work, travel, and avoid the rigid schedule of in-center HD. PD was utilized in about 14%-15% of dialysis patients from the early 1980s through the early 1990s and was an attractive option during those years when physicians faced multiple barriers to start outpatient HD programs. For many reasons, some of which remain enigmatic, PD use subsequently declined to about 6% of all dialysis patients in 2008 (US Renal Data System, 2010).

As in HD patients infections also represents a serious complication for PD patients. Reducing the risk of PD-related infections should be a primary goal of every PD program. Quality improvement programs with continuous monitoring of infections and root-cause analysis of each infectious episode are critical to decrease PD-related infections (Borg *et al.*, 2003). Very low rates of infection can be achieved if close attention is continuously paid to training and retraining, equipment, and protocols to prevent infections.

8   Peritonitis

Peritonitis, infection of the peritoneal cavity, remains the Achilles' heel of PD. In these patients, peritonitis is the most common reason for hospitalisation and for discontinuation of PD (Bloembergen & Port, 1996). A major route of spread of infection is as a consequence of intraluminal contamination associated with frequent manipulations of the catheter (Nolph, 1988). The overall incidence of peritonitis in CAPD patients during the 1980s and early 1990s had averaged 1.1–1.3 episodes per year in the United States, but the introduction of Y-set and double-bag systems has reduced this to approximately one episode every 24 months (Monteon *et al.*, 1998). The incidence rate in CAPD patients in the U. S. is now comparable to that seen in APD patients. The same flush-before-fill methodology used in CAPD Y sets may also be used effectively in APD (Leehey & Lentino, 2003).

Peritonitis etiology is determine by using appropriate culture techniques, an organism can be isolated from the peritoneal fluid in over 90% of cases in which symptoms and signs of peritonitis and an elevated peritoneal fluid neutrophil count are present. The responsible pathogen is almost always a bacterium, usually of the Gram-positive variety (Table 3). Gram-positive organisms account for two thirds of all episodes of peritonitis (Band, 1999). However, unlike to HD-related infections, coagulase-negative staphylococci, especially *S. epidermidis*, are more common that *S. aureus* in PD-related peritonitis. Moreover, peritonitis caused by *S. aureus* are more severe. It has been well documented that patients who are nasal carriers of *S. aureus* are at increased risk of infection and are prone to recurrent infection (Lazar *et al.*, 1990; Swartz *et al.*, 1991). Like occurs in HD patients, elimination of nasal carriage in patients on PD decreased the ESI rate, but the effect on the incidence of peritonitis is unclear. Other less common, but accounting significant number of episodes Gram-positive infective agents, are non-enterococcal streptococci and enterococci. Patients receiving outpatient PD are at a low risk for acquiring VRE because these patients receive less intravenous vancomycin than HD patients (Ng *et al.*, 1999). Among all the Gram-negative organisms, the genus *Pseudomonas* and the *Enterobacteriaceae*, have become an increasingly recognized cause of infective peritoneal complications. Within the Enterobacteriaceae group, *E. coli*, *Klebsiella spp.*, and *Enterobacter* sp. are the most prevalent PD-infection-related organisms. At this point, the production of extended-spectrum β-lactamases (ES βLs) in Enterobacteriaceae must be commented. There are few reports on ESβLs-producing Enterobacteriaceae in haemodialysis patients. However, the presence of ESβLs-producing *Escherichia coli* infections in PD-patients has been associated with a higher risk of dialysis failure (Yip *et al.*, 2006). In addition, *Pseudomonas* species isolates account for a few episodes of and anaerobes are rarely if ever isolated. Probably, *Pseudomonas aeruginosa* is the most important peritonitis-causal agent of this genus (Krothapalli *et al.*, 1982). The infection is severe and frequently associated with exit site or tunnel infection (Bernardini *et al.*, 1987), loss of peritoneal space, and abscess formation (Kaczmarski *et al.*, 1988), and is the main reason for the excess catheter removal rate in *P. aeruginosa*-caused peritonitis compared with rates in peritonitis of other etiology (Bernardini *et al.*, 1987). Less common are reported infections by *Acinetobacter* spp. (Ruiz *et al.*, 1988). The occurrence of fungal peritonitis (e.g., *Candida*) is uncommon but by no means rare. Infection with *Mycobacterium tuberculosis* or other type of mycobacteria has been reported but is unusual.

Common	Uncommon
Staphylococcus aureus	Aerobic gram-negative bacilli
Coagulase-negative staphylococci	- *Acinetobacter*
- *Staphylococcus epidermidis*	- *Alcaligenes*
Enterococcus faecium	- *Aeromonas*
Enterococcus faecalis	- *Achromobacter*
Klebsiella pneumoniae	- *Flavobacterium*
Escherichia coli	- *Proteus*
Nonenterococcal streptococci	- *Pseudomonas aeruginosa*

Table 3: Bacterial pathogens causing infections in Dialysis Patients

9   Exit Site Infections

Proportionally to the decline in the incidence of peritonitis because of improvements in PD, there has been an increase in the incidence of exit site infections (ESIs). Habitually, the incidence of ESI is directly proportional to the size of the exit wound. Approximately one-fifth of peritonitis episodes are temporally associated with exit site and tunnel infections (Piraino *et al.*, 1987). The incidence of exit site infections is approximately one episode every 24–48 patient-months. Patients with previous infections tend to have a higher frequency of occurrence.

Exit site infections are predominantly due to *S. aureus* or Gram-negative organisms. In contrast to peritonitis, *S. epidermidis* is the causative organism in less than 20% of patients. *S. aureus* infections appear to have a distinct pathogenesis as they are associated with nasal and or skin carriage of the organism (Luzar, 1990). Therefore, eradication of the carrier state is very helpful to effective management. Exit site infections due to Gram-negative bacilli (enteric and pseudomonal organisms are most common) are also a source of considerable morbidity.

10   Staphyloccoci Resistance to Antibiotics in Dialysis

10.1   Methicillin

Methicillin resistance in staphylococci is conferred by the *mecA* gene, which is easily transferred horizontally and encodes for an altered penicillin-binding protein (PBP2a) that has a low binding affinity for all lactam-β antibiotics. The progressive spread of methicillin-resistant *S. aureus* (MRSA) is daunting. Twelve to 30% (2006 through 2007 European data), 33% (1994 through 2001 U.S. data), and up to 65% (most recent U.S. data) of patients on hemodialysis are colonized with MRSA (Lederer *et al.*, 2007). The proportion of infections that are caused by MRSA varies strongly with local epidemiology and according to the year of surveillance. A recent report from Taiwan demonstrated a colonization rate with MRSA as low as 2.4% (Lu *et al.*, 2008). In North America, conversely, community-acquired MRSA infections are rapidly emerging, accounting for 60 to 75% of all isolates in the community (Moellering *et al.*, 2008). The risk for invasive MRSA infections is 100-fold higher in dialysis patients than in the general population (45.2/1000 *versus* 0.2 to 0.4/1000) (Centers for Disease Control and Prevention, 2007). Dialysis patients currently account for up to 15.4% of all invasive MRSA infections (Centers for Disease Control and Prevention, 2007). As for methicillin-sensitive *S. aureus* (MSSA) infections, molecular typing suggests that colonization of MRSA strains precedes clinical infection (Lu *et al.*, 2008). Data regarding the role of methicillin resistance in outcome are conflicting, although most data suggest a higher mortality and recurrence rate. A small, single-center, case-control study found a 38% case fatality rate for the MRSA group *versus* 28% for the MSSA group, but the difference lost significance after adjustment for major confounders (Harbarth *et al.*, 1998). A large cohort study of 908 consecutive SAB episodes did not find an increased adjusted mortality risk in the MRSA group (Soriano *et al.*, 2000). In contrast, a large, single-center cohort study of 385 episodes of SAB reported that methicillin resistance resulted in a 2.59 times higher mortality in the elderly (McClelland *et al.*, 1999). Despite the use of appropriate antibiotics in the majority of patients, a large (504 episodes of SAB) retrospective cohort study demonstrated a significantly higher mortality rate in the MRSA than in the MSSA group (18.6 *versus* 12.9%) (Selvey *et al.*, 2000). A steady increase over time of the minimal inhibitory concentration (MIC) for vancomycin is observed in the staphylococcal population (Boucher *et al.*, 2007). MRSA strains with an increased MIC for vancomycin (> 1 to 2 µg/ml) impart a higher risk for death (Hidayat *et al.*, 2006). MRSA strains with MIC for vancomycin of >2 and <16 µg/ml are referred to as vancomycin intermediate *S. aureus* (VISA) (Tenover *et al.*, 2007). VISA strains predispose to treatment failure, even when high dosages of vancomycin are used. Some patients are infected with heteroresistant MRSA (hVISA), defined by the presence of subpopulations with reduced susceptibility to vancomycin. Heteroresistant MRSA are easily missed by commercial automated tests and predispose to treatment failure (Jones, 2006).

10.2 Vancomycin

Recently, vancomycin-resistant *S. aureus* (VRSA) was reported in seven patients from the United States. All patients had chronic colonization with MRSA and vancomycin-resistant enterococci, and most of them had received prolonged therapy with vancomycin for MRSA infection. Of note, three of seven patients had ESRD. All VRSA had acquired the *vanA* gene from vancomycin-resistant enterococci, and the median vancomycin MIC was 512 µg/ml. The mechanism of resistance in VRSA is quite different from VISA. The *vanA* gene results in the replacement of D-Ala-D-Ala-ending peptidoglycan precursors with D-alanyl-D-lactate termini, causing a decreased binding affinity for vancomycin and an almost 1000-fold increase in MIC (Sievert *et al.*, 2008). Vancomycin tolerance refers to an inhibition of growth without bacterial killing (and thus cure) and is defined as a MBCMIC ratio of >32, or a MBC-MIC ratio of >16 in case of a MIC $\geq$32 µg/ml (Jones, 2006). Vancomycin tolerance is highly prevalent (74 to 100%) in hVISA, VISA, and VRSA strains and causes clinical treatment failure (Jones, 2006).

10.3 Mupirocin

Mupirocin resistance has been reported (Annigeri *et al.*, 2001; Lobbedez *et al.*, 2004; Pérez–Fontán *et al.*, 2002). Resistance to mupirocin can be classified as "low" if the minimal inhibitory concentration is greater than or equal to 8 µg/mL, or "high" if the minimal inhibitory concentration is greater than or equal to 512 µg/mL. It is expected that high-level resistance will eventually result in clinical failure or a high relapse rate. Resistance to mupirocin does not yet appear to have eliminated the efficacy of that agent, but that consequence is likely with longer periods of individual exposure and with more patients being exposed. Pérez–Fontán et al. have observed a greater incidence of exit-site infections in patients colonized with mupirocin-resistant *S. aureus* than in those colonized with sensitive organisms, suggesting that the development of mupirocin resistance may have adverse clinical consequences and lead to treatment failures (Pérez–Fontán *et al.*, 2002).

10.4 Oxazolidinone

Oxazolidinone is a bacteriostatic oxazolidin that has high oral bioavailability and inhibits bacterial protein synthesis by binding to the 50S ribosomal subunit in Gram-positive bacteria and mycobacterial species (Moellering, 2003). On the basis of several randomized, controlled trials, oxazolidinone has been approved for complicated and non-complicated skin and skin-structure infections and for community-acquired and nosocomial pneumonia in a dosage of 600 mg twice daily, intravenously or orally (Moellering, 2003, 2008). No dosage adjustment is necessary in chronic kidney disease, but a strict monitoring for adverse effects is recommended (Moellering, 2008). Several case reports and smaller series suggested a place for oxazolidinone in the treatment of MRSA osteoarticular infections (Moellering, 2008). Only limited data demonstrated activity of oxazolidinone in MRSA sepsis (mainly in secondary bacteremia), and the antibiotic is not approved for this indication (Lentino et al., 2008). The use of oxazolidinone for a period beyond 2 to 3 weeks is associated a dosage- and time-dependent myelosuppression and risk for lactic acidosis that is caused by a depletion of several mitochondrial proteins (Moellering, 2002).

11   Dialysis Associated Infections in Diabetic Patients: A Molecular Approach

One of the most worrisome examples about pathogenic bacteria infections in the hospital setting is rising incidence in patients with CKD and particularly in those patients undergoing HD and PD. Dialysis-related infections (including peritonitis and VA infections) are the second leading cause of death in dialysis patients (Sarnak & Jaber, 2000). Moreover, as for other types of infections, microorganisms causing dialysis-related infections are becoming more resistant to antimicrobials (D'Agata, 2005). Several factors converge to convert infections by far the most common complications affecting ESRD patients. Dialysed patients are extremely vulnerable to infections because of the presence of an access susceptible to be colonized by many infective agents (Butterly & Schwab, 2000). Even more, this population is hospitalised with greater frequency than the general population, which is correlated with higher infection rates (Foley, 2007). To this situation, a greater risk of infection in this population partially caused by impaired host immunity must be added. It has been found that the uremic state interferes with T-cell and B-cell dysfunction, macrophage phagocytosis, and antigen presentation (Ryan et al., 2004).

Patients with diabetes, which is the most common cause of treated ESRD (US Renal Data System, 2006), often face unique challenges when it comes to infection. They may have additional immune defects as well as vascular disease which may further increase the risk of certain types of infections. Dialysed patients with diabetes can be more prone to infection because of related conditions related to diabetes. In example, the excess of glucose in blood may prevents white blood cells, which are one of the main defences against infection, from doing their jobs (Minnaganti & Cunha, 2001). It is important to achieve a good glycaemia control.

Staphylococci and other Gram-positive bacteria are the agents most commonly involved in such dialysis infections, accounting for 20% – 40% of the cases of PD–related peritonitis (Zelenitsky et al., 2001), and at lesser extent, different species of aerobic Gram-negative bacilli (Sullivan et al., 2007).

11.1   Molecular approach for dialysis infections

Although the conventional phenotypic method is still popular to identify common bacteria in clinical microbiology laboratories, it is difficult to use this method when bacteria reveal uncommon phenotypes, grow slowly, or are not included in commercial kit databases (Petti *et al.*, 2005; Shin *et al.*, 2005). In addition, we cannot detect uncultivable or fastidious microorganisms or organisms in patients who have recently received antibiotic therapy, even when bacteria are present in the clinical samples (Yoo *et al.*, 2006). To overcome these problems, many molecular techniques have been adopted. In this section, we will comment different methods which is used to detect infection's causative pathogen or methods that might be useful to typing the isolates.

HD patients with MRSA infections face high morbidity and mortality. Nasal carriage of *S. aureus* is known to play an important role as an endogenous source for HD-access-related infections that contribute significantly to morbidity, mortality and cost of ESRD management (Lederer *et al.*, 2007). Pulsed-field gel electrophoresis (PFGE) with *SmaI* digestion of chromosomal DNA has been used for the genotyping of MRSA isolates from haemodialysis patients.

Since the chromosome is the most fundamental component of identity of the cell, methods measuring this molecule represent a preferred approximation for assessing strain interrelatedness. Restriction patterns originated after chromosomal DNA enzymatic digestion generates a restriction fragment length polymorphism (RFLP), after PFGE, which efficiently and accurately allows the differentiation of strains and compare following conventional agarose gel electrophoresis. PFGE methods have been used to evaluate the spread of various antimicrobial resistant bacteria. The finding of isolates that have identical or related restriction endonuclease patterns suggests spread from single strains.

The accuracy and reliability of this technique have led to be considered as the reference method for typing MRSA isolates. Several studies have used this technique to typing isolates from haemodialysis patients (Taylor *et al.*, 2002).

Actually, PFGE is being more widely replaced by sequence-based methods that allow for unambiguous identification of isolates, easy data accumulation and comparison. Multi-locus sequence typing (MLST) is the molecular method with highest discriminatory capability and is based in characterizing the sequences of internal fragments of different housekeeping genes. In the case of *S. aureus* MLST, these are *carbamate kinase (arcC)*, *shikimate 5-dehydrogenase (aroE)*, *glycerol kinase (glpF)*, *guanylate kinase (gmk)*, *phosphate acetyltransferase (pta)*, *triose-phosphate isomerase (tpi)* and *acetyl-CoA C-acetyltransferase (yqiL)*. The sequences obtained are assigned to allele numbers after comparison with a DNA sequences database. The allele numbers at each of the seven *loci* define the allelic profile or sequence type (ST). Novel alleles and STs not found on the MLST website are confirmed by repeating both the Polymerase Chain Reaction (PCR) and sequencing (Peacock *et al.*, 2002).

Peritonitis is one of the most common complications of CAPD, and rapid and accurate identification of the causative pathogen is essential for diagnosis and selection of the appropriate therapy. However, conventional culture takes at least 2 or 3 days to provide the final identification, and we would be in a difficult situation if there were small numbers of bacteria or fastidious bacteria in the CAPD fluid. It would be valuable to use supplementary molecular methods such for detection and identification of pathogens.

A number of novel diagnostic techniques have been explored for the early diagnosis of peritonitis (Akman *et al.*, 2005; Park *et al.*, 2005) reported that leukocyte esterase reagent strip has excellent accuracy for the diagnosis of peritonitis. Various commercially available strips have been tested to diagnose non-PD peritonitis but the results vary enormously; more studies are required before this can be applied in a routine setting (Nguyen-Khac *et al.*, 2008).

Broad-spectrum PCR with RNA sequencing and quantitative bacterial DNA PCR assays may also complement culture methods in the diagnosis of CAPD peritonitis, especially in patients with previous or current antibiotic use. The latter technique may also help to identify those patients likely to relapse despite apparent clinical improvement with standard antibiotic therapy. Another study suggests that the matrix metalloproteinase-9 test kit may be a reliable method for early diagnosis of PD peritonitis (Ro *et al.*, 2004). The role of rapid detection of the causative pathogen of peritonitis using *in situ* hybridization has also been explored (Ota *et al.*, 2007).

Amplification and sequencing conserved genes of bacterial genomic DNA are used for identification of staphylococcal species and their genotypes. In *S. aureus* the genes encoding 16S rRNA, factor A essential for methicillin resistance (*femA*), and staphylococcal thermonuclease (*nuc*) (among others) are frequently used for identification at the species level. Moreover, antibiotic resistance is a troubling phenomenon very extended. Another important use of PCR is to determine resistance phenotype based on the holding of genes encoding related factors. Pasqual et al. (2012) reviewed the records of 62 *S. aureus* peritonitis episodes that occurred between 1996 and 2010 in the dialysis unit of a single university hospital and evaluated the host and bacterial (gene resistance) factors influencing peritonitis outcome by PCR (*mec*A gene). Another study could detect and identify bacterial pathogens directly from CAPD culture fluids by application of broad-range PCR using 16S rDNA (Si *et al.*, 2012).

Many other genotyping techniques are applied to support epidemiological methods described in order to characterize infection causal agents from dialysis like *spa* typing (Moremi *et al.*, 2012; Turlej *et al.*, 2011).

In conclusion, catheters are inherently vulnerable to luminal and extra luminal infection and have high rates of associated bacteremia. On the other hand, *S. aureus* peritonitis is a common and serious complication of PD and is associated with a high rate of relapse (20%) and repeat episodes (29%) (Govindarajulu *et al.*, 2010). As a result of that, early recognition and treatment of dialysis-related bacteremia minimizes morbidity and mortality from complications.

12   Cardiovascular Risk Associated to Infections

CV morbidity and mortality have always been major concerns for nephrologists managing patients on dialysis, and it has been shown that reduced residual renal function, inflammation, valvular calcification and left ventricular hypertrophy are predictors of CV mortality in patients on peritoneal dialysis. The interaction between infection and CV disease, however, seems to be a new concern. Although the mechanisms linking infection, chronic inflammation and cardiovascular disease have been elusive, this phenomenon of infection being a harbinger of future CV events and death has been repeatedly investigated and confirmed in observational and epidemiological studies (Foley *et al.*, 2004; Ishani *et al.*, 2005). In a historical cohort study of 393.451 patients on HD or PD, septicemia was identified as a precursor to the development of cardiovascular events and death (Foley *et al.*, 2004). Septicemia was associated with the development of myocardial infarction, congestive heart failure, stroke and peripheral vascular disease, and the adjusted risk ratio of these events remained approximately double that expected for up to 5 years after the initial infection (Foley *et al.*, 2004). These observations have been confirmed in another prospective study—the Dialysis Morbidity and Mortality Wave 2 study—in which septicemia or bacteremia were associated with a nearly twofold increase in the risk of myocardial infarction or stroke (Ishani *et al.*, 2005).

Although mechanisms linking infection, chronic inflammation, and CV disease in the general population are incompletely understood, this is an active area of basic and clinical research (Ross, 1999). It is known that macrophages and T cells are prominent in fatty streaks and homeostatic abnormalities of lipid metabolism and inflammatory pathways may be synergistically involved in the pathogenesis of fatty streaks. In addition, immune cells are present in early atherosclerotic lesions and effector molecules from these immune cells seem to facilitate progression of these lesions. Inflammation is also thought negatively to affect the stability of established plaques, enhancing the risk of acute coronary syndromes (Hansson, 2005). Acute bacterial infections are prototypical inflammatory events, and are typified by abnormal endothelial function, oxidative stress, and disequilibrium between pro-coagulant and anticoagulant systems, cardiac dysfunction, and diminished cellular oxygen availability (Hotchkiss & Karl, 2003). One further considers that low-grade inflammation and high-grade CV disease are typical features of CKD (Kaysen & Eiserich, 2003). It seems natural to suspect that common macro-inflammatory events in dialysis patients (like pneumonia and septicemia) may contribute to the sizeable burden of CV in this population. Whether infection can be considered a risk factor for atherogenesis and cardiovascular disease, however, remains unclear.

13   Conclusions

Kidney disease represents one of the leading causes of death in the western world and the total cost of treating ESRD patients with dialysis therapies is continuously increasing. Much of the dialysis treatment is provided in the outpatient setting; however the number of hospitalizations for associated conditions, such as diabetes, CVD and infections, is substantial. Dialysis places patients at high risk of infection because of patient comorbidities and numerous human, environmental and procedural factors. Among pathogens gram positive bacteria, mainly *S. aureus*, represents the major cause of infections morbidity and mortality in CKD patients. These agents cause a wide variety of clinical manifestations ranging from colonizing without any sign of disease to localize or invasive bloodstream infections and septicemia. These effects are related to the circumstance that *S. aureus* is provided by several virulence factors permitting rapid tissue invasion and dissemination throughout the body and its genetic plasticity that permits a constant adaptation to changing environmental conditions together with the development of several antibiotic resistance patterns. Invasive devices for vascular and peritoneal procedures for dialysis access represent the leading predisposing factor for infections in dialysis patients. Thus central venous catheters related infections in hemodialysis and peritonitis in peritoneal dialysis are the most frequent type of infections in patients undergoing dialysis treatment. Moreover, infection in patients on either form of dialysis is also associated with an increasing risk of subsequent CV events. The presence of infection in a patient on dialysis has a substantial effect on CV mortality and morbidity, and should influence decisions regarding the use of therapies and strategies intended to minimize that risk (i.e. arterio-venous fistula as permanent vascular access). Establishing an infection prevention and control program which includes a bundle of strategies and interventions that are consistently performed will reduce the infection risk and associated conditions for both health personnel and patients.

Establishing an infection prevention and control program which includes a bundle of strategies and interventions that are consistently performed will reduce the infection risk for both health personnel and patients. The control and treatment of infectious agents such as *Staphylococcus* spp. , especially methicillin resistant strains, and other Gram-positive bacteria need for developing reliable and rapid methods of detection and characterization of these microorganisms. Nowadays, new insights into the diagnostic and epidemiology of MRSA and other pathogenic staphylococci have been developed employing molecular methods. This has meant an important advance in the diagnostic and treatment plans of such infective bacteria.

Acknowledgements

This work was partially supported by grant FIS10/00125 from INSTITUTO DE SALUD CARLOSIII (Spanish Health Ministry) to S.M.-A and from FEDER founds.

References

Abbott KC, Agodoa LY. 2002. *Hospitalizations for bacterial endocarditis after initiation of chronic dialysis in the United States. Nephron 91: 203–209.*

Adler AI, Stevens RJ, Manley SE et al. 2003. *Development and progression of nephropathy in type 2 diabetes: the United Kingdom Prospective Diabetes Study (UKPDS 64). Kidney Int 63: 225–232.*

Akman S, Uygun V, Guven AG. 2005. *Value of the urine strip test in the early diagnosis of bacterial peritonitis. Pediatr Int 47:523-527*

Annigeri R, Conly J, Vas S, Dedier H, Prakashan KP, Bargman JM. *Emergence of mupirocin-resistant Staphylococcus aureus in chronic peritoneal dialysis patients using mupirocin prophylaxis to prevent exit-site infection. Perit Dial Int 2001; 21:554–9*

ANZDATA Registry Report. 2008. *Appendix II. pp 1–97. In: McDonald S, Excell L, Livingston B (eds). Australia and New Zealand Dialysis and Transplant Registry: Adelaide. Australia.*

Band JD. 1999. *Nosocomial infections associated with peritoneal dialysis. In: Hospital Epidemiology and Infection Control, Mayhall CG (ed), 2nd ed. Lippincott Williams & Wilkins, PAIS.*

Bernardini, J., B. Piraino, M. Sorkin. 1987. *Analysis of continuous ambulatory peritoneal dialysis-related Pseudomonas aeruginosa infections. Am. J. Med. 83: 829-832.*

Bloembergen WE, Port FK. 1996. *Epidemiological perspective on infections in chronic dialysis patients. Adv Ren Replace Ther 3:201.*

Boelaert JR, Van Landuyt HW, De Baere YA, Deruyter Clin J Am Soc Nephrol 4: 1388–1400, 2009 S. aureus Bacteremia in Hemodialysis 1395 MM, Daneels RF, Schurgers ML, Matthys EG, Gordts BZ. Staphylococcus aureus infections in *haemodialysis patients: Pathophysiology and use of nasal mupirocin for prevention. J Chemother 7 [Suppl 3]: 49-53, 1995*

Borg D, Shetty A, Williams D, Faber MD. Fivefold reduction in peritonitis using a multifaceted continuous quality initiative program. Adv Perit Dial 2003; 19: 202–5

Boucher HW, Sakoulas G: Perspectives on daptomycin resistance, with emphasis on resistance in Staphylococcus aureus. Clin Infect Dis 45: 601-608, 2007

Butterly D.W., Schwab S.J. 2000. Dialysis access infections. Curr. Opin. Nephrol. Hypertens. 9: 631-635.

Centers for Disease Control and Prevention (CDC). 2007. Invasive methicillin-resistant Staphylococcus aureus infections among dialysis patients-United States, 2005. Morb. Mortal. Wkly. Rep. 56: 197-1999.

Cosgrove S.E., Sakoulas G., Perencevich E.N.,et al. 2003. Comparison of mortality associated with methicillin-resistant and methicillin-susceptible Staphylococcus aureus bacteremia: a meta-analysis. Clin. Infect. Dis. 36, 53-59.

D'Agata E.M. 2005. Antimicrobial-resistant, Grampositive bacteria among patients undergoing chronic hemodialysis. Clin. Infect. Dis. 35, 1212-1218, 2002; Salzer W. Antimicrobial-resistant gram-positive bacteria in PD peritonitis and the newer antibiotics used to treat them. Perit. Dial. Int. 25: 313-319:

Dancer SJ. Importance of the environment in methicillin-resistant Staphylococcus aureus acquisition: The case for hospital cleaning. Lancet Infect Dis 8: 101–113, 2008

Descamps-Latscha B, Herbelin A, Nguyen AT, et al. 1994. The immune system in end-stage renal disease. Semin Nephrol 14: 253.

Diaz-Granados C.A., Zimmer S.M., Klein M., et al. 2005. Comparison of mortality associated with vancomycin-resistant and vancomycin-susceptible enterococcal bloodstream infections: a metaanalysis. Clin. Infect. Dis. 41: 327-333.

Diekema D.J., BootsMiller B.J., Vaughn T.E., et al. 2004. Antimicrobial resistance trends and outbreak frequency in United States hospitals. Clin. Infect. Dis. 38: 78-85.

Diskin CJ, Stokes TJ, Dansby LM, Radcliff L, Carter TB. 2007. Is systemic heparin a risk factor for catheter-related sepsis in dialysis patients? An evaluation of various biofilm and traditional risk factors. Nephron Clin Pract 107: c128–c132.

Eknoyan G, Hostetter T, Bakris GL et al. 2003. Proteinuria and other markers of chronic kidney disease: A position statement of the national kidney foundation (NKF) and the national institute of diabetes and digestive and kidney diseases (NIDDK) Am J Kidney Dis 42: 617-622.

Ena J, Boelaert JR, Boyken LD, Van Landuyt HW, Godard CA, Herwaldt LA: Epidemiology of Staphylococcus aureus infections in patients on hemodialysis. Infect Control Hosp Epidemiol 15: 78-81, 1994

Foley R.N. 2007. Infections in patients with chronic kidney disease. Infect. Dis. Clin. North Am. 21, 659-672.

Foley, R. N., Guo, H., Snyder, J. J., Gilbertson, D. T. & Collins, A. J. 2004. Septicemia in the United States dialysis population, 1991 to 1999. J. Am. Soc. Nephrol. 15: 1038–1045.

Girndt M, Kohler H, Schiedhelm-Weick E, et al. 1993. T cell activation defect in hemodialysis patients: evidence for a role of the B7/CD28 pathway. Kidney Int 44:359–365.

Girndt M, Sester U, Sester M, et al. 1999. Impaired cellular immune function in patients with end stage renal failure. Nephrol Dial Transplant 14: 2807–2810.

Golper T.A., Schulman G., D'Agata E.M. 2000. Indications for vancomycin in dialysis patients. Semin. Dial. 13: 389-392.

Govindarajulu S, Hawley CM, McDonald SP, Brown FG, Rosman JB, Wiggins KJ, Bannister KM, Johnson DW. 2010. Staphylococcus aureus peritonitis in Australian peritoneal dialysis patients: predictors, treatment, and outcomes in 503 cases. Perit Dial Int. 30: 311-319.

Graham PL III., Lin SX, Larson EL. A U.S. population-based survey of Staphylococcus aureus colonization. Ann Intern Med 144: 318–325, 2006

Hansson GK. 2005. Inflammation, atherosclerosis, and coronary artery disease. N Engl J Med 352: 1685–1695.

Harbarth S, Rutschmann O, Sudre P, Pittet D. Impact of methicillin resistance on the outcome of patients with bacteremia caused by Staphylococcus aureus. Arch Intern Med 158: 182-189, 1998

Hidayat LK, Hsu DI, Quist R, Shriner KA, Wong-Beringer A. High-dose vancomycin therapy for methicillin-resistant Staphylococcus aureus infections: Efficacy and toxicity. Arch Intern Med 166: 2138-2144, 2006

Himmelfarb J, and Ikizler T. Alp. Hemodialysis N Engl J Med 2010; 363:1833-1845

Hoen B, Paul-Dauphin A, Hestin D, Kessler M. 1998. EPIBACDIAL: A multicenter prospective study of risk factors for bacteremia in chronic hemodialysis patients. J Am Soc Nephrol 9: 869–876.

Hotchkiss RS, Karl IE. 2003. The pathophysiology and treatment of sepsis. N Engl J Med 348:138–150.

Inrig JK, Reed SD, Szczech LA, Engemann JJ, Friedman JY, Corey GR, Schulman KA, Reller LB, Fowler VG Jr. 2006. Relationship between clinical outcomes and vascular access type among hemodialysis patients with Staphylococcus aureus bacteremia. Clin J Am Soc Nephrol 1: 518–524.

Ishani, A., Collins, A. J., Herzog, C. A. & Foley, R. N. 2005. Septicemia, access and cardiovascular disease in dialysis patients: the USRDS Wave 2 study. Kidney Int. 68: 311–318.

Jevons M.P. 1961. "Celbenin-resistant" staphylococci. Brit. Med. J. 1: 124-125.

Jones RN: Microbiological features of vancomycin in the 21st century. Minimum inhibitory concentration creep, bactericidal/static activity, and applied breakpoints to predict clinical outcomes or detect resistant strains. Clin Infect Dis 42[Suppl 1]: S13–S24, 2006

Kaczmarski, E. B., J. A. Tooth, E. Anastassiades, J. Manos, and R. Gokal. 1988. Pseudomonas peritonitis with continuous ambulatory peritoneal dialysis: a six-year study. Am. J. Kidney Dis. 11: 413-417.

Kamalakannan D, Pai RM, Johnson LB, Gardin JM, Saravolatz LD. 2007. Epidemiology and clinical outcomes of infective endocarditis in hemodialysis patients. Ann Thorac Surg 83: 2081–2086.

Kaysen GA, Eiserich JP. 2003. Characteristics and effects of inflammation in end-stage renal disease. Semin Dial 16:438–446.

King H, Aubert R, Herman W. 1998. Global burden of diabetes, 1995–2025: prevalence, numerical estimates, and projections. Diabetes Care 21: 1414–1431.

Kluytmans J, van Belkum A, Verbrugh H. 1997. Nasal carriage of Staphylococcus uureus: Epidemiology, underlying mechanisms, and associated risks. Clin Microbiol Rev 105-20.

Kohler H, Arnold W, Renschin G, et al. 1984. Active hepatitis B vaccination of dialysis patients and medical staff. Kidney Int 25:124–128.

Krothapalli, R., W. B. Duffy, C. Lacke, W. Payne, H. Patel, V. Perez, and H. 0. Senekjian. 1982. Pseudomonas peritonitis and continuous ambulatory peritoneal dialysis. Arch. Intern. Med. 142: 1862-1863.

Laupland KB, Gregson DB, Zygun DA, Doig CJ, Mortis G, Church DL. 2004. Severe bloodstream infections: A population-based assessment. Crit Care Med 32: 992–997.

Lazar MA, Brown CB, Bull D et al. 1990. Exit site care and exit site infections in continuous ambulatory peritoneal dialysis: Results of a randomized multicenter trial. Perit Dial Int 10: 25-9

Lederer S R, Riedelsdorf G, Schiffl H. 2007. Nasal carriage of meticillin resistant Staphylococcus aureus: the prevalence, patients at risk and the effect of elimination on outcomes among outclinic haemodialysis patients. Eur J Med Res. 12:284-288.

Leehey DJ, Lentino, JR. Peritonite e Infecção do Local de Saída. In: Daurgidas JT, Blake PG, Ing TS. Manual de Diálise. 3 ed. Rio de Janeiro: Medsi, 2003, pp. 385-408.

Lentino JR, Narita M, Yu VL. New antimicrobial agents as therapy for resistant gram-positive cocci. Eur J Clin Microbiol Infect Dis 27: 3-15, 2008

Lewis SL. 1992. Fever: Thermal regulation and alterations in end stage renal disease patients. ANNA J 19:13.

Lobbedez T, Gardam M, Dedier H, Burdzy D, Chu M, Izatt S. Routine use of mupirocin at the peritoneal catheter exit site and mupirocin resistance: still low after 7 years. Nephrol Dial Transplant 2004; 19:3140–3)

Lu PL, Tsai JC, Chiu YW, Chang FY, Chen YW, Hsiao CF, Siu LK. Methicillin-resistant Staphylococcus aureus carriage, infection and transmission in dialysis patients, healthcare workers and their family members. Nephrol Dial Transplant 23: 1659-1665, 2008

Luzar MA. Exit-site infection in CAPD: a review. Contrib Nephrol. 1990;85:57-66. Review.

Lysaght M. 2002. Maintenance dialysis population dynamics: current trends and long-term implications. J Am Soc Nephrol 13: S37–S40.

Marr KA, Kong L, Fowler VG, Gopal A, Sexton DJ, Conlon PJ, Corey GR. 1998. Incidence and outcome of Staphylococcus aureus bacteremia in hemodialysis patients. Kidney Int. Nov;54(5):1684-1689.

McClelland RS, Fowler VG Jr, Sanders LL, Gottlieb G, Kong LK, Sexton DJ, Schmader K, Lanclos KD, Corey R. Staphylococcus aureus bacteremia among elderly vs younger adult patients: Comparison of clinical features and mortality. Arch Intern Med 159: 1244-1247, 1999

Melzer M., Eykyn S.J., Gransden W.R., Chinn S. 2003. Is methicillin-resistant Staphylococcus aureus more virulent than methicillin-susceptible S. aureus? A comparative cohort study of British patients with nosocomial infection and bacteremia. Clin. Infect. Dis. 37: 1453-1460

Minnaganti VR, Cunha BA. 2001. Infections associated with uremia and dialysis. Infect Dis Clin North Am. 15:385-406.

Moellering RC Jr. Current treatment options for community-acquired methicillin-resistant Staphylococcus aureus infection. Clin Infect Dis 46: 1032-1037, 2008

Moellering RC. Linezolid: The first oxazolidinone antimicrobial. Ann Intern Med 138: 135-142, 2003

Monteon F, Correa-Rotter R, Paniagua R et al. Prevention of peritonitis with disconnect systems in CAPD: a randomized controlled trial. The Mexican Nephrology Collaborative Study Group. Kidney Int 1998; 54:2123-38.

Moremi N, Mshana SE, Kamugisha E, Kataraihya J, Tappe D, Vogel U, Lyamuya EF, Claus H. 2012. Predominance of methicillin resistant Staphylococcus aureus -ST88 and new ST1797 causing wound infection and abscesses. J Infect Dev Ctries. 21: 620-625

Moss AH. 2001. Shared decision-making in dialysis: the new RPA/ASN guideline on appropriate initiation and withdrawal of treatment. Am J Kidney Dis 37: 1081-1091.

Murtagh FE, Marsh JE, Donohoe P, Ekbal NJ, Sheerin NS, Harris FE. 2007. Dialysis or not? A comparative survival study of patients over 75 years with chronic kidney disease stage 5. Nephrol Dial Transplant 22: 1955-1962.

Nassar GM, Ayus JC. 2001. Infectious complications of the hemodialysis access. Kidney Int 60: 1–13.

Ng R, Zabetakis PM, Callahan C. 1999. Vancomycin-resistant Enterococcus infection is a rare complication in patients receiving PD on an outpatient basis. Perit Dial Int 19: 273.

Nguyen-Khac E, Cadranel JF, Thevenot T, Nousbaum JB. 2008. The utility of reagent strips in the diagnosis of infected ascites in cirrhotic patients. Aliment Pharmacol Ther 28:282-288

Ninomiya T, Perkovic V, de Galan BE et al. 2009. Albuminuria and kidney function independently predict cardiovascular and renal outcomes in diabetes. J Am Soc Nephrol 20: 1813–1821.

Nolph KD. 1988. Current status of CAPD and CCID. Dial Transplant 17:457.

Nsouli KA, Lazarus JM, Schoenbaum SC, et al. 1979. Bacteremic infection in hemodialysis. Arch Intern Med 139:1255.

Ota K, Maruyama H, Iino N, Nakamura G, Shimotori M, Tanabe Y, et al. 2007. Rapid detection of causative pathogen of peritonitis using in-situ hybridization in a patient with continuous ambulatory peritoneal dialysis. J Infect Chemother 13: 273-275.

Park SJ, Lee JY, Tak WT, Lee JH. 2005. Using reagent strips for rapid diagnosis of peritonitis in peritoneal dialysis patients. Adv Perit Dial 21:69-71.

Pasqual Barretti, Taíse M. C. Moraes, Carlos H. Camargo, Jacqueline C. T. Caramori, Alessandro L. Mondelli, Augusto C. Montelli, Maria de Lourdes R. S. da Cunha. 2012. Peritoneal Dialysis-Related Peritonitis Due to Staphylococcus aureus: A Single-Center Experience over 15 Years. PLoS One. 7: e31780.

Peacock SJ, de Silva GD, Justice A, Cowland A, Moore CE, Winearls CG, Day NP. 2002. Comparison of multilocus sequence typing and pulsed-field gel electrophoresis as tools for typing Staphylococcus aureus isolates in a microepidemiological setting. J Clin Microbiol. 40: 3764-3770.

Pérez–Fontán M, Rosales M, Rodríguez–Carmona A, Falcón TG, Valdés F. Mupirocin resistance after long-term use for Staphylococcus aureus colonization in patients undergoing chronic peritoneal dialysis. Am J Kidney Dis 2002; 39:337–41)

Petti C. A., Polage C. R., Schreckenberger P. 2005. The Role of 16S rRNA Gene Sequencing in Identification of Microorganisms Misidentified by Conventional Methods J Clin Microbiol. 43: 6123–6125.

Piraino B, Bernardini J, Sorkin M. A five-year study of the microbiologic results of exit site infections and peritonitis in continuous ambulatory peritoneal dialysis. Am J Kidney Dis. 1987 Oct;10(4):281-6.

Retnakaran R, Cull CA, Thorne KI et al. 2006. Risk factors for renal dysfunction in type 2 diabetes: U.K. Prospective Diabetes Study 74. Diabetes 55: 1832–1839.

Reutens AT, Prentice L, Atkins R. 2008. The epidemiology of diabetic kidney disease. In: Ekoé J-M, Rewers M, Williams R, Zimmet P (eds). The Epidemiology of Diabetes mellitus. John Wiley & Sons Ltd. UK.

Ro Y, Hamada C, Io H, Hayashi K, Hirahara I, Tomino Y. 2004. Rapid, simple, and reliable method for the diagnosis of CAPD peritonitis using the new MMP-9 test kit. J Clin Lab Anal 18: 224-230.

Ross R. 1999. Atherosclerosis: an inflammatory disease. N Engl J Med 340: 115–126.

Ruiz, A., B. Ramos, D. Burgos, M. A. Grutos, and E. Lopez de Novales. 1988. Acinetobacter calcoaceticus peritonitis in continuous ambulatory peritoneal dialysis (CAPD) patients. Peritoneal Dialysis Int. 8: 285-286.

Ryan S.V., Calligaro K.D., Dougherty M.J. 2004. Management of hemodialysis access infections. Semin. Vasc. Surg. 17: 40-44.

Sarnak MJ, Jaber BL: Mortality caused by sepsis in patients with end-stage renal disease compared with the general population. Kidney Int 58: 1758–1764, 2000

Selvey LA, Whitby M, Johnson B. Nosocomial methicillin resistant Staphylococcus aureus bacteremia: Is it any worse than nosocomial methicillin-sensitive Staphylococcus aureus bacteremia? Infect Control Hosp Epidemiol 21: 645-648, 2000

Shin JH, Kim HR, Lee JN. 2005. Clinical significance and species identification of rapidly growing mycobacteria isolated from routine blood cultures. Korean J Lab Med 26:162-167

Si Hyun Kim, M.S., Haeng Soon Jeong, Yeong Hoon Kim, Sae Am Song. 2012. Evaluation of DNA Extraction Methods and Their Clinical Application for Direct Detection of Causative Bacteria in Continuous Ambulatory Peritoneal Dialysis Culture Fluids from Patients with Peritonitis by Using Broad-Range PCR. Ann Lab Med. 32: 119–125.

Sicree R, Shaw J, Zimmet P. 2006. Diabetes and impaired glucose tolerance. In: Gan D (ed). Diabetes Atlas, 3rd edn. International Diabetes Federation. Brussels, pp 15–109.

Sievert DM, Rudrik JT, Patel JB, McDonald LC, Wilkins MJ, Hageman JC: Vancomycin-resistant Staphylococcus aureus in the United States, 2002-2006. Clin Infect Dis 46: 668-674, 2008

Soriano A, Martinez JA, Mensa J, Marco F, Almela M, Moreno-Martinez A, Sanchez F, Munoz I, Jimenez de Anta MT, Soriano E. Pathogenic significance of methicillin resistance for patients with Staphylococcus aureus bacteremia. Clin Infect Dis 30: 368-373, 2000

Stevenson KB, Hannah EL, Lowder CA, Adcox MJ, Davidson RL, Mallea MC, Narasimhan N, Wagnild JP. 2002. Epidemiology of hemodialysis vascular access infections from longitudinal infection surveillance data: Predicting the impact of NKF-DOQI clinical practice guidelines for vascular access. Am J Kidney Dis 39:549–555.

Sullivan R., Samuel V., Le C. 2007. Hemodialysis vascular catheter-related bacteremia. Am. J.Med. Sci. 334: 458-465.

Sunder-Plassmann G, Patruta SI, Horl WH. 1999. Pathobiology of the role of in infection. Am J Kidney Dis 34: S25.

Swartz R, Messana J, Starmann B. 1991. Preventing Staphylococcus aureus infection during chronic peritoneal dialysis. J Am SOC Nephrol 23: 085-91.

Taylor G, Gravel D, Johnston L, Embil J, Holton D, Paton S. 2002. Prospective surveillance for primary bloodstream infections occurring in Canadian hemodialysis units. Infect Control Hosp Epidemiol 23: 716–720.

Teehan GS, Bahdouch D, Ruthazer R, Balakrishnan VS, Snydman DR, Jaber BL. 2004. Iron storage indices: Novel predictors of bacteremia in hemodialysis patients ca

Vandecasteele SJ, Boelaert JR, De Vriese AS. Staphylococcus aureus infections in hemodialysis: what a nephrologist should know. Clin J Am Soc Nephrol. 2009 Aug;4(8):1388-400. 2009 Jul 9.

Vanholder R, Van Loo A, Dhondt AM. 1996. Influence of uremia and haemodialysis on host defense and infection. Nephrol Dial Transplant 11: 593.

Vascular Access 2006 Work Group. 2006. Clinical practice guidelines for vascular access. Am. J. Kidney Dis. 48: S176–S247.

von Eiff C, Becker K, Machka K, Stammer H, Peters G. Nasal carriage as a source of Staphylococcus aureus bacteremia. Study Group. N Engl J Med 344: 11–16, 2001

Wertheim HF, Melles DC, Vos MC, van Leeuwen W, van Belkum A,Verbrugh HA, Nouwen JL. The role of nasal carriage in Staphylococcus aureus infections. Lancet Infect Dis 5: 751–762, 2005

Wertheim HF, Vos MC, Ott A, van Belkum A, Voss A, Kluytmans JA, van Keulen PH, Vandenbroucke-Grauls CM, Meester MH, Verbrugh HA. Risk and outcome of nosocomial Staphylococcus aureus bacteraemia in nasal carriers versus non-carriers. Lancet 364: 703-705, 2004

Whitby M., McLaws M.L., Berry G. 2003. Risk of death from methicillin-resistant Staphylococcus aureus bacteraemia: a meta-analysis. Med. J. Aust. 175: 264-267.

Yamagata K, Iseki K, Nitta K et al. 2008. Chronic kidney disease perspectives in Japan and the importance of urinalysis screening. Clin Exp Nephrol 12: 1–8.

Yip T., Tse K.C., Lam M.F., et al. 2006. Risk factors and outcomes of extended-spectrum beta-lactamase-producing E. coli peritonitis in CAPD patients. Perit. Dial. Int. 26: 191-197.

Yoo TH, Chang KH, Ryu DR, Kim JS, Choi HY, Park HC, et al. 2006. Usefulness of 23S rRNA amplification by PCR in the detection of bacteria in CAPD peritonitis. Am J Nephrol 26:115-120

Yoon JW, Gollapudi S, Pahl MV, et al. 2006. Native and central memory T-cell lymphopenia in end-stage renal disease. Kidney Int 70: 371–376.

Yoon K, Lee JH, Kim JW et al. Epidemic obesity and type 2 diabetes in Asia. Lancet 2006; 368: 1681–1688.

Zelenitsky S, Barns L, Findlay I, Alfa M, Ariano R, Fine A. 2000. Analysis of microbiological trends in peritoneal dialysis-related peritonitis from 1991 to 1998. Am J Kidney Dis 36: 1009–1013

Zimmet P, Alberti K, Shaw J. 2001. Global and societal implications of the diabetes epidemic. Nature 414: 782–787.

Cardiovascular Effects of Diabetes Mellitus in Paediatrics

Mohammed Al-Biltagi
Pediatric Department, Faculty of Medicine
Tanta University, Egypt

1   Introduction

Diabetes mellitus (DM) is a chronic metabolic disorder which affects in one way or another all the stages of childhood. Diabetes effects start in utero and affect neonates, infants, children and adolescent. Its cardiovascular complications constitute a considerable portion of morbidity in such an active age because of the metabolic derangement, associated dyslipidemia, atherosclerosis, hypertension and autonomic dysfunction. Gestational diabetes (GD) may have overwhelming effects on the embryonic heart as well as the infant born to a diabetic mother (IDM). The neonates and infants who may suffer this metabolic disease may also have considerable cardiovascular effects. Both types of diabetes can occur in children and it can affect various cardiac functions as well as cardiac remodelling in adolescents and young youth. In this chapter we will shed some light on the pathogenesis and the various cardiovascular effects of diabetes in the pediatric population (Abraha *et al.*, 1999; Rodriguez *et al.*, 2006; Gillian *et al.*, 2009).

2   Pathogenesis

Vascular dysfunction is present in children with both types of diabetes and is a critical precursor of atherosclerosis. The cardiovascular mortality rate is higher in diabetic patients than non diabetic with the same cardiovascular risk factors. Diabetes has an additive role when combined with one or more risk factors. It is usually associated with one or more of cardiovascular risk factors like increased low density lipids (LDL), decreased high density lipids (HDL) increased glycosylated haemoglobin (Hb A1c), elevated systolic blood pressure, hyperglycaemia, hyperinsulinemia and insulin resistance, dyslipidemia, increased plasma oxidative stress, enhanced fibrinolysis and abnormal vasodilator function. Type 2 diabetes (T2 DM) has more cardiovascular risk than type 1. T2 DM has early occurrence of cardiovascular diseases with a higher rate of multi-vessel disease and poorer outcomes than in type 1 diabetes (T1 DM). The pathogenesis of diabetic vascular diseases is complex, incompletely understood and still in need for a thorough investigation. Table 1 showed summary of the different pathogenesis mechanisms of diabetic vascular diseases.

Endothelial cell dysfunction	Peipheral neuropathy
Vascular smooth muscle dysfunction	Cardiac autonomic neuropathy
Thickening of the basement membranes and medial calcification	Disturbance of thrombosis, and coagulation process
Insulin resistance and compensatory Hyperinsulinemia	Associated Autoimmune disorders (e.g. hypothyroidism, hyperthyroidism etc.)
Inflammation	Angiogenesis
Diabetes-associated- Hypoglycaemia	

Table 1: Summary of the different pathogenesis mechanisms of diabetic vascular diseases.

2.1   Endothelial Cell Dysfunction

The vascular endothelium is a single cell layer lining of the intimal surface of the blood vessels. This active layer acts as a controlling barrier between the circulation and body tissues. It secretes a variety of substances that cause vasodilatation (e.g. Nitric oxide [NO], prostanoids, endothelin, and angiotensin II).

It controls the vascular tone and blood flow and maintains a balance between vasodilatation and vasoconstriction. It also controls the nutrient delivery and waste removal, controls local inflammation, inhibits leucocyte migration and influences the platelet activation. So, disturbance of the endothelial functions will lead to increased vasoconstriction, inflammation, thrombosis, impaired platelet function and abnormal coagulation (Wheaton & Pinkstaff, 2006; Kampoli *et al.*, 2009; Goligorsky, 2005).

The diabetes-induced endothelial dysfunction results from the oxidative stress that arises from the abnormal cluster of hyperglycemia, elevated free fatty acids, increased production of glycosylated endproducts; and insulin resistance which characterizes DM. All act together in a harmony to target the endothelial cell (Aljada, 2003). Elevated levels of free fatty acids also reduce NO production, and promote the formation of oxidized low-density lipoproteins (Ox-LDL), which can damage endothelial cells and induce the expression of adhesion molecules such as P-selectin as well as chemotactic factors such as monocyte chemoattractant protein-1 and macrophage colony stimulating factor which increase endothelial dysfunction in DM and hence initiate the process of atherosclerosis. (Hsueh & Quinones, 2003; Hsueh *et al.*, 2004) Nitric oxide (NO) is produced by endothelial nitric oxide synthase (eNOS). Endothelial Nitric Oxide is an anti- inflammatory, anti-oxidant, and potent vasodilator that counteracts smooth muscle cell proliferation and decreases platelet adhesiveness (Moncada & Higgs 2002).

Chronic hyperglycemia induced endothelial damage result from glucose auto-oxidation, activation of poly-alcohol pathway with production of sorbitol, production of diacylglcerol and activation of protein kinase enzyme; with production of glycation end products. All these changes will increase the oxidative stress and cause endothelial damage (Du *et al.*, 2003). In diabetes associated endothelial dysfunction; there is a decrease in nitric oxide (NO) production and release and increased NO inactivation especially with presence of insulin resistance. The decrease in the vasodilator function of nitric oxide (NO) together with the increased secretion of the vasoconstrictor endothelin-1 cause dysregulation of vascular tone; hyper-constrictive state; hypertension and its concomitant complications that result from vasoconstriction (Koh *et al.*, 2005). So, endothelial dysfunction provides an environment that allows the development of vascular disease, offering a link between DM and microvascular and macrovascular disease.

2.2 Vascular Smooth Muscle Dysfunction

Vascular smooth muscle is an important component of the blood vessel and contracts and relaxes in response to certain stimuli. Its main function is to regulate the blood flow inside the blood vessel. The endothelial nitric oxide is the main vasodilator stimulus while the endothelin-1 is the main vasoconstrictor stimulus (Clark & Pyne-Geithman, 2005). Alteration of vascular smooth muscle functions is an important mechanism for the development of cardiovascular complications in diabetes. Hyperglycemia can cause vascular smooth muscle dysfunction by increased oxidative stress and abnormal apoptosis in the same way of endothelial damage. Hyperglycemia increases also Angiotensin II which causes vasoconstriction and smooth muscle proliferation (Amiri *et al.*, 1999). There is a decrease in vascular smooth muscle response to the relaxing effect of nitric oxide, as well as presence of an exaggerated contractility response to nor-epinephrine. These changes may be due to an enhanced intracellular Ca2 + signaling of the vascular smooth muscle cells to contractile stimuli as a result of changes in subcellular Ca2+ distribution on cell activation (Fleischhacker *et al.*, 1999). Patients with T2 DM show decreased vasoconstriction in response to infusion of endothelin-1 and Angiotensin. The degree of alterations in vascular reactivity to vasoconstrictor phenylephrine is significantly influenced by the duration of diabetes (Suzuki *et al.*, 2001; Hassan *et al.*, 2011). Role of vascular smooth muscle cells in the development of atherosclerosis is essential. When macrophage-rich fatty streak forms, the vascular smooth muscle cells in the medial layer of the arteries start to migrate into the nascent intimal lesion, replicate, and lay down a complex extracellular matrix, important steps in the progression to advanced atherosclerotic plaque. Arterial vascular smooth muscle cells cultured from patients with T1 DM demonstrate enhanced migration (Beckman *et al.*, 2002).

2.3   Thickening of the Basement Membranes (BM) and Medial Calcification

The vascular basement membrane is a specialized extracellular matrix secreted by endothelial cells to provide support -cell regulatory- and filtering sieving functions. Capillary BM thickening is an ultra-structural hallmark in diabetic patients which occurs with prolonged hyperglycaemia and since 1970's to 1980's; diabetes was considered as a basement membrane disease (Melvin *et al.*, 2005). Thickening of BM affects its ability and selectivity to transport the metabolic products and nutrients between the circulation and the tissue (Hayden *et al.*, 2005). Various high glucose-induced mechanisms have been investigated and excess synthesis of BM components has been identified as a major contributing factor to BM thickening. Several vascular BM components have been identified whose expression is up-regulated in diabetes. Hyperglycaemia cause altered extracellular matrix (ECM) synthesis and accumulation due to increase cellular fibronectin and type IV collagen fragments which ends by thickening of vascular basement membrane. Enzymes responsible for the degradation of BM components have been reported to exhibit reduced activity. Thickening of capillary BM is integrally involved with profound cardiovascular and microvascular complications of diabetes (Chronopoulos *et al.*, 2011; Roy & Sato, 2000).

2.4   Insulin Resistance and Compensatory Hyperinsulinemia

Insulin resistance was first described by Reaven as "syndrome X". The complete form of this syndrome includes hyperinsulinaemia, glucose intolerance, dyslipidaemia, elevated blood pressure and fibrinolytic impairment (Fontbonne, 1996). Insulin resistance commonly precedes hyperglycemia in diabetic patients. Insulin resistance and compensatory hyperinsulinemia may increase atherogenic risk through several different mechanisms. In insulin resistance, the ability of insulin to induce vasodilation is low, suggesting an impairment or inactivation of nitric oxide. The insulin resistance-associated hyperinsulinemia induces smooth- muscle cell hypertrophy and hyperplasia and increased extracellular proteins which is an important factor contributing to atherogenesis. Studies have indicated a connection between hyperinsulinaemia and activation of both atherogenic and anti-atherogenic pathways (Nigro *et al.*, 2006). Also; insulin per se seems to have the capacity to both increase and decrease vascular tone (Muniyappa *et al.*, 2007).

2.5   Inflammation

Inflammation is a process by which the body try to heal itself or fight off infection in response to tissue injury or pathogen exposure. This response engages activation of leukocytes and release of certain inflammatory cytokines and chemokines. Inflammation seems to fuel the atherogenic process and is strongly linked to DM and insulin resistance. Immune activation in diabetes initiates state of chronic low-level inflammation which even may precede insulin resistance in diabetic and pre-diabetic states and is an important risk factor for the diabetes-associated cardiovascular complications. The reason for this chronic state of inflammation may be due to the reduced production of the potent vasodilator NO and an increased secretion of the vasoconstrictor and growth factor endothelin-1. These changes enhances the release of pro-inflammatory cytokines which cause or exacerbate injury by a variety of mechanisms including enhanced vascular permeability, programmed cell death (apoptosis), recruitment of invasive leukocytes, and the promotion of reactive oxygen species (ROS) production (Pradhan *et al.*, 2001; Festa *et al.*, 2000).

Association of obesity in diabetic patients also plays a role in triggering inflammation. Obesity is associated with increased levels of a number of adipokines (cytokines released from adipose tissue), including tumor necrosis factor-α, interleukin 1β, interleukin 6, and plasminogen activator inhibitor 1 (PAI-1); all linked to the inflammatory response. On the other hand, adipokine adiponectin, which has anti-inflammatory properties; is decreased in obese subjects, exacerbating the chronic inflammatory nature of obesity (Dokken, 2008; Trayhurn & Wood, 2005). Both hyperglycemia and insulin resistance are correlated directly with markers of inflammation and hence the poor vascular outcomes. In the same way, improvements in insulin resistance and glycemic control reduce inflammation and consequently the cardiovascular complications. These benefits are translated to the vasculature. Reductions in inflammation through medication or by reducing visceral adiposity, improve endothelial function and soluble markers of endothelial cellular activation (Yatagai *et al.*, 2004).

2.6 Diabetes-associated-Hypoglycaemia

With the intense glycemic control; there is an increased rate of hypoglycemia in diabetic patients. The body responds by release of counter-regulatory hormones and substance to return blood glucose to the normal non-pathologic levels. There is an excess secretion of glucagon, epinephrine, nor-epinephrine, cortisol, pancreatic polypeptide, growth hormone, corticotrophin, as well as activation of the autonomic nervous system in response to hypoglycemia. The level of this excess is directly proportional to the severity of hypoglycaemia. Hypoglycemia was linked to the development of cardiac and cerebral ischemia and cardiac arrhythmias (Wright & Frier, 2008). It can induce significant several acute inflammatory thrombotic, and fibrinolytic and increases the oxidative-stress which may further contribute to atherosclerotic processes. Hypoglycemia significantly increases soluble vascular cell adhesion molecule 1, soluble intercellular adhesion molecule 1, soluble E-selectin and soluble P-selectin (a marker of platelet activation). Hypoglycemia increases plasminogen activator inhibitor 1, (a major inhibitor of fibrinolysis), while plasma tissue plasminogen activator concentrations does not change, with the result that hypoglycaemia induced acute reductions in fibrinolytic balance. Hypoglycaemia also is related to impaired vascular endothelial function in children with type 1 diabetes. (Joy *et al.*, 2010; Wright *et al.*, 2010; Younk & Davis, 2011; Boulton *et al.*, 2005)

2.7 Peripheral Neuropathy

Pryce described the degenerative lesions of the peripheral nerves in the extremities of diabetic patients for the first in 1887. It occurs as a micro-vascular complication of diabetes. Peripheral neuropathy may be a cause or a result of the cardiovascular changes that occur in diabetes. Endothelial dysfunction has also been considered an important event in the development of diabetic neuropathy. Vascular endothelial dysfunction results in vascular damage of the small blood vessels supplying the peripheral nerves causing peripheral neuropathy. Injury to the peripheral nerves can result from polyol accumulation, injury from advance glycation end products (AGEs), and oxidative stress (Kalani, 2008). Arteriovenous shunting leading to impaired blood flow through nutritive capillaries results in sympathetic neuropathy due to both hemodynamic and metabolic disturbances. Microvascular dysfunction is seen at an early stage in the peripheral nerve, which contributes to impaired endoneural blood flow, leading to destruction of neuronal and Schwann cells and, and finally, nerve degeneration (Bhowmik *et al.*, 2009). In diabetic peripheral neuropathy; there may be loss of normal vascular tone that can cause severe venous swelling and even leads to ulceration and infection with lack of healthy blood flow. Diabetic peripheral neuropathy can induce autonomic dysfunction which can be manifested by orthostatic hypotension or fainting when standing up (Peña *et al.*, 2012).

2.8   Cardiac Autonomic Neuropathy

The autonomic nervous system adjusts the cardiac electrical and contractile activity through the balance between sympathetic and parasympathetic activity. Cardiac autonomic neuropathy occurs in parallel to the development of peripheral neuropathy as a part of the neuropathy which begins distally and progressing proximally. Diabetic associated cardiovascular autonomic neuropathy causes abnormalities in heart rate control, as well as defects in central and peripheral vascular dynamics. (Maser & Lenhard, 2005) The degree of cardiac autonomic neuropathy depends on degree of glycemic control, disease duration, age-related neuronal attrition, and systolic and diastolic blood pressure (Witte *et al.*, 2005). There are different pathogenic mechanisms which help to developed cardiac autonomic neuropathy. These include: formation of AGEs, increased oxidative/nitrosative stress with increased free radical production, activation of the polyol and protein kinase C pathways, activation of polyADP ribosylation, and activation of genes involved in neuronal damage (Edwards *et al.*, 2008).

2.9   Disturbance of Thrombosis and Coagulation Process

Diabetes is often associated with a hypercoagulable state which increases the risk of ischemic cardiovascular events as well as cerebrovascular events which are the cause of death in about 80% of diabetic patients (Gu *et al.*, 1998). In diabetes; there is an increased platelet aggregation, increased plasma levels of platelet coagulation products and clotting factors including fibrinogen, factor VII, factor VIII, factor XI, factor XII, kallikrein, and von Willebrand factor. Platelet hyperactivity is indicated by higher plasma levels of beta-thromboglobulin, platelet factor 4, and thromboxane B2. Coagulation activation markers, such as prothrombin activation fragment 1+2 and thrombin–anti-thrombin complexes are also elevated in diabetes. Another cause of disturbance of thrombosis, and coagulation process is the diminished fibrinolytic activity due to abnormal clot structures that are more resistant to degradation, and also because of an increase in PAI-1. The increase in coagulation and thrombosis potentiates thrombus formation after plaque rupture and makes the development of arterial occlusion and clinical events more likely (Carr, 2001).

2.10   Autoimmune Disorders (e.g. Hypothyroidism and Hyperthyroidism)

Type 1 diabetes results from the body's failure to produce insulin due to autoimmune or idiopathic destruction of cells. There is an increased frequency of other autoimmune diseases in T1 DM e.g. thyroid dysfunction, vitamin B12 deficiency, or celiac disease. Auto-immune thyroid disease is the most common autoimmune disorder associated with diabetes, occurring in 17–30% of patients with T1 DM. The presence of thyroid auto-antibodies is predictive of thyroid dysfunction, generally hypothyroidism but less commonly hyperthyroidism. Plus the increased risk cardiovascular complications in diabetic patients; the presence of these autoimmune disorders further increases this risk (Gerstein, 2007; Nathan *et al.*, 2007).

2.11   Disturbances of Angiogenesis

Angiogenesis is a physiological process of new vessel formation (neo-vascularisation). A balanced angiogenesis is important for both embryonic and postembryonic vascular development. It is essential for embryological growth, tissue development, and wound healing in damaged tissues. Defect in angiogenesis could affect the body ability to grow or to regenerate the damaged tissue while increased angiogenesis is also an important step in the transition of tumors from a confined locale to malignancy (Carmeliet, 2000). There are numerous mechanisms for aberrant angiogenesis in diabetes. Reduced angiogenesis and the ability of collateral formation are due to reduced vascular endothelial growth factor-A (VEGF), fibroblast growth factor (FGF), endothelial progenitor cells (EPC) circulation, cytokines, the extracellular matrix (ECM)/vascular basement membrane (BM) {ECM/BM} degradation; and increased AGEs and matrix metalloproteinase (MMP). Angiogenesis also is reduced by vascular occlusion and inflammation which occur due to increased free fatty acids, polyol pathway, cytokines, ICAM, and VCAM. Impaired angiogenesis also reduces wound healing probably due to reduced VEGF and growth factors; sorbitol-inositol imbalance; increased ACE, Ang-II and tissue factor mRNA. In gestational diabetes, embryonic vasculopathy with anomalous vasculogenesis and angiogenesis; occurs due to reduced VEGF, IL-1, and transforming growth factor beta (TGF-β). On the other hand excessive angiogenesis can also occur in diabetic patients. Retinal capillary occlusion occurs due to elevated intraocular pressure. Increased VEGF can cause increased vascular permeability while vascular remodelling occurs due to increased laminin, fibronectin, collagen IV, ECM components, and lipidosis. Capillary sprouting also can occurs due to elevated levels of VEGF, FGF, PDGF; cytokines (TGF-β); and integrins (Kolluru, 2012).

3   Fetal Effects of Maternal Diabetes

The fetal heart is a target organ for the congenital effects of pre-existing as well as gestational maternal diabetes. Cardiac anomalies and myocardial hypertrophy are about three times more prevalent in the offspring of women with DM. Maternal DM significantly affect the fetal heart and fetal–placental circulation in both structure and function. The diversity of cardiac abnormalities in foetuses of diabetic mothers suggests a complex pathogenesis, though it is similar to the general pathogenetic mechanisms of cardiovascular effects of diabetes but with some specific fetal effects. The teratogenic effect of DM is likely to be multi-factorial. The higher is the maternal Hb A1C values during early pregnancy, the more the risk of malformations. Glycosylated haemoglobin (Hb A1C) > 6.3% in the first trimester is associated with a significant increased risk of congenital heart abnormalities. Hyperglycaemia and hyperketonemia are toxic factors for the developing embryo and can induce and modify multiple biochemical and signal transduction pathways which include reduction in cellular levels of myoinositol and arachidonic acid and increase in production of reactive oxygen species. Hyperglycaemia induces proliferation and migration of neural crest cells which are critical to heart and brain development. High plasma triglycerides, ketones, branched chain amino acids, and creatinine increase resorption rates and malformation rates among affected pregnancies (Kumar, et al., 2007).

Maternal DM increases the expression of certain placental genes concerned with chronic stress and inflammation which play major role in evolution of maternal diabetes-induced embryopathy (Suhonen et al., 2000). Down-regulation of genes involved in development of cardiac neural crest could contribute to pathogenesis of maternal diabetes-induced congenital heart defects (Hornberger, 2006). Hypoglycemia is a common side effect of diabetes therapy and is a potential teratogen. Hypoglycaemia interferes with normal cardiogenesis and alters morphology, function, metabolism, and expression of certain proteins in the developing heart. It is likely that these factors contribute to heart defects observed in the diabetic embryopathy, but the definitive link has yet to be made (Smoak, 2002). Intrauterine hyperglycemia that occurs in type-I diabetic pregnancies are associated with congenital cardiac malformations, fetal cardiomyopathy, fetal venous thrombosis, altered placental villi vascularization, and pathological fetal heart rates even with tight maternal glucose control. Hyperglycaemia exerts its teratogenic effects during the period of organogenesis—the first 42 days of pregnancy. Intrauterine hyperglycemia induces reflex fetal hyper-insulinemia. Chronic fetal hyperinsulinemia can cause increased total body weight and selective organo-megaly as a result of hypertrophy of insulin-sensitive tissues including the heart and increased expression and affinity of insulin receptors. Chronic fetal hypoxemia is also common in foetuses of diabetic mothers due to relative immaturity of the placenta, with an increased distance over which oxygen diffusion has to occur from maternal to fetal side. Chronic fetal hypoxemia is commonly seen in cases of increased ma-ternal and fetal glucose levels. This chronic fetal hypoxemia causes higher haemoglobin levels in new-borns of diabetic mothers and elevated number of nucleated red blood cells which in turn causes compen-satory changes in fetal circulation (Lisowski *et al.*, 2003).

In presence of diabetic associated fetal macrosomia, there is an increase in the cardiac mass due to a larger mass of myocardial nuclei, increased cell number and hypertrophy of myocardial fibers. Reduced left ventricular filling was also observed in infants of mothers with gestational diabetes. Underdevelop-ment of ventricular compliance in foetuses of diabetic mothers occurs secondary to cardiac wall thicken-ing or other factors which can influence diastolic function as a result of DM (e.g. hypoxemia, polycythe-mia and altered in utero metabolic environment). This decrease of ventricular compliance can present with impairment of cardiac diastolic function as expressed by the ratio between early and late diastolic ventricular filling at the level of both mitral and tricuspid valves (Tsyvian, 1998). Interventricular septal hypertrophy may be associated with functional cardiac changes during pregnancy as well as in the neona-tal period and seems to normalize within the first 6 months after birth. Ventricular hypertrophy can occur as early as before 20 weeks of gestation. However there is accelerated growth of the fetal heart in the mid and third trimesters when compared to foetuses of non-diabetic pregnancies. Lisowski *et al.* found that the expected decrease of the ratio of the right to left ventricular output that usually takes place with the progress of pregnancy does not occur which indicates a dominant role for the right ventricle until the end of pregnancy, whereas in normal pregnancy right and left ventricles transport half each of the cardiac output until the end of gestation. They explained this right ventricle dominance because the head of the foetuses of women with diabetes is relatively smaller than the body. As a result of the placental immaturi-ty, more blood has to be transported to the placenta and the right ventricle is responsible for delivery of blood to the placenta. These changes in fetal circulation may suggest the existence of a compensatory mechanism which increases cardiac output and causes cardiac hypertrophy (Lisowski *et al.*, 2003).

3.1   Pre-Gestational Diabetes

The prevalence of pre-gestational DM among women early in their reproductive years is increasing. The fetal effect of pre-gestational DM begins during the early embryonic development in the first trimester, with altered cardiac morphogenesis and placental development. It continues to affect the fetal circulation through the second and third trimesters and into the perinatal and neonatal period (Hornberger, 2006). Turan *et al* showed that foetuses of poorly controlled diabetic mothers had significant decrease in first-trimester diastolic myocardial function and myocardial performance than in non-diabetic controls. The decrease in myocardial performance is more marked with increasing HbA1c and appears to be independ-ent of preload and after load (Turan, 2011). Good glycemic control in foetuses of diabetic mothers results in normal cardiac growth and ventricular diastolic filling. Progression of diastolic filling is abnormally delayed, however, and is presumably more exaggerated in poorly controlled diabetics (Weber *et al.*,

1994). The ability to document these cardiac functional changes early in pregnancy opens potential new avenues to understand the consequences of maternal glycemic status.

3.2   Gestational Diabetes

Gestational diabetes mellitus (GDM) is diabetes which diagnosed during pregnancy and is not clearly overt diabetes. Chu *et al* showed that foetuses of GDM mothers have some cardiac function impairments. In GDM foetuses; cardiac ventricular walls were thicker and left atrial shortening fraction was smaller than foetuses of non-diabetic mothers. Left atrial shortening was negatively correlated with thicknesses of left ventricular walls and interventricular septum in foetuses of diabetic mother with poor glycemic control. However; good maternal glycemic control may delay the impairments, but cannot reduce the degree. Some cardiac changes in GDM foetuses were similar to those in pre-gestational diabetic pregnancies except for several parameters and their changing time. (Chu, *et al*., 2012)

3.3   Types of Cardiac Anomalies Associated with Gestational Diabetes

There is a wide range of cardiac anomalies observed in foetuses in pregnant diabetic women. Most types of cardiac structural lesions have been associated with diabetes mellitus, ranging from small septal defects to major heart disease. Table 2 summarizes the most encountered cardiac anomalies observed in foetuses of pregnant diabetic mothers.

Hypertrophic cardiomyopathy (adaptive hypertrophy)	Transposition of the great vessels
Pericardial effusion (15%)	Coarctation
Intermittent or persistent bradycardia	Single umbilical artery
Cardiomegaly	Hypoplastic left ventricle
Patent ductus arteriosus	Persistent truncus arteriosus
Patent foramen ovale	Visceral heterotaxia
Ventricular septal defect	Single ventricle
Atrial septal defect	Diabetic fetopathy associated heart failure
Tetralogy of Fallot	

Table 2: The most encountered cardiac anomalies observed in foetuses of pregnant diabetic mother

3.4   Fetal ECG Signs in Diabetes Mellitus

Gestational diabetes mellitus has a noticeable impact on the fetal heart rate and ECG. The alteration is slight but evident and reflects fetal wellbeing and correlate with neonatal reactivity. Only cCTG may allow detecting those slight but significant differences. Fetal ECG during delivery showed that significant ST depression is more prevalent in foetuses of diabetic mothers during delivery than in foetuses of non-diabetic mothers. These changes probably are not indicating hypoxia but an altered ability of the myocardium to respond to the stress of labour. Presence of these changes could give a significant add on information to predict moderate fetal acedemia (Yli *et al*., 2011; Veille *et al*., 1992).

3.5   Fetal Echocardiography Features in Diabetes Mellitus

The effectiveness of routine fetal echocardiographic screening in diabetic mothers has been thoroughly studied. However; selective fetal echocardiography should be considered after an abnormal detailed anatomic survey as a screening strategy for cardiac defects in pregnant diabetics. It can be done as early as in the first trimester of pregnancy which can help to alleviate a lot of anxiety the parents could have if the fetus is at high risk of having cardiac abnormalities such as in diabetic pregnancy. In most patients the resolution of images is sufficient to allow assessment of basic cardiac anatomy, when normal, or detection of complex malformations, when present. Fetal echocardiography can show structural defects in the fetal heart as well as the ability to look at rhythm abnormalities and other functional aspects of the fetal heart. In fetal echocardiography, the four-chamber view and the outflow-tract view are usually used to diagnose cardiac anomalies. Four-chamber view is technically very easy to obtain.

M-mode and 2-D echocardiography can show cardiomegaly (30%), asymmetric septal hypertrophy and fetal ventricular walls thickness. It may be manifested similar to idiopathic hypertrophic subaortic stenosis and increase progressively with advancing gestation. A diabetic cardiomyopathy has been proposed as a unique entity that is characterised by localised septal hypertrophy and accompanying cardiac dilatation (Veille *et al.*, 1992). This is in contrast to the prenatal symmetrical hypertrophy of the ventricular walls and may be explained by peri-natal changes of ventricular geometry. Fetal cardiac systolic function indicated by ejection fraction (EF) may be significantly increased in the presence of GDM independently of maternal glycemic control (Ren *et al.*, 2011). However, one disadvantage of the conventional M-mode derived cardiac function is that ventricular minor axis function is usually preserved in the fetal heart until there is overt myocardial dysfunction. Furthermore, ventricular filling velocities are affected by heart rate, packed cell volume, and myocardial thickness, all of which may be increased in foetuses of diabetic mothers (FDM) (Rizzo *et al.*, 1994). Doppler echocardiography can detect ventricular inflow and outflow velocities and altered fetal myocardial function in foetuses of diabetic mothers from the late first and mid trimesters. There is an accelerated increase in maximum and mean temporal velocities across atrioventricular valves through gestation relative to normal pregnancies with increased left and right ventricular output adjusted for fetal weight (Lisowski *et al.*, 2003). Lowered E/A wave ratio was observed in poor maternal glycaemic control, which may be indirectly due to changes in fetal heart rate, ventricular wall thickness and haematocrit (Rizzo *et al.*, 1994).

Tissue Doppler is a better technique to assess long-axis atrial and ventricular function than the conventional methods. Gardiner *et al* found that the absolute age related values of ventricular systolic and diastolic long-axis function is greater in foetuses of diabetic mothers than in foetuses of non- diabetic mothers which may reflect improved age-related cardiac performance. They demonstrated a significant increase in myocardial shortening velocities and long-axis amplitude of motion of the LV and septal free wall. Late lengthening myocardial velocities in the LV and RV free walls were also significantly increased, possibly in keeping with improved ventricular diastolic performance, despite the presence of increased ventricular and septal wall thickness. So, they considered this increase in cardiac function associated with cardiac hypertrophy as a form of functional adaptation. So; they suggest to rename the ''fetal diabetic cardiomyopathy'' as ''adaptive hypertrophy (Gardiner *et al.*, 2006).

4   Effect of Diabetes on Neonates and Infants

Neonates and infants could be the victim of maternal diabetes or they could suffer from the effects of diabetes that primarily affects them. The increased risk of cardiovascular problems associated with maternal diabetes is well recognised with an incidence of 1.7–4.0%. These problems can be categorized in 3 main groups which include cardiovascular mal-adaptation to extra-uterine life, congenital heart defects and hypertrophic cardiomyopathy. It is essential to be able to differentiate between these categories as the treatment is different for each one. Which could be helpful for one category may be harmful for another. For example using digoxin may be helpful in case of heart failure due to structural heart defects but harmful if used in cases with hypertrophic cardiomyopathy. The incidence of malformations is highest in mothers who were on insulin at the time of conception. (Day & Insley, 1976)

4.1 Cardiovascular Mal-adaptation to Extra-uterine Life

Adaptation to the extra-uterine life is a critical process in the neonatal life. Full-term healthy newborns demonstrate a predictable pattern of physiologic adaptations during the first 6 to 8 hours of life which is referred to as the transitional period during which the newborn makes dramatic adaptations to extra-uterine life required for neonatal survival. The most important changes are seen in the cardiovascular system that occurs when the fetal bypass shunts close and blood begins to circulate normally. Lungs filled with alveolar fluid must clear the fluid and adjust to the mechanics of breathing air with improving lung compliance. The pressure and concentration of blood gases and the binding properties of haemoglobin must also adjust, as well as the acid-base balance established by those factors. In addition, the newborn must gain the feedback mechanisms for respiratory control. The myocardial wall tension acutely increases because of the high systemic arterial pressure. During the fetal life the myocardium contracts against a low systemic pressure, whereas after delivery the systemic arterial pressure increase immediately due to obliteration of the umbilical blood flow and initiation of respiration (Þimßek et al., 1999).

Adaptations to each of these aspects of respiration occur during prenatal, natal and postnatal periods. Each stage is characterized by specific pulmonary physiology to which certain adjustments are made. Right ventricular systolic time intervals have been used in neonates to demonstrate both normal and abnormal cardiovascular adaptation to extra-uterine life. It was noted that IDM who presented with respiratory distress had prolonged isometric contraction phase of RV with elevated RV pre-ejection period (RVPEP)/RV ejection time (RVET) ratio (RVPEP/ RVET Ratio). This ratio correlates closely with pulmonary vascular resistance (PVR) and pulmonary artery diastolic pressure. This may suggests an abnormality of the transitional pulmonary circulation. There were also delayed closure of the ductus arteriosus and delayed postnatal decrease in pulmonary artery pressure in these neonates which could explain the increased frequency of respiratory disorders as well as the delay in the recovery of such infants. Primary pulmonary hypertension may be due to increased muscularization of small pulmonary arteries. It also associated with and aggravated by polycythemia which is frequently present in these neonates (Narchi & Kulaylat, 2000).

4.2 Congenital Heart Defects (CHD)

Infants of diabetic mother (IDM) are at a significant risk for CHD which occur in about 5% of them. "Overt" diabetes was present in 0.5% of mothers of babies with CHD. The highest relative risk for major cardiovascular defects occurs if the mother has gestational diabetes and develops insulin resistance in the 3rd trimester. The most frequent CHD in IDMs include ventricular septal defect (VSD), transposition of great arteries (TGA) and aortic stenosis. Defects involving the great arteries, including truncus arteriosus and double outlet right ventricle (DORV), are also more prevalent in IDMs (Narchi & Kulaylat, 2000). Mills and colleagues reported a number of cardiac malformations in infants of diabetic mothers in 1988. The abnormalities included anomalous origin of the left coronary artery from the pulmonary artery, co-arctation of the aorta, and atrial septal defect (ASD), malformations that are not usually apparent at this early age (Mills et al., 1988). Abu-Sulaiman and Subaih found in study included 100 consecutive IDMs that the most common echocardiographic findings were patent ductus arteriosus (PDA; 70%), patent foramen ovale (68%), ASD (5%), small muscular VSD (4%), mitral valve prolapse (2%), and pulmonary stenosis (1%). Hypertrophic cardiomyopathy (HCMP) was observed in 38% of cases, mainly hypertrophy of the interventricular septum. Severe forms of CHD encountered were D-transposition of great arteries, Tetralogy of Fallot (TOF), and hypoplastic left heart syndrome (1% each). Isolated aortic stenosis and coarctation of aorta were not encountered in this series. Overall incidence of congenital heart disease was 15% after excluding PDA and HCMP (Abu-Sulaiman & Subaih, 2004). Maternal diabetes increases the risk of having "conotruncal" defects (that included truncus arteriosus, TOF, TGA, and DORV) than in normal population. (Becerra *et al.*, 1990) These "conotruncal" malformations are dependent upon neural-crest-cell-derived ectomesenchymal tissues; these are precisely the conotruncal abnormalities that result from experimental ablation of the neural crest in chick embryos.

4.3   Hypertrophic Cardiomyopathy (HCMP)

Hypertrophic cardiomyopathy has been well documented in infants of diabetic mothers (IDMs). It was first observed in a stillborn infant of a diabetic mother by Maron *et al* (Maron *et al.*, 1978). Clinically manifest HCMP is present in 12.1% of IDMs, but the ratio rises up to 30% when routinely searched for with an echocardiographic scan. The severity of IDM-HCMP can vary from an incidental finding on echocardiography to an infant with severe symptoms of congestive heart failure. Fatal cases HCMP may occur in an infant of a diabetic mother. HCMP is a condition characterised by stiff, hypertrophied ventricular muscle, predominant thickening of the ventricular septum, impaired relaxation, and powerful but in-coordinate contraction. Functional subaortic obstruction may occur in severe cases and this is referred to as idiopathic hypertrophic subaortic stenosis (IHSS). Previous reports have suggested that a unique form of IHSS may occur transiently in infants of diabetic mothers and when it occurs it is generally benign and transient (Sheehan *et al.*, 1986). Natural history of IDM-HCMP appears to be benign, with a resolution of symptoms within 2-4 weeks and a resolution of septal hypertrophy within 2- 12 months. Most of the infants need only supportive care. If pharmacologic intervention is deemed necessary, propranolol appears to be the drug of choice. Natural history of this entity is that of spontaneous regression of symptoms and septal hypertrophy irrespective of therapy (Way *et al.*, 1979). However, fatal cases of HCMP were observed in cases with diabetic fetopathy. In the diabetic fetopathy; the affected neonates are macrosome, suffer from respiratory distress syndrome due to delayed lung maturity, acidosis, hypoglycaemia, electrolyte-imbalances and polycythaemia. Severe hypertrophy of the right ventricle is associated with intrauterine heart failure. However; HCMP could normalize within 6 weeks after birth without further treatment (Krautzig *et al.*, 1979). Echocardiography in such cases can demonstrate cardiomegaly, increases in thickness of the interventricular septum and RV and LV free wall with disproportionate septal hypertrophy in about one quarter of cases.

This increased myocardial thickness cannot be simply explained by being macrosomic infants because this thickness was also observed in small infants born to diabetic mothers and because the myocardial thickness in the large normal babies never exceeded the upper limit of normal value (Deorari *et al.*, 1999). Neonatal asymmetric septal hypertrophy is not specific for any disorder. It may present in normal infants when the ratio of septum:ventricular posterior wall >1.3. This can be distinguished from other pathological causes because there is no absolute increase in septal thickness. Asymmetric septal hypertrophy may be observed in familial cases, glycogen storage disease (type II), and any cause of right ventricular hypertension. In diabetes; the hypertrophy may be asymptomatic and regress over months. In Pompe's disease it presents at about 3-4 months of age. (Maron *et al.*, 1974)

4.4 Neonatal Diabetes Mellitus

Neonatal DM, defined as insulin-requiring hyperglycemia within the first month of life. Neonatal DM was also described in association with CHD. Permanent neonatal DM due to pancreatic Partial agenesis/hypoplasia with congenital heart defects has been reported. Pancreatic agenesis can be associated with intra-uterine growth retardation, dysmorphic features, non-specific immunodeficiency, and malformations of the heart, the biliary tract, and the cerebellum. Transient neonatal DM is caused by over expression of a gene cluster at 6q24. CHD may be one of the anomalies associated with transient neonatal DM; plus severe intrauterine growth retardation, structural brain anomalies, macroglossia, developmental delay, and umbilical hernia (Balasubramanian *et al*., 2008; Taha *et al*., 2010).

5 Effect of Diabetes on Childhood and Adolescence

Diabetes mellitus is one of the most severe chronic diseases of childhood and adolescence. Most pediatric patients with diabetes are of T1 DM. For the age between 10-19 years; T1 DM is more common than T2 DM. The prevalence rate is 2.28 per 1,000 for T1 DM and 0.42 per 1,000 for those with T2 DM (Faulkner, 2010). In the United States; each year more than 13,000 children are diagnosed with T1 DM. Fifty percent of subjects with T1 DM are diagnosed within the first 15 years of life. While most new pediatric diabetic cases are of T1 DM, there are increasing numbers of older children and adolescents with T2 DM in response to childhood obesity and sedentary life with increasing detection of more cases of T2 DM among children (Krishnan & Short, 2009). With the increasing number of children and young youth being diagnosed with DM; there is an increasing incidence of premature heart disease in early adulthood. Both types of diabetes often coexists with other multiple cardiovascular risk factors, including hyperlipidemia, hypertension, and obesity and may be associated with poor cardiovascular outcome.

5.1 Cardiovascular Complications Associated with Childhood and Adolescent's Diabetes

The following cardiovascular complications are usually associated with childhood and adolescent's diabetes:

5.1.1 Impaired Vascular Functions and Accelerated Atherosclerosis

Endothelial dysfunction in children with DM is an indicator of future cardiovascular events and atherosclerotic changes were observed to occur much earlier than the appearance of clinical diabetes. Children and adolescents with T1 DM have more rate of endothelial dysfunction than non-diabetic age-matched control children, as measured by flow-mediated dilation (FMD) in the brachial artery. These children have adverse carotid remodelling which increase the future cardiovascular risk (Järvisalo *et al*., 2004). Early signs of abnormal vascular homeostasis including impaired endothelial function; increased carotid intima-media thickness; and increased markers of systemic inflammation may appear in prepubertal children with T1 DM. So, diabetic children are at increased risk of early asymptomatic atherosclerosis, and cardiovascular morbidity and mortality are substantially increased in this group of patients. The atherosclerotic process starts in childhood and proceeds silently over a long period of time before clinical events occur. Several studies in children and adolescents with T1 DM have consistently reported increased carotid artery intima-media thickness (c-IMT) compared with healthy control subjects. cIMT is a reliable surrogate marker of generalized atherosclerosis because it correlates to coronary artery disease and predicts future cardiovascular events. cIMT correlates well with cardiovascular risk factors and coronary atherosclerosis and is an independent predictor of future cardiovascular disorders (CVD) (Margeirsdottir *et al.*, 2010). With the limited available data about markers of subclinical atherosclerosis in pediatric populations, there is a need for more studies, including those of a longitudinal design.

Dyslipidemia is a disorder of lipoprotein metabolism that results in increased total cholesterol, high low density lipoprotein cholesterol (LDL-C), low high-density lipoprotein cholesterol (HDL-C), and high triglycerides (TG). Although dyslipidemia is an established risk factor for CVD in adults, no long-term studies directly link dyslipidemia in childhood with subsequent CVD (Hong, 2010). There was a trend of increased HDL cholesterol levels and significantly reduced cholesterol–to– HDL cholesterol ratios in preadolescent children with T1 DM. Despite the athero-protective effect of the higher plasma HDL cholesterol levels but in the setting of T1 DM, this HDL cholesterol may be dysfunctional in combating the adverse, pro-inflammatory, and pro-atherogenic effects of oxidized LDL cholesterol.   The presence of dysfunctional HDL cholesterol would make type 1 diabetic subjects more vulnerable to oxidative vascular damage despite higher absolute levels (Babar *et al.*, 2011).

These atherosclerotic changes affect both small and large blood vessels. Small vessel affection increases the risk for tissue injury in organs supplied by an endarterial system due to microangiopathy. These microvascular complications include nephropathy, retinopathy, and neuropathy while macrovascular disease including heart disease and stroke (Moore *et al.*, 2009). Improved glycaemic control obtained by intensive insulin treatment is associated with delayed atherosclerosis development and fewer cardiovascular events. Prevention and screening for vascular complications are important in the care of children and adolescents with T1DM. Target levels to reduce the risk of microvascular and macrovascular complications in children and adolescents with T1 DM are the following: HbA1c <7.5%, lipids in normal range, blood pressure <90th percentile by age, sex and height, BMI <95th percentile, no smoking and adequate physical activity (Fröhlich-Reiterer & Borkenstein, 2010).

5.1.2   Hypertension

Hypertension is considered as a major cardiovascular risk factor in young patients with T1 DM. Both pre-hypertension and hypertension are common disorders in young patients with diabetes. The prevalence of pre-hypertension is associated with older age, longer duration of diabetes and the shift of the sympatho-vagal balance toward sympathetic activation (Szadkowska *et al.*, 2006). Hypertension is 2–3 times more frequent in children and adolescent with diabetes compared with the general population especially nocturnal hypertension when compared to diurnal hypertension. Persistently elevated blood pressures can induce serious complications on both the micro- and macrovascular level. On the other hand; children with T2 DM often have several risk factors for elevated blood pressures, such as obesity, family history, and generally poor cardiovascular health. Nocturnal hypertension is a risk factor of diabetic nephropathy. It is related to higher BMI and triglycerides and with lower HDL cholesterol. Type I diabetic patients have high incidence of non-dipping hypertension which related to increase in target organ damage such as diabetic nephropathy and cardiovascular events. The onset of renal pathology seen in diabetes is usually noted around the time when blood pressure elevations begin. In diabetic nephropathy; the patients initially develop microalbuminuria which progress to gross proteinuria with widespread microvascular nephropathy. Elevated blood pressure occurs with development of glomerular damage. However, it has also been shown that increases in systolic blood pressure during sleep can precede the onset of microalbuminuria in patients with T1 DM which may denote other mechanisms implicated in the pathogenesis of hypertension other than diabetic nephropathy (Moore *et al.*, 2009; Basiratnia *et al.*, 2012).

Lee *et al* showed significant increase in carotid intima-media thickness (c-IMT) and daytime blood pressure in diabetic children and adolescents with nocturnal hypertension. c-IMT is a good measure for identifying subclinical atherosclerosis. This means that subclinical atherosclerosis is another possible mechanism for the diabetes-associated hypertension (Lee *et al.*, 2011). Children with T1 DM and hypertension have a higher level of vascular endothelial growth factor (VEFG) in serum compared with Children with T1 DM without hypertension, and the healthy control group. The VEGF may have an important function in the modification of tissue damage and its acceleration. It induces vascular endothelial cell proliferation and migration and increases the permeability of renal glomerular and retinal capillaries. So; measurement of VEGF serum levels allows for the identification of groups of patients who have the highest risk of hypertension and, subsequently, progression of vascular complications (Zorena *et al.*, 2011). Also children with diastolic hypertension have higher level of E-selectin which is an early atherosclerosis biomarker. Diastolic BP z-scores were associated with E-selectin level in children with T1 DM. Polymorphism of angiotensin-converting enzyme (ACE) gene was observed in some T1 DM children with pre-hypertension or with nocturnal BP abnormalities even if they are normotensive and normo-albuminuric. (Maggio *et al.*, 2012) Poor glycaemic control and male gender are risk factors for abnormal systolic BP as measured by 24-hour ambulatory blood pressure monitoring. So, it is important to evaluate renal function and BP even when they are in normal range to minimize the deleterious effects of hypertension in the development of nephropathy and cardiovascular disease.

5.1.3 Cardiac Dysfunction and Diabetic Cardiomyopathy

Diabetes mellitus can induce a pattern of myocardial pathology known as specific diabetic cardiomyopathy, even if this is not clearly specified. Diabetic cardiomyopathy is responsible for the increased incidence of heart failure in diabetic patients even in absence of coronary atherosclerosis or arterial hypertension. This diabetic cardiomyopathy has been suggested to cause systolic and/or diastolic dysfunction. The cause of this cardiomyopathy is debatable. The dysfunction of autonomic nervous system can cause higher heart rate in diabetic patients than observed in normal subjects and may affect the cardiac haemodynamics. Hypertrophy, increased diastolic stiffness and noncompliance of LV with increased LV wall thickness and mass are other possible causes of diastolic dysfunction which occurs early in the course of T1 DM even in absence of hypertension. There is reduction of LV end-systolic wall stress which is used as an indicator of LV after-load which can be roughly approached by certain non-invasive measurements, including systolic blood pressure and aortic pulse wave velocity, which are related to LV after-load. Also, the impairment of ventricular relaxation may be related to cardiac fibrosis, abnormal calcium transport in the sarcoplasmic reticulum, and the increased levels of advanced glycation end products, formed by non-enzymatic glycation of proteins or lipids. These advanced glycation end products can increase the cross linking of proteins like collagen and elastin, causing reduced tissue elasticity and decreased protein turnover (Tavares *et al.*, 2012; Suys *et al.*, 2004).

Even with normal systolic ventricular functions, the diabetic children may suffer diastolic dysfunction as expressed by reduced LV compliance which could serve as an early marker of diabetic cardiomyopathy even before clinical symptoms appear. The degree of diastolic dysfunction correlates with the severity of the diabetic complications. More pronounced diastolic dysfunction was found in presence of severe vascular complications. Girls are more liable to diabetic cardiomyopathy and more significant changes in LV dimensions than boys. These sex differences may be related to the significant higher BMI or HbA1c in girls or related to the role of hormonal changes. However, some studied showed no correlation of diabetes duration and HbA1c with the cardiovascular changes. Children and young adolescents rarely have good health education and proper insight regarding their disease, and their diet is accordingly difficult to control. Therefore, alteration of myocardial function induced by diabetes may begin earlier than is generally thought and these changes may be accelerated when glycemic control is poor. Early manifestations of diabetic cardiomyopathy have been suggested to contribute to depressed levels of aerobic fitness described in children and adolescents with this disease. These early manifestations produce certain echocardiographic abnormalities in asymptomatic young diabetic adolescents and can be elucidated by post-exercise echocardiography. This test is a non-invasive procedure that can easily be done in the adolescent population and is useful for evaluating subclinical cardiomyopathy. Diabetic cardiomyopathy could occur in both types of diabetes. However, Adolescent-onset T2 DM is often coexists with multiple other cardiovascular risk factors, including hyperlipidemia, hypertension, and obesity and is associated with poor cardiovascular outcome. This explains the more prevalence of diabetic cardiomyopathy in children and adolescents with T2 DM than those with T1 DM. ACE inhibitors and non-selective B-blockers have been proposed to prevent or treat diabetic cardiomyopathy (Baum *et al.*, 1987; Eun *et al.*, 2010; Gillian *et al.*, 2009).

5.1.4   Cardiac Autonomic Dysfunction

Cardiac autonomic neuropathy (CAN) is a common complication in T1 DM and is frequent in subclinical stages. Its prognostic value has been demonstrated and is associated with an increased morbidity and mortality. Sudden death and cardio-respiratory arrest in patients with T1 DM and T2 DM have been attributed to cardiac autonomic dysfunction. It is a part of the well studied diabetic autonomic neuropathy which is a well recognized complication of T1 DM. It can induce different functional cardiac changes, especially a reduction in LV contractility and changes in ventricular repolarisation. It is also associated with changes in the daily variations in blood pressure (Valensi, 2000). Cardiac autonomic neuropathy involves both parasympathetic and sympathetic systems. There is an early parasympathetic impairment that may raise the heart rate, but as the duration of the diabetes increases, sympathetic involvement occurs that may relatively slow the heart rate (Elamin *et al.*, 2009).

The development of autonomic complications depends on the diabetes duration, glycemic control and patient age. Rapid progression of the diabetic autonomic neuropathy could occur with the pubertal spurt. Chronic hyperglycemia and microvascular abnormalities induce certain enzymes activation that play important roles in the progressive nerve fibers damage in patients with longstanding T1 DM. Early neuropathic changes as endoneural edema or intra-axonal sodium accumulation could be reversed by intensified glycaemic control. Hormonal changes during puberty and prolonged periods of poor metabolic control could induce irreversible neuropathic changes which emphasize for the importance of early detection of cardiac autonomic dysfunction and motivation of the patients to improve their diabetes control that hopefully could delay the development of complications with strict follow up especially during the puberty stage (Massin *et al.*, 1999).

Clinically; diabetic cardiac autonomic neuropathy could be detected early by the increased resting heart rate, decreased heart rate variation to deep breathing (deep breathing test), and diminished heart rate response to standing or sustained handgrip tests. There was impairment of the parasympathetic control of heart rate in young patients with diabetes as detected by deep breathing test. Study of heart rate variations during deep respiration (which test parasympathetic function), active orthostatism (which test sympathetic function) or Valsalva manoeuvre, is still the reference. Heart rate variability (HRV) is a sensitive, reproducible, non-invasive method and is able to determine early cardiac autonomic neuropathy independent of the patient's cooperation. It depends on the influence of sympathetic and vagal activity on the sinus node and can easily be determined from 24-h Holter recordings. It is one of the first indices of cardiac dysautonomia observed in young diabetic patients. Squat test (1-min standing, 1-min squatting, 1-min standing) can be used with continuous monitoring of HR and BP, using a Finapres device. This active test imposes greater postural stress than the passive head-up tilt test, and provokes large changes in BP and HR that can be analyzed to derive indices of cardiac autonomic neuropathy. In healthy subjects, squatting is associated with increase in BP and decrease in HR, whereas the squat-stand transition is accompanied by a deep but transient drop in BP associated with sympathetic-driven tachycardia. In diabetic patients with cardiac autonomic neuropathy, BP increases are accentuated during squatting whereas reflex brady-cardia is reduced. When standing from squatting position, the fall in BP tends to be more pronounced and orthostatic hypotension is more prolonged, while reflex tachycardia is markedly dampened (Philips *et al.*, 2011). Another sign of cardiac autonomic neuropathy is a reduced gain of the baroreflex regulation of the heart period. Prolonged Q-Tc intervals were also found in presence of cardiac autonomic neuropathy. Impaired circadian blood pressure (BP) variation with impaired nocturnal BP reduction has been associated with autonomic dysfunction. Orthostatic hypotension is a late sign of sympathetic nervous system disease. Spectral analysis of blood pressure variations on orthostatism or the study of cutaneous blood flow during activating the sympathetic system can help in identifying autonomic neuropathy. Diabetic children also showed reduced baroreceptor sensitivity (BRS). The degree of BRS impairment was related to the degree of autonomic imbalance and with positively correlated with the disease duration (Dalla Poz-za, Bechtold *et al.*, 2007).

Microalbuminuria is an independent predictive of autonomic dysfunction as same pathological processes, such as microvascular complications may lead to both neuropathy and nephropathy. Pupillom-etry and studying urinary bladder function may indicate presence of autonomic dysfunction in type 1 dia-betic child but do not reflect cardiac autonomic dysfunction. However, there is a high risk of development of diabetic cardiac autonomic neuropathy in children with T1 DM in the presence of the autonomic dys-function syndrome (Manukian *et al.*, 2011). It has been shown that the early treatment of functional dis-turbances of the autonomic nervous system using transcranial magnetic stimulation is necessary to pre-vent the manifestation of diabetic cardiac autonomic neuropathy.

5.1.5   Impaired Physical fitness and Cardiovascular Endurance

There is a reciprocal relationship between glucose tolerance, physical fitness and cardiovascular endur-ance. Higher levels of fitness at baseline are protective against the development of impaired glucose tol-erance. Also, impairments in glucose regulation are associated with lower fitness levels. The protective effect of fitness on glucose homeostasis could be due to exercise induced alterations in skeletal muscle substrate metabolism with specific adaptations to skeletal muscle such as increased mitochondrial volume and density and oxidative enzyme capacity which in turn lead to improvements in glucose metabolism. Physical activity directly improves insulin sensitivity through increased skeletal muscle glucose uptake, and indirectly through improvements in body composition. Despite the fact that exercise stimulates glu-cose uptake, a certain amount of insulin is required. In children with T1 DM, exercise occasionally may result in a worsening of their glucose control if the endogenous insulin is not enough. However, patients with T2 DM have sufficient endogenous insulin available and very rarely develop hyperglycemia with ketosis in response to exercise. Children with good metabolic control should respond well to exercise. (Shaibi *et al.*, 2006; Kollipara & Warren-Boulton, 2004)

Children and adolescents with T1 DM may have some impaired fitness-related components and al-terations in their cardio-respiratory responses to exercise. The maximal aerobic power and physical work capacity are reduced especially with fair to poor metabolic control. This may be due to reduced level of habitual activity, a smaller body stature, or impairment in cardio-respiratory or skeletal muscle function. Other possible causes may be due to associated high systolic blood pressure, lower O_2 pulse, a thickening of capillary basement membrane in skeletal muscle, impairments in the regulation of skeletal muscle blood flow and impaired nerve conduction velocity (Riddell & Iscoe, 2006). On the other side; low cardiorespiratory fitness is observed in patients with impaired glucose tolerance and T2 DM. Despite the education on the importance of increased physical activity for diabetes management given to the diabetic youth; they spent nearly 60% less time per day in moderate to vigorous activities compared to their non-diabetic counterparts. Lower fitness was observed in overweight and severely insulin resistant diabetic adolescents. This lower fitness is due to impairments in oxidative capacity of skeletal muscle as a result of mitochondrial dysfunction and hence impaired oxidative metabolism and because of the circulatory defects which limit oxygen delivery to exercising muscle. However; children with T1 DM have better cardio-respiratory fitness than those with type 2 (Shaibi et al., 2006).

Gender, BMI, metabolic control, and physical activity were strong predictors of cardiovascular endurance, regardless of type of DM. Females are exhibiting at least 20% lower capacity than males. This decrease in the levels of cardiovascular endurance in females versus males increases as they age into later adolescence. There is a significant inverse relationship between cardiovascular endurance and most lipid profile's components and systolic blood pressure in poor controlled T1DM children and adolescents; found independently of body adiposity (Lobstein et al., 2004). American Diabetes Association (2010) presently recommends that Hb A1C values to be maintained below 7.5% to improve long-term health outcomes (American Diabetes Association, 2010). The Physical Activity Guidelines for (2008) and the Exercise in Medicine initiative of the American College of Sports Medicine (2010) emphasize at least 60 minutes of moderate to vigorous activity on most days for adolescents (Group SfDiYS,2006). Physically fit adolescents with T1 DM can have better overall glucose control and a reduction in serum lipids (Miculis et al., 2012).

5.1.6   Cardiac Effects of Diabetes-associated Obesity

Diabetes and obesity are related to each other. Adolescents with T2 DM have a higher tendency towards obesity and obese children are more prone to develop T2 DM. The increased risk of T2 DM in obese children is not well understood. It could be due to the increased body fat; and possibly specific depots of body fat such as visceral fat which have unique effects on insulin resistance. The increased frequency of obesity in T2 DM may be due to poor cardiorespiratory fitness coupled with a sedentary lifestyle. Obese diabetic children are associated with various risk factors for cardiovascular disease and early development of atherosclerotic lesions. They are 4.5 times more likely to have adverse levels of cholesterol, LDL-cholesterol, HDL-cholesterol, triglycerides, and blood pressure, respectively, than normal weight subjects. In addition, obese children have elevated levels of hemostatic and inflammatory factors, including fibrinogen, plasminogen activator inhibitor 1, and C-reactive protein which contribute to endothelial dysfunction and early atherosclerosis. Syndrome X or the Insulin Resistance Syndrome is a combination of obesity, hyperglycemia, hyperinsulinemia, dyslipidemia, and hypertension. This collection of risk factors increases the chance of developing heart disease (Goran et al., 2003). With the increasing level of insulin in insulin resistant syndrome; the insulin will stimulate renal sodium retention while increasing free water clearance. Insulin resistance is also associated with increased sympathetic nervous system activity and stimulation of vascular smooth muscle growth which is an important risk factor for hypertension and early atherosclerosis (Steinberger et al., 2003).

5.2   Risk Factors for Cardiac Complications in Childhood and Adolescent Diabetes

5.2.1   Type of Diabetes Mellitus

Children and adolescents with T2 DM have more cardiovascular risk factors than those with T1 DM. Rodriguez *et al* showed that about 14% of youths with T1 DM and about 92% of youths with T2 DM have two or more traditional cardiovascular disease (CVD) risk factors present in addition to glucose intolerance (Rodriguez *et al.*, 2006). Faulkner conducted a study on 151 diabetic adolescents which showed significantly greater body mass index and age-adjusted BMI percentile for adolescents with type 2 than for those with T1 DM, denoting more characteristic overweight noted with the former group. Systolic and diastolic blood pressure and triglycerides were significantly higher in those with T2 DM; whereas, HDL-c, CV fitness, and physical activity expenditure (METS) were significantly lower than for those with T1 DM (Faulkner, 2010). Cardiovascular endurance and heart rate variability were significantly lower in adolescents with T2 DM in comparison to those with T1 DM. (Faulkner *et al* 2005)

5.2.2   Age at Onset of the Disease

Pozza *et al* found a direct correlation between the cIMT and risk factors for CVD with the age at onset of diabetes. The earlier the onset of T1 DM is, the more the intima-media thickness (Dalla Pozza, *et al.*, 2007). Also Schwab *et al* showed in a study involved more than 27,000 German children and young adults with T1 DM that the presence of cardiovascular risk factors increased with age, suggesting the need for early screening and counselling to prevent their occurrence and early treatment if present (Schwab *et al.*, 2006).

5.2.3   Gender Difference

Girls with T1 DM had significantly increased mean Hb A1C levels, body mass index, LDL cholesterol, and C-reactive protein, compared with boys who have the disease. In a study done by Zhou *et al*, the male group showed that BMI z–scores have significant positive correlations with insulin resistance and diastolic blood pressure while in the female group, BMI z–scores showed significant positive correlations with insulin resistance and systolic blood pressure (Zhou *et al.*, 2010). Study performed in adults with T1 DM, showed unexpected increased female risk for microvascular complications in T1 DM (Monti *et al.*, 2007). Also female adolescents showed lower levels of cardiovascular endurance than male adolescents (Faulkner *et al* 2005). Girls with T1 DM are particularly at risk of being overweight. They need larger insulin dose, and their HbA1c and cholesterol levels are higher than boys with T1 DM suggesting that girls are at increased insulin resistance and cardiovascular risk (Davis *et al.*, 2012).

5.2.4   Puberty

Puberty is another risk factor that enhances development of vascular complications in diabetic children and the majority of the complications initially present or become more significant after the onset of puberty. This increased risk is due to numerous factors associated with puberty as impaired compliance with treatment during adolescent stage, the increase in blood pressure, and the effect of the increasingly produced sex steroids on hyperglycemia (Moore *et al.*, 2009).

5.2.5   Body Mass Index

There is an increased prevalence of obesity among diabetic children and adolescent especially those with T2 DM. Obesity itself is associated with increased cardiac dimensions and higher LV mass. Adolescent obesity has been previously associated with increased LV volumes and mass (Chinali *et al.*, 2006). It is also associated with diastolic dysfunction and may independently lead to heart failure (Kenchaiah *et al.*, 2002). Obesity is an important factor contributing to structural changes in the heart augmenting the cardiovascular changes that occur in diabetes as impaired diastolic and systolic function, increased LV filling pressure, as well as increase left atrial volume which is used as a marker of long-standing diastolic disease. The higher LV mass in obese diabetic children and adolescents may reflect normal physiological growth in response to higher fat-free mass (FFM) as LV mass is related to body composition, in particular FFM. There is also increase risk of hypertension among the obese children. Patients with a higher BMI had a higher systolic and diastolic BP, and also higher total and LDL cholesterol levels. A significant thickening of the endothelial wall has been demonstrated in obese children. Obesity increases the risk of insulin resistance in the young diabetics which increases the risk of hypertension, and abnormal lipid profile. So; it is reasonable to suggest that lifestyle modification and weight control in childhood could reduce the risk of developing the insulin resistance syndrome, T2 DM, and cardiovascular disease. As obesity is associated with hypertension and dyslipidemia, a patient's poor nutritional status is of high risk of developing diabetic vascular complications. (Whalley *et al.*, 1999; August *et al.*, 2008; Villa *et al.*, 2000)

5.2.6   Metabolic Control (HbA1c)

Poor metabolic control among adolescents is related to their changing physiology (pubertal growth and development) as well as to behavioral and adherence issues. Young diabetics with poorer metabolic control tended to have lower levels of cardiovascular endurance (Faulkner *et al.*, 2005). Poor metabolic control can lead to early onset of diabetic neuropathy and development of severe consequences including cardiovascular autonomic dysfunction and ventilatory dysfunction during sleep. Good metabolic control is crucial for the prevention of long- term diabetic complications. Good metabolic control and intensified insulin therapy are associated with a better health-related quality of life (Wagner *et al.*, 2005). Lower HbA1c was significantly associated with better adolescent-rated quality of life (Hoey *et al.*, 2001). Metabolic control is an important determinant of lipid profile in diabetic children. Metabolic control may contribute to the subsequent risk of cardiovascular disease and possibly the development of incipient diabetic nephropathy (Abraha *et al.*, 1999).

5.2.7   Exercise Beliefs and Physical Activity

Cardiovascular fitness is the direct measure of maximal oxygen uptake during a participant's exercise of progressive intensity. Exercise is an essential component in blood glucose regulation for T1 DM patients, along with insulin management. Adolescents with T1 DM, being more physically fit can lead to better overall glucose control and a reduction in serum lipids. Exercise fitness was associated with improved lipids, Hb A1c, health perception, cardiovascular fitness, and athletic competence in adolescents with T1 DM (Faulkner, 2010). Physical activity is a strong predictor of cardiovascular fitness and exercise beliefs consistently predicted both frequency and time domain heart rate variability (HRV) measures (Faulkner *et al.*, 2005). Early findings of poor physical fitness; lower HRV; fewer positive beliefs about exercise, and less active lifestyles highlight the importance of developing culturally sensitive interventions for assisting youth to make lifelong changes in their physical activity routines. Females, those with poorer metabolic control, and minority youth with T2 DM may be particularly vulnerable to later cardiovascular disease (Faulkner *et al.*, 2005).

5.3   Electrocardiography (ECG) Finding in Diabetic Children

5.3.1   Heart Rate Variability

Heart rate variability (HRV) is good tool to measure the cardiac autonomic control, and disturbances in HRV have been documented in patients with diabetic autonomic neuropathy. HRV can be determined using 24-h Holter recordings. HRV depends on the balanced effects of both sympathetic and vagal activity on the sinus node. HRV analysis can characterize and quantify variations in sympathetic and vagal activity and has been used to foster a better understanding of physiological and pathological processes in adults and children (Massin *et al.*, 1999). In diabetic children with mean Hb A1c >10%; a reduction in HRV was predictive for onset of symptomatic autonomic neuropathy (Rollins *et al.*, 1992). Therefore, all T1 DM patients should be screened by HRV analysis for that complication beginning at the first stage of puberty regardless of illness duration, microalbuminuria, and level of metabolic control.

5.3.2   P wave Dispersion

Another tool to evaluate the cardiovascular autonomic function is P wave dispersion. P wave dispersion is an ECG index that measures the difference between the longest and the shortest P wave duration recorded from multiple different ECG surface leads. It shows a diurnal variation in healthy subjects such as shortest in summer and longest in winter. It has a good predictive value for assessment the risk of having atrial fibrillation (AF) in various subclinical cardiac disorders (Kose *et al.*, 2002). In diabetic children; there was an increase in the dispersion of the p wave that could reveal the onset of cardiac electrophysiological heterogeneity before it is possible to detect autonomic (both parasympathetic and sympathetic) dysfunction with other tests (Imamoglu *et al.*, 2008).

5.3.3   Corrected QT interval (QTc)

Prolonged QTc interval and a larger QTc dispersion were found in a significant proportion of children and adolescents with diabetes. QT interval was found to be prolonged in diabetic children and adolescents, with no interrelationship in patients between Hb A1c, diabetes duration and length of QTc. However, moderate correlation was found between dose of insulin administered in 24 hours and length of QTc (Riabykina *et al.*, 2007). The same finding was confirmed by Shiono *et al* who studied children and adolescents aged 7-20 years with poor glycaemic control (Hb A1c > 10%) with signal-averaged ECG; they found a prolonged filtered QRS duration and a significantly low root mean square voltage, demonstrating subclinical cardiac impairment (Shiono *et al.*, 2001). In difficult controlled diabetes, hyperinsulinemia-induced hypoglycaemia can prolong the QTc interval and decrease T-wave area and amplitude. Murphy *et al* showed that young subjects with T1 DM had prolonged QTc which occurred frequently with spontaneous overnight hypoglycaemia which may be related to insulin-induced hypokalaemia. Prolonged QTc also occurs frequently during DKA and is correlated with ketosis. This abnormal cardiac repolarisation occurs consistently during insulin-induced hypoglycaemia. Potassium infusion or beta-blockade prevents increased QT dispersion but only partially prevents QT lengthening (Murphy *et al.*, 2004).

5.4   Echocardiographic Finding in Diabetic Children

Children and early adolescents with DM rarely have insight on the significance of DM, and their diet is difficult to control. An alteration of myocardial function induced by DM may begin earlier than generally thought, and these changes are accelerated when glycaemic control is poor. These impose the need for early detection of the cardiac dysfunction among those children. Doppler echocardiography is a reliable simple non-invasive and reproducible tool to assess early impairment of cardiac function and for serial follow up of such patients. Diastolic dysfunction was twice as common as systolic dysfunction. The diabetes induced myocardial damage affects diastolic function before systolic function. Diastolic abnormalities could be observed even in absence of other complication but both diastolic and systolic dysfunction usually observed in presence of severe cardiac complications. Early diastolic dysfunction showed an early impairment of LV filling and is expressed by reduced LV compliance. Diastolic dysfunction is manifested by significant reduction of E wave and E/A ratio with more contribution of atrial component to the LV filling greater than 0.25. Diastolic dysfunction is also associated significant prolongation of isovolumic relaxation time. These changes are more evident during isometric exercise.

Stress Doppler echocardiography is a reliable tool to detect early diastolic dysfunction in diabetic patients. The diastolic dysfunction related to diabetes duration, cardiac autonomic dysfunction and genetic factors but its relation to glycaemic control or microvascular complications is controversial. A reduced LV cavity size and increased atrial ejection were noted in children with insulin-dependent diabetes even in absence of hypertension, nephropathy or ischaemic heart disease, suggesting the existence of a metabolically-induced cardiomyopathy. Using M-mode echocardiography, morphological parameters and systolic time-intervals (fractional shortening; ejection fraction) could be determined. M-mode echocardiography showed a high prevalence of echocardiographic abnormalities in diabetic patients that increased with age. Mean dimensions of the left atrium, RV, and LV (systolic and diastolic) could be increased significantly in diabetic individuals. Hypertrophy of the interventricular septum was present in some patients older than 12 yr of age. Echocardiographic abnormalities in asymptomatic young diabetic adolescents can be elucidated by post-exercise echocardiography (Kim *et al*., 2010; Baum *et al*., 1987).

6   Prevention of Complications of Diabetes Mellitus

6.1   Measures to Decrease Effects of Diabetes on Fetal Cardiovascular System

If the pregnancy is planned, the most important aim is to achieve the best possible glycaemic control in women entering their reproductive years before pregnancy to prevent major forms of cardiac and non-cardiac anomalies. Implementation of preconception counselling, emphasizing strict glycaemic control before and throughout pregnancy reduces the rate of perinatal mortality and malformations. Intensive glucose management should be initiated with a goal to keep Hb A1C around 6.1%. Dietary and diabetic counselling should be offered with daily multivitamin with at least 400 g of folic acid. Unfortunately; unplanned pregnancy occurs in about two-thirds of women with diabetes leading to a persistent excess of malformations in their infants (Vargas *et al*., 2010). Counselling against pregnancy should be done in patients with Hb A1C ≥10%. Comprehensive ophthalmologic examination and thyroid function tests should be performed with strict follow up of renal functions. Pre-pregnancy care from specialised multi-disciplinary clinics, involving optimisation of glycaemic control and prescription of folic acid, could considerably decrease the observed rates of malformation. It is now routine practice to advice women to take 5 mg of folic acid daily before conception and for the first trimester (Taylor & Davison., 2007).

During pregnancy; adequate glycaemic control should be maintained. Fluctuations in glucose values rather than basal state may be more important determinants of fetal cardiac and general somatic growth in maternal diabetes. Diabetic counselling should be readily available to help manage rapidly changing insulin requirements. Insulin pump should be considered if proper glycaemic control is not attainable. Repeating ophthalmologic assessment should be done at 16-18 weeks if baseline retinal examination was abnormal and at 28 weeks if ophthalmologic assessment was normal at baseline. Fetal anatomy scan with 4-chamber cardiac imaging should be performed at 18-20 weeks for early detection of major cardiac anomalies. Monthly fetal ultrasound to assess growth and amniotic fluid levels should be performed after 28 weeks of gestation with daily fetal movement counts. Biweekly fetal monitoring (NST) can be started at 32 weeks of gestation, or earlier if needed. Maternal immune-stimulation and maternal antioxidant therapy in fetal protection against exposure to teratogens such as DM are not yet completely elucidated and are worth research attention (Punareewattana *et al.*, 2004). Delivery at about 38 weeks' gestation is advised for women with DM to minimise the risk of unexplained late fetal death. The timing and mode of delivery should be determined on an individual basis based on best possible assessments of risk to mother and baby.

6.2 Measures to Decrease Effects of Diabetes on Neonates and Infants

Strict diabetes control before and during pregnancy may reduce the severity of HCMP. However, other studies found no relationships between the echocardiographic results and the metabolic control of pregnancy or fetal characteristics, suggesting that strict maternal diabetes control may not prevent accelerated fetal cardiac growth and abnormal development of cardiac function (Sheehan *et al.*, 1986). The high incidence of the cardiac manifestations in IDM and the risk of occurrence of some severe problems, require a complete cardiac examination from the first few days of life and a follow-up schedule until the normalization of the cardiac parameters (Dimitriu *et al.*, 2004).

6.3 Measures to Decrease Effects of Diabetes on Children and Adolescents

Controlling weight gain, and enhancing physical activity, and improvement in glycemic control are important aspects to decrease the cardiovascular complication in diabetic children and adolescents. It is important to keep LDL-cholesterol in diabetic children and adolescents less than 100 mg/dl. They have to follow a meal plan developed by a registered dietician, diabetes educator, or physician. Those children need to practice regular physical activity, ideally a total of 60 minutes each day. Physical activity helps to lower blood glucose levels and increase insulin sensitivity, especially in children with type II. It is important to monitor hypertension among those children. ACE inhibitors should be considered for the treatment of hypertension in children as they have beneficial effects on slowing progression or preventing diabetic nephropathy (Rosenbloom *et al.*, 2009).

References

Abraha A, Schultz C, Konopelska-Bahu T, James T, Watts A, Stratton IM, Matthews DR, Dunger DB. (1999) *Glycaemic control and familial factors determine hyperlipidaemia in early childhood diabetes. Oxford Regional Prospective Study of Childhood Diabetes. Diabet Med. 16(7):598-604.*

Abu-Sulaiman RM, Subaih B. (2004) Congenital heart disease in infants of diabetic mothers: echocardiographic study. Pediatr Cardiol. 25(2):137-40.

Aljada A. (2003) Endothelium, Inflammation and Diabetes. Metab Syndr Relat Disord; 1: 3-21.

American Diabetes Association. (2010) Standards of medical care in diabetes--2010. Diabetes Care. 33(1): S11–S61.

Amiri F, Venema VJ, Wang X, Ju H, Venema RC, Marrero MB. (1999) Hyperglycemia enhances angiotensin II-induced janus-activated kinase/STAT signaling in vascular smooth muscle cells. J Biol Chem. 5; 274 (45):32382-6.

August GP, Caprio S, Fennoy I, Freemark M, Kaufman FR, Lustig RH, Silverstein JH, Speiser PW, Styne DM, Montori VM; Endocrine Society. (2008) Prevention and treatment of pediatric obesity: an endocrine society clinical practice guideline based on expert opinion. J Clin Endocrinol Metab. 93(12): 4576–4599.

Babar GS, Zidan H, Widlansky ME, Emon Das, Hoffmann RG, Daoud M, Alemzadeh R. (2011) Impaired Endothelial Function in Preadolescent Children With Type 1 Diabetes. Diabetes Care. 34(3): 681–685.

Balasubramanian M, Shield JP, Acerini CL, Walker J, Ellard S, Marchand M, Polak M, Vaxillaire M, Crolla JA, Bunyan DJ, Mackay DJ, Temple IK. (2010) Pancreatic hypoplasia presenting with neonatal diabetes mellitus in association with congenital heart defect and developmental delay. Am J Med Genet A. 152A(2):340-6.

Basiratnia M, Abadi SF, Amirhakimi GH, Karamizadeh Z, Karamifar H. (2012) Ambulatory blood pressure monitoring in children and adolescents with type-1 diabetes mellitus and its relation to diabetic control and microalbuminuria. Saudi J Kidney Dis Transpl. 23(2):311-5.

Baum VC, Levitsky LL, Englander RM. (1987) Abnormal cardiac function after exercise in insulin-dependent diabetic children and adolescents. Diabetes Care. 10(3):319-23.

Becerra JE, Khoury MJ, Cordero JF, Erickson JD. (1990) Diabetes mellitus during pregnancy and the risks for specific birth defects: a population-based case-control study. Pediatrics. 85:1–9.

Beckman JA, Creager MA, Libby P. (2002) Diabetes and atherosclerosisepidemiology, pathophysiology, and management. JAMA. 287(19):2570-2581.

Bhowmik D, Chiranjib.B, Yadav J, Chandira M R. (2009) Role of community pharmacist in management and prevention diabetic foot ulcer and infections. Journal of Chemical and Pharmaceutical Research. 1 (1): 38-53

Boulton AJ, Vinik AI, Arezzo JC, Bril V, Feldman EL, Freeman R, Malik RA, Maser RE, Sosenko JM, Ziegler D. (2005) Diabetic neuropathies: a statement by the American Diabetes Association. Diabetes Care 28:956-962.

Carmeliet P. (2000) "Mechanisms of angiogenesis and arteriogenesis," Nature Medicine.. 6(4). 389–395.

Carr ME. (2001) Diabetes: a hypercoagulable state. J Diabetes Comp 15:44–54.

Chinali M, de Simone G, Roman MJ, Lee ET, Best LG, Howard BV, Devereux RB. (2006) Impact of obesity on cardiac geometry and function in a population of adolescents: the Strong Heart Study. J Am Coll Cardiol.47:2267–73.

Chronopoulos A, Trudeau K, Roy S, Huang H, Vinores SA, Roy S. (2011) High glucose-induced altered basement membrane composition and structure increases trans-endothelial permeability: implications for diabetic retinopathy. Curr Eye Res. 36(8):747-53.

Chu C, Gui YH, Ren YY, Shi LY. (2012) The Impacts of Maternal Gestational Diabetes Mellitus (GDM) on Fetal Hearts. Biomed Environ Sci. 25 (1):15-22.

Clark JF, Pyne-Geithman G. (2005) Vascular smooth muscle function: The physiology and pathology of vasoconstriction. Pathophysiology. 12: 35-45.

Dalla Pozza R, Bechtold S, Bonfig W, Putzker S, Kozlik-Feldmann R, Netz H, Schwarz HP. (2007) Age of onset of type 1 diabetes in children and carotid intima medial thickness. J Clin Endocrinol Metab. 92(6):2053-7.

Dalla Pozza R, Bechtold S, Bonfig W, Putzker S, Kozlik-Feldmann R, Schwarz HP, Netz H. (2007) Impaired short-term blood pressure regulation and autonomic dysbalance in children with type 1 diabetes mellitus. Diabetologia. 50(12):2417-23.

Davis NL, Bursell JD, Evans WD, Warner JT, Gregory JW. (2012) Body composition in children with type 1 diabetes in the first year after diagnosis: relationship to glycaemic control and cardiovascular risk. Arch Dis Child. 97(4):312-5.

Day RE, Insley J. (1976) Maternal diabetes mellitus and congenital malformation. Survey of 205 cases. Arch Dis Child. 51:935–8.

Deorari AK, Saxena A, Singh M, Shrivastava S. (1989) Echocardiographic assessment of infants born to diabetic mothers. Arch Dis Child. 64(5):721-4.

Dimitriu AG, Russu G, Stamatin M, Jităreanu C, Streangă V. (2004) Clinical and developmental aspects of cardiac involvement in infant of diabetic mother. Rev Med Chir Soc Med Nat Iasi. 108(3):566-9.

Dokken BB. (2008) The Pathophysiology of Cardiovascular Disease and Diabetes: Beyond Blood Pressure and Lipids. Diabetes Spectrum. 21:3, 160-65.

Du X, Matsumura T, Edelstein D, Rossetti L, Zsengellér Z, Szabó C, Brownlee M. (2003) Inhibition of GAPDH activity by poly(ADP-ribose) polymerase activates three major pathways of hyperglycemic damage in endothelial cells. J Clin Invest. 112(7):1049-57.

Edwards JL, Vincent AM, Cheng HT, Feldman EL. (2008) Diabetic neuropathy: mechanisms to management. Pharmacol Ther. 120:1–34.

Elamin A, Rajesh K, Tuvemo T. (2007) Cardiac Autonomic Dysfunction in Children and Adolescents with Type 1 Diabetes Mellitus. Sudan JMS. 2(2), 95-100.

Eun Ha Kim, Yeo Hyang Kim. (2010) Left Ventricular Function in Children and Adolescents With Type 1 Diabetes Mellitus. Korean Circ J. 40(3): 125–130.

Faulkner MS, Quinn L, Rimmer JH, Rich BH. (2005) Cardiovascular endurance and heart rate variability in adolescents with type 1 or type 2 diabetes. Biol Res Nurs. 7(1):16-29.

Faulkner MS. (2010) Cardiovascular fitness and quality of life in adolescents with type 1 or type 2 diabetes. J Spec Pediatr Nurs. 15(4):307-16.

Festa A, D'Agostino Jr R, Howard G, Mykkänen L, Tracy RP, Haffner SM. (2000) Chronic subclinical inflammation as part of the insulin resistance syndrome. Circulation 102:42–47.

Fleischhacker E, Esenabhalu VE, Spitaler M, Holzmann S, Skrabal F, Koidl B, Kostner GM, Graier WF. (1999) Human diabetes is associated with hyperreactivity of vascular smooth muscle cells due to altered subcellular Ca2+ distribution. Diabetes. 48(6):1323-30.

Fontbonne A. (1996) Insulin-resistance syndrome and cardiovascular complications of non-insulin-dependent diabetes mellitus. Diabetes Metab. 22(5):305-13.

Fröhlich-Reiterer EE, Borkenstein MH. (2010) Microvascular and macrovascular complications in children and adolescents with type 1 diabetes mellitus. Wien Med Wochenschr. 160(15-16):414-8.

Gardiner HM, Pasquini L, Wolfenden J, Kulinskaya E, Li W, Henein M. (2006) Increased periconceptual maternal glycated haemoglobin in diabetic mothers reduces fetal long axis cardiac function. Heart. August; 92(8): 1125–1130.

Gerstein HC. (2007) Point: If it is important to prevent type 2 diabetes, it is important to consider all proven therapies within a comprehensive approach. Diabetes Care. 30:432–434.

Gillian A. Whalley, Silmara Gusso, Paul Hofman, Wayne Cutfield, Katrina K. Poppe, Robert N. Doughty, J. Chris Baldi. (2009) Structural and Functional Cardiac Abnormalities in Adolescent Girls with Poorly Controlled Type 2 Diabetes. Diabetes Care. 32(5): 883–888.

Goligorsky MS. (2005) Endothelial cell dysfunction: can't live with it, how to live without it," American Journal of Physiology. 288(5) 871–80.

Goran MI, Ball GD, Cruz ML. (2003) Obesity and Risk of Type 2 Diabetes and Cardiovascular Disease in Children and Adolescents. J Clin Endocrinol Metab. 88(4):1417-27.

Group SfDiYS. (2006) The Burden of Diabetes Mellitus Among US Youth: Prevalence Estimates From the SEARCH for Diabetes in Youth Study. Pediatrics. 118:1510–8.

Gu K, Cowie CC, Harris ML. (1998) Mortality in adults with and without diabetes in a national cohort of the US population, 1971–1993. Diabetes Care 21:1138–1145.

Hassan Z, Dewa A, Asmawi MZ, Sattar MZA. (2011) Assessment of vascular reactivity at different time-course on streptozotocin-induced diabetic rats. J Exp Integr Med. 1(3): 175-183.

Hayden MR, Sowers JR, Tyagi SC. (2005) The central role of vascular extracellular matrix and basement membrane remodeling in metabolic syndrome and type 2 diabetes: the matrix preloaded. Cardiovasc Diabetol 4:9–29.

Hoey H, Aanstoot HJ, Chiarelli F, Daneman D, Danne T, Dorchy H, Fitzgerald M, Garandeau P, Greene S, Holl R, Hougaard P, Kaprio E, Kocova M, Lynggaard H, Martul P, Matsuura N, McGee HM, Mortensen HB, Robertson K, Schoenle E, Sovik O, Swift P, Tsou RM, Vanelli M, Aman J. (2001) Good metabolic control is associated with better quality of life in 2,101 adolescents with type 1 diabetes. Diabetes Care. 24(11):1923-8.

Hornberger L K. (2006) Maternal diabetes and the fetal heart. Heart. 92:1019–1021.

Hsueh WA, Lyon CJ, Quinones MJ. (2004) Insulin resistance and the endothelium. Am J Med; 117: 109-117.

Hsueh WA, Quinones MJ. (2003) Role of endothelial dysfunction in insulin resistance. Am J Cardiol; 92: 10J-17J.

Imamoglu EY, Oztunc F, Eroglu AG, Onal H, Guzeltas A. (2008) Dispersion of the P wave as a test for cardiac autonomic function in diabetic children. Cardiol Young. 18(6):581-5.

Järvisalo MJ, Raitakari M, Toikka JO, et al. (2004) Endothelial dysfunction and increased arterial intima-media thickness in children with type 1 diabetes. Circulation. 109:1750–1755.

Joy NG, Hedrington MS, Briscoe VJ, Tate DB, Ertl AC, Davis SN. (2010) Effects of acute hypoglycemia on inflammatory and pro-atherogenic biomarkers in individuals with type 1 diabetes and healthy individuals. Diabetes Care.33:1529–35.

Kalani M. (2008) The importance of endothelin-1 for microvascular dysfunction in diabetes. Vasc Health Risk Manag. 4(5): 1061–1068.

Kampoli A, Tousoulis D, Marinou K, Siasos G, Stefanadis C. (2009) Vascular Effects of Diabetes Mellitus. Vascular Disease Prevention. 6, 85-90.

Kenchaiah S, Evans JC, Levy D, Wilson PWF, Benjamin EJ, Larson MG, Kannel WB, Vasan RS. (2002) Obesity and the risk of heart failure. N Engl J Med. 347:305–313.

Kim EH, Kim YH. (2010) Left ventricular function in children and adolescents with type 1 diabetes mellitus. Korean Circ J. 40(3):125-30.

Koh KK, Han SH, Quon MJ. (2005) Inflammatory markers and the metabolic syndrome. J Am Coll Cardiol 46:1978–1985.

Kollipara S, Warren-Boulton E. (2004) Diabetes and Physical Activity in School. School Nurse News. 21:12–16.

Kolluru GK, Bir SC, Kevil CG. (2012) Endothelial dysfunction and diabetes: effects on angiogenesis, vascular remodeling, and wound healing. Int J Vasc Med. 2012:918267.

Kose S, Aytemir K, Can I, Iyisoy A, Kilic A, Amasyali B, Kursaklioglu H, Isik E, Oto A, Demirtas E. (2002) Seasonal variation of P wave dispersion in healthy subjects. J Electrocardiol. 35:307-311.

Krautzig A, Christoph J, Kattner E. (1999) Heart failure caused by myocardial hypertrophy in diabetic fetopathy. Z Geburtshilfe Neonatol. 203(5):221-4.

Krishnan S, Short KR. (2009) Prevalence and significance of cardiometabolic risk factors in children with type 1 diabetes. J Cardiometab Syndr. 4(1): 50–56.

Kumar, S.D.; Dheen, S.T. & Tay, S.S.W. (2007) Maternal diabetes induces congenital heart defects in mice by altering the expression of genes involved in cardiovascular development. Cardiovascular Diabetology, (6)34, 1475-2840.

Lee SH, Kim JH, Kang MJ, Lee YA, Won Yang S, Shin CH. (2011) Implications of nocturnal hypertension in children and adolescents with type 1 diabetes. Diabetes Care. 34(10):2180-5.

Lisowski LA, Verheijen PM, De Smedt MM, Visser GH, Meijboom EJ. (2003) Altered fetal circulation in type-1 diabetic pregnancies. Ultrasound Obstet Gynecol. 21(4):365-9.

Lobstein T, Baur L, Uauy R. (2004) Obesity in children and young people: a crisis in public health. Obesity Reviews. 5:4–85.

Maggio AB, Farpour-Lambert NJ, Montecucco F, Pelli G, Marchand LM, Schwitzgebel V, Mach F, Aggoun Y, Beghetti M. (2012) Elevated E-selectin & diastolic blood pressure in diabetic children. Eur J Clin Invest. 42(3):303-9.

Manukian VIu, Bolotova NV, Aver'ianov AP, Filina NIu, Raĭgorodskiĭ IuM. (2011) Autonomic dysfunction syndrome and diabetic cardiac autonomic neuropathy in children with diabetes mellitus type I. The correction method. Zh Nevrol Psikhiatr Im S S Korsakova. 111(1):33-7.

Margeirsdottir HD, Stensaeth KH, Larsen JR, Brunborg C, Dahl-Jørgensen K. (2010) Early signs of atherosclerosis in diabetic children on intensive insulin treatment: a population-based study. Diabetes Care. 33:2043–2048.

Margeirsdottir HD, Stensaeth KH, Larsen, JR, Brunborg C, Dahl-Jørgensen K. (2010) Early Signs of Atherosclerosis in Diabetic Children on Intensive Insulin Treatment: A population-based study. Diabetes Care. 33(9): 2043–2048.

Maron BJ, Edwards JE, Henry WL, Clark CE, Bingle GJ, Epstein SE. (1974) Asymmetric septal hypertrophy in infancy. Circulation. 50:809-20.

Maron BJ, Verter J, Kapur S. (1978) Disproportionate ventricular septal thickcning in the developing normal human heart. Circulation. 57:520-6.

Maser RE, Lenhard MJ. REVIEW. (2005) Cardiovascular Autonomic Neuropathy Due to Diabetes Mellitus: Clinical Manifestations, Consequences, and TreatmentJ Clin Endocrinol Metab. 90(10):5896–5903.

Massin MM, Derkenne B, Tallsund M, Rocour-Brumioul D, Ernould C, Lebrethon MC, Bourguignon JP. (1999) Cardiac Autonomic Dysfunction in Diabetic Children. Diabetes Care. 22(11):1845-50.

Melissa Spezia Faulkner, Laurie Quinn, James H. Rimmer, Barry H. Rich. (2005) Cardiovascular Endurance and Heart Rate Variability in Adolescents With Type 1 or Type 2 Diabetes. Biol Res Nurs. 7(1): 16–29.

Melvin R Hayden, James R Sowers, Suresh C Tyagi. (2005) The central role of vascular extracellular matrix and basement membrane remodeling in metabolic syndrome and type 2 diabetes: the matrix preloaded. Cardiovasc Diabetol. 4: 9.

Miculis CP, de Campos W, Gasparotto GS, Silva MP, Mascarenhas LP, Boguszewski MC. (2012) Correlation of cardiorespiratory fitness with risk factors for cardiovascular disease in children with type 1 diabetes mellitus. J Diabetes Complications. Jun 18.

Mills JL, Knopp RH, Simpson JL, Jovanovic-Peterson L, Metzger BE, Holmes LB, Aarons JH, Brown Z, Reed GF, Bieber FR, Allen MV, Holzman I, Ober C, Peterson CM, Withiam MJ, Duckles A, Mueller-Heubach E, Polk BF, (1988) Lack of relation of increased malformation rates in infants of diabetic mothers to glycaemic control during organogenesis. N Engl J Med. 318:671–6.

Moncada S, Higgs A. (1993) The L-Arginine-Nitric Oxide Pathway. N Engl J Med;329(27):2002-12.

Monti MC, Lonsdale JT, Montomoli C, Montross R, Schlag E, Greenberg DA. (2007) Familial risk factors for microvascular complications and differential male-female risk in a large cohort of American families with type 1 diabetes. J Clin Endocrinol Metab. 92(12):4650-5.

Moore DJ, Gregory JM, Kumah-Crystal YA, Simmons JH. (2009) Mitigating micro-and macro-vascular complications of diabetes beginning in adolescence. Vasc Health Risk Manag. 5: 1015–1031.

Muniyappa R, Montagnani M, Koh KK, Quon MJ. (2007) Cardiovascular actions of insulin. Endocrine Reviews. 28 463–491.

Murphy NP, Ford-Adams ME, Ong KK, Harris ND, Keane SM, Davies C, Ireland RH, MacDonald IA, Knight EJ, Edge JA, Heller SR, Dunger DB. (2004) Prolonged cardiac repolarisation during spontaneous nocturnal hypoglycaemia in children and adolescents with type 1 diabetes. Diabetologia. 47(11):1940-7.

Narchi H, Kulaylat N. (2000) Heart disease in infants of diabetic mothers. Images Paediatr Cardiol. 2(2): 17–23.

Nathan DM, Davidson MB, DeFronzo RA, Heine RJ, Henry RR, Pratley R, Zinman B, American Diabetes Association. (2007) Impaired fasting glucose and impaired glucose tolerance: implications for care. Diabetes Care. 30:753–759.

Nigro J, Osman N, Dart AM, Little PJ. (2006) Insulin resistance and atherosclerosis. Endocrine Reviews. 27 242–259.

Peña AS, Couper JJ, Harrington J, Gent R, Fairchild J, Tham E, Baghurst P. (2012) Hypoglycemia, but not Glucose Variability, Relates to Vascular Function in Children with Type 1 Diabetes. Diabetes Technol Ther. Feb 7.

Philips JC, Marchand M, Scheen AJ. (2011) Squatting, a posture test for studying cardiovascular autonomic neuropathy in diabetes. Diabetes Metab. 37(6):489-96.

Þimßek E, Ozturk MA, Þenel F. (1999) The Role of Atrial Natriuretic Peptide in Adaptation To Extra-uterine Life and Physiological Weight Loss of the Newborn. Turk Jem. 3: 143-147.

Ping Zhou, Ronak S. Chaudhari, Zoltan Antal. (2010) Gender Differences in Cardiovascular Risks of Obese Adolescents in the Bronx. J Clin Res Pediatr Endocrinol. 2(2): 67–71.

Pradhan AD, Manson JE, Rifai N, Buring JE, Ridker PM. (2001) C-reactive protein, interleukin 6, and risk of developing type 2 diabetes mellitus. JAMA. 286(3):327-34.

Punareewattana K, Holladay SD.(2004) Immunostimulation by complete Freund's adjuvant, granulocyte macrophage colony-stimulating factor, or interferon-gamma reduces severity of diabetic embryopathy in ICR mice. Birth Defects Res A Clin Mol Teratol. 70(1):20-27.

Ren Y, Zhou Q, Yan Y, Chu C, Gui Y, Li X. (2011) Characterization of fetal cardiac structure and function detected by echocardiography in women with normal pregnancy and gestational diabetes mellitus. Prenat Diagn. May;31(5):459-65.

Riabykina GV, Laptev DN, Seid-Guseĭnov AA. (2007) Changes of QT-interval duration in children and adolescents suffering from type 1 diabetes mellitus. Kardiologiia. 47 (12):35-8.

Riddell MC, Iscoe KE. (2006) Physical activity, sport, and pediatric diabetes. Pediatr Diabetes. 7(1):60-70.

Rizzo G, Pietropolli A, Capponi A, Cacciatore C, Arduini D, Romanini C. (1994) Analysis of factors influencing ventricular filling patterns in fetuses of type I diabetic mothers. J Perinat Med. 22(2):149-57.

Rodriguez BL, Fujimoto WY, Mayer-Davis EJ, Imperatore G, Williams DE, Bell RA, Wadwa RP, Palla SL, Liu LL, Kershnar A, Daniels SR, Linder B. (2006) Prevalence of cardiovascular disease risk factors in U.S. children and adolescents with diabetes: the SEARCH for diabetes in youth study. Diabetes Care. 29(8):1891-6.

Rollins MD, Jenkins JG, Carson DJ, McClure BG, Mitchell RH, Imam SZ. (1992) Power spectral analysis of the electrocardiogram in diabetic children. Diabetologia. 35: 452–455.

Rosenbloom AL, Silverstein JH, Amemiya S, et al. ISPAD Clinical Practice Consensus Guidelines 2009 Compendium - Type 2 diabetes in children and adolescents. Pediatric Diabetes 2009;10(Suppl. 12):17-32.

Roy S, Sato T. (2000) Role of vascular basement membrane components in diabetic microangiopathy. Drug News Perspect. 13(2):91-8.

Schwab KO, Doerfer J, Hecker W, Grulich-Henn J, Wiemann D, Kordonouri O, Beyer P, Holl RW; DPV Initiative of the German Working Group for Pediatric Diabetology. (2006) Spectrum and Prevalence of Atherogenic Risk Factors in 27,358 Children, Adolescents, and Young Adults With Type 1 Diabetes: Cross-sectional data from the German diabetes documentation and quality management system (DPV). Diabetes care. 29:218–225.

Shaibi GQ, Ball GD, Cruz ML, Weigensberg MJ, Salem GJ, Goran MI. (2006) Cardiovascular fitness and physical activity in children with and without impaired glucose tolerance. Int J Obes (Lond). 30(1):45-9.

Shaibi GQ, Faulkner MS, Weigensberg MJ, Fritschi C, Goran MI. (2008) Cardiorespiratory Fitness and Physical Activity in Youth with Type 2 Diabetes. Pediatr Diabetes. 9(5): 460–463.

Sheehan PQ, Rowland TW, Shah BL, McGravey VJ, Reiter EO. (1986) Maternal diabetic control and hypertrophic cardiomyopathy in infants of diabetic mothers. Clin Pediatr (Phila). 25(5):266-71.

Shiono J, Horigome H, Kamoda T, Matsui A. (2001) Signal-averaged electrocardiogram in children and adolescents with insulin-dependent diabetes mellitus. Acta Paediatr. 90 (11):1244-8.

Smoak IW. (2002) Hypoglycemia and embryonic heart development. Front Biosci. 1;7:d307-18.

Steinberger J, Daniels SR; American Heart Association Atherosclerosis, Hypertension, and Obesity in the Young Committee (Council on Cardiovascular Disease in the Young); American Heart Association Diabetes Committee (Council on Nutrition, Physical Activity, and Metabolism). (2003) Obesity, insulin resistance, diabetes, and cardiovascular risk in children: an American Heart Association scientific statement from the Atherosclerosis, Hypertension, and Obesity in the Young Committee (Council on Cardiovascular Disease in the Young) and the Diabetes Committee (Council on Nutrition, Physical Activity, and Metabolism). Circulation. 18;107(10):1448-53.

Suhonen L, Hiilesmaa V, Teramo K. (2000) Glycaemic control during early pregnancy and fetal malformations in women with type I diabetes mellitus. Diabetologia. 43:79–82.

Suys BE, Katier N, Rooman RP, Matthys D, Op De Beeck L, Du Caju MV, De Wolf D. (2004) Female Children and Adolescents With Type 1 Diabetes Have More Pronounced Early Echocardiographic Signs of Diabetic Cardiomyopathy. Diabetes Care. 27(8):1947-53.

Suzuki LA, Poot M, Gerrity RG, Bornfeldt KE. (2001) Diabetes accelerates smooth muscle accumulation in lesion of atherosclerosis. Diabetes. 50: 851-860.

Szadkowska A, Pietrzak I, Mianowska B, Czerniawska E, Bodalska-Lipińska J, Chrul S, Markuszewski L, Bodalski J. (2006) Prehypertension in type 1 diabetic children and adolescents. Endokrynol Diabetol Chor Przemiany Materii Wieku Rozw. 12(4):286-91.

Taha D, Bardise J, Hegab A, Bonnefond A, Marchand M, Drunat S, Vaxillaire M, Polak M. (2008) Neonatal diabetes mellitus because of pancreatic agenesis with dysmorphic features and recurrent bacterial infections. Pediatr Diabetes. 9(3 Pt 1):240-4.

Tavares AC, Bocchi EA, Guimarães GV. Clinics (Sao Paulo). Endothelial function in pre-pubertal children at risk of developing cardiomyopathy: a new frontier. 2012;67(3):273-8.

Taylor R, Davison JM. (2007) Type 1 diabetes and pregnancy. BMJ. 7; 334(7596): 742–745.

Trayhurn P, Wood IS. (2005) Signalling role of adipose tissue: adipokines and inflammation in obesity. Biochem Soc Trans 33:1078–1081.

Tsyvian P, Malkin K, Artemieva O, Wladimiroff JW. (1998) Assessment of left ventricular filling in normally grown fetuses, growth-restricted fetuses and fetuses of diabetic mothers. Ultrasound Obstet Gynecol. 12(1):33-8.

Turan S, Turan OM, Miller J, Harman C, Reece EA, Baschat AA. (2011) Decreased fetal cardiac performance in the first trimester correlates with hyperglycemia in pregestational maternal diabetes. Ultrasound Obstet Gynecol. 38(3):325-31.

Valensi P. (2000) Blood pressure and heart rate regulation in diabetics. Arch Mal Coeur Vaiss. 93 Spec No 4:51-8.

Vargas R, Repke JT, Ural SH. (2010) Type 1 Diabetes Mellitus and Pregnancy. Rev Obstet Gynecol. 3(3): 92–100.

Veille JC, Sivakoff M, Hanson R, Fanaroff AA.. (1992) Interventricular septal thickness in fetuses of diabetic mothers. Obstet Gynaecol.79:51–4.

Villa MP, Multari G, Montesano M, Pagani J, Cervoni M, Midulla F, Cerone E, Ronchetti R. (2000) Sleep apnoea in children with diabetes mellitus: effect of glycaemic control. Diabetologia. 43(6):696-702.

Wagner VM, Müller-Godeffroy E, von Sengbusch S, Häger S, Thyen U. (2005) Age, metabolic control and type of insulin regime influences health-related quality of life in children and adolescents with type 1 diabetes mellitus. Eur J Pediatr. 164(8):491-6.

Way GL, Wolfe RR, Eshaghpour E, Bender RL, Jaffe RB, Ruttenberg HD. (1979) The natural history of hypertrophic cardiomyopathy in infants of diabetic mothers. J Pediatr. 95(6):1020-5.

Weber HS, Botti JJ, Baylen BG. (1994) Sequential longitudinal evaluation of cardiac growth and ventricular diastolic filling in fetuses of well controlled diabetic mothers. Pediatr Cardiol. 15(4):184-9.

Whalley GA, Gamble GD, Doughty RN, Culpan A, Plank L, MacMahon S, Sharpe N. (1999) Left ventricular mass correlates with fat-free mass but not fat mass in adults. J Hypertens. 17:569–574.

Wheaton J, Pinkstaff S. (2006) Aspects of Diabetes Mellitus: Atherosclerotic vascular Disease and Diabetes in the Older Adult; Part I: Understanding Pathogenic Mechanisms and Identifying Risk Factors. Clin Geriatr; 14: 17-25.

Witte DR, Tesfaye S, Chaturvedi N, Eaton SE, Kempler P, Fuller JH, EURODIAB. (2005) Prospective Complications Study Group. Risk factors for cardiac autonomic neuropathy in type 1 diabetes mellitus. Diabetologia. 48:164–171.

Wright RJ, Frier BM. (2008) Vascular disease and diabetes: is hypoglycemia an aggravating factor? Diabetes Metab Res Rev. 24:353– 63.

Wright RJ, Newby DE, Stirling D, Ludlam CA, Macdonald IA, Frier BM. (2010) Effects of acute insulin induced hypoglycemia on indices of inflammation: putative mechanism for aggravating vascular disease in diabetes. Diabetes Care. 33:1591–7.

Yatagai T, Nakamura T, Nagasaka S, Kusaka I, Ishikawa SE, Yoshitaka A, Ishibashi S. (2004) Decrease in serum C-reactive protein levels by troglitazone is associated with pretreatment insulin resistance, but independent of its effect on glycemia, in type 2 diabetic subjects. Diabetes Res Clin Pract. 63(1):19-26.

Yli BM, Källen K, Khoury J, Stray-Pedersen B, Amer-Wåhlin I. (2011) Intrapartum cardiotocography (CTG) and ST-analysis of labor in diabetic patients. J Perinat Med. 39(4):457-65.

Yli BM, Kallen K, Stray-Pederson B, Amer-Wahlin I. (2008) Intrapartum fetal ECG and diabetes. J Matern Fetal Neonatal Med. 21:231–238.

Young Mi Hong. (2010) Atherosclerotic Cardiovascular Disease Beginning in Childhood. Korean Circ J. 40(1): 1–9.

Younk LM, Davis SN. (2011) Hypoglycemia and vascular disease. Clin Chem. 57(2):258-60.

Zorena K, Myśliwska J, Myśliwiec M, Rybarczyk-Kapturska K, Malinowska E, Wiśniewski P, Raczyńska K. (2010) Association between vascular endothelial growth factor and hypertension in children and adolescents type I diabetes mellitus. J Hum Hypertens. 24(11):755-62.

Significant Risk Factors for Atherosclerotic Vascular Disease in Diabetes Mellitus as Measured by Carotid Intima Media Thickness

Basil N. Okeahilam, Benjamin A. Alonge
Department of Medicine
Jos University Teaching Hospital, Jos, Nigeria

Ayuba I. Zoakah
Department of Community Medicine
Jos University Teaching Hospital, Jos, Nigeria

Stephen D. Pam
Department of Radiology
Jos University Teaching Hospital, Jos, Nigeria

Fabian H. Puepet
Department of Medicine
Jos University Teaching Hospital, Jos, Nigeria

1   Introduction

Diabetes mellitus especially the type 2 variety is increasingly being seen as a cardiovascular disease that manifests as hyperglycaemia (Yki Jarvinen, 2000). It is therefore not surprising that cardiovascular disease accounts for 80% of mortality in diabetic patients (United Kingdom Prospective Diabetic Study, 2002). Most of the time, these cardiovascular diseases are atherosclerotic by nature (Treatment Options for Type 2 Diabetes Mellitus, 2000). Even before the time of diagnosis as cases of diabetes mellitus, these individuals are known to have established cardiovascular disease (Morrish *et al*, 1990). Following from this, all studies of cardiovascular disease risk factors in diabetics compared to non-diabetics in any locality show a two- fold burden in the former compared with the latter (Keen *et al*, 1999).

Intima media thickness is a measure of atherosclerotic vascular disease, considered to capture comprehensively all perturbations caused by several risk factors over time on the arterial walls (Grobbee & Bots, 1994). Though values differ by race, it is a robust measure of sub-clinical development of atherosclerosis (Lazdan *et al*, 2010). That being the case, any risk factor that correlates significantly with intima media thickness could be considered critical in the development of atherosclerosis; and therefore amenable to treatment to ameliorate cardiovascular disease morbidity. Traditional and some newer cardiovascular disease risk factors have shown a positive association with intima media thickness in epidemiological studies of patients and the general population (Bolinde *et al*, 1997; Lee *et al*, 1998; Bots *et al*, 1997). A cardiovascular disease risk factor is a term coined by Dr. William Kannel, the first director of the Framingham study; and refers to any condition associated with an increased tendency to developing cardiovascular disease (Black, 1992). They are divided into major(cigarette smoking, elevated blood pressure, elevated total and low density lipoprotein cholesterol, low high density lipoprotein cholesterol, diabetes mellitus and advancing age), predisposing (obesity, abdominal obesity, physical inactivity, family history of premature coronary heart disease, ethnic characteristics and psychosocial factors) and conditional (hypertriglyceridaemia, small low density lipoprotein particles, hyperhomocysteinaemia, increased serum lipoprotein(a), prothrombotic factors, left ventricular hypertrophy, hyperuricaemia, short stature, microalbuminuria, oral contraceptive use, hormone replacement therapy and menopause) (Grundy *et al*, 1999). We therefore sought to use carotid media intima thickness to determine those modifiable cardiovascular risk factors critical to the development of atherosclerotic vascular disease in a diabetic cohort seen in our healthy facility.

2   Methodology

This was part of a larger study on cardiovascular risk factors and carotid atherosclerosis in non-hypertensive type 2 Diabetes Mellitus in Jos University Teaching Hospital, Jos, Nigeria (Alonge, 2007). The protocol was approved by the hospital ethics committee and each patient provides a written consent to be part of the study after careful explanation by BAA.

Seventy non-hypertensive type 2 Diabetes Mellitus patients were recruited from the Diabetes Clinic of the hospital in a consecutive manner. They were all equal to or above 30 years of age, an age chosen to remove the likelihood of including type 1 (insulin dependent diabetes mellitus) which is more common in the younger age group. They were patients who developed classical symptomatology of diabetes mellitus with a fasting plasma glucose (FPG) greater than or equal to 7.0 mmol/l or 2 hour post-prandial glucose (2HPPBG)of greater than or equal to 11.1 mmol/l. Known diabetes mellitus patients whose plasma glucose had been controlled on physician prescribed oral hypoglycaemic or who in the course of treatment came to require insulin for control of plasma glucose (Alberti & Zimmet, 1998). Other than hypertension (blood pressure greater than or equal to 140/90 mmHg or history of physician prescribed anti-hypertensives) and age less than 30 years, the following also served as exclusion criteria: history of ketosis, treatment with drugs capable of affecting serum lipid profile, pregnancy, puerperium, thyroid diseases, heart disease with or without heart failure, and unwillingness to participate in the study.

At enrolment each participant was interviewed with regard to age (as at last birthday), age at diagnosis, duration of disease, occupation, civil status, educational background, family history of diabetes mellitus, alcohol and tobacco use. Degree of physical activity was also sought. They were then examined physically. Weight was recorded in kilograms (to the nearest 0.1 kg) using a flat scale on a firm horizontal plane with patients clad in light clothing only. Height was measured using a stadiometer (to the nearest centimeter) without food or head gear. Both of these conform to the standard prescription (Dowse & Zimmet, 1992). From the height and weight, Body Mass Index (BMI) was determined as the quotient of weight in kilograms and the square of height in metres. Waist circumference was measured using a dress maker's tape placed horizontally at the mid- point between the iliac crest and lower costal margin (National Institute of Health, 1998). Using the same tape, placed horizontally at the maximum circumference over the buttocks posteriorly and the symphysis pubis anteriorly, the hip circumference was determined in the same centimeter unit as the waist circumference. The waist to hip ratio (WHR) was determined from the two values, the former as the numerator and the latter as denominator.

Blood pressure was then measured, first on both arms with a five minute rest in-between. The arm with the higher value was used for two subsequent measurements separated by at least five minutes. The average of the last two measurements was used for systolic and blood pressure (SBP) and diastolic blood pressure (DBP). Korotkoff sounds 1 and 5 from standard mercury sphygmomanometry using appropriate sized cuff determined systolic and diastolic blood pressures respectively. Measurements were taken with patients supine and standing. The standing values were used for analysis, since diabetics are prone to orthostatic hypotension; and being ambulant, the erect blood pressures would be more representative. Thereafter, blood samples were taken after an overnight fast and two hours after food in appropriate (fluoride oxalate) bottles. Plasma glucose was measured by the glucose oxidase method (Caraway & Watts, 1998) on both the fasting and post prandial samples. Glycosylated haemoglobin (HbA1c) was determined on the fasting sample using the DCA 2000 ® ANALYSER. The analysis is based on a latex immune agglutination inhibition methodology. Total cholesterol (TC) and High density lipoprotein cholesterol (HDL – C)were determined on the fasting sample by the same enzymatic end point method (Trinder, 1981) using reagent contained in a kit supplied by Randox Laboratories Ltd. U.K. Serum creatinine (Cr) was determined by the Jaffe method (Spencer, 1986), and uric acid (UA) by the phosphotungstic acid method (Newman & Price).

The patients then underwent echocardiography using SONOS 1500 ultrasound system (Hewlett Packard USA) with a 3.5 mHz transducer except in obese patients when a 2.5 mHz transducer was used. The index of interest here was the left ventricular mass (LVM) which was given automatically by the machine from interventricular septal thickness in diastole, left ventricular posterior wall thickness in diastole and left ventricular internal diameter in diastole. These values were determined in standard fashion from a 2D mode guided M mode image of the left ventricle at the level of the chordae tendinae; just beyond the tip of the mitral valve. Finally they underwent carotid ultrasonography using a 7.5 mHz linear array transducer of the SONOS 1500 ultrasound system (Hewlett Packard USA) with the patients in the supine position. Both carotids (left and right) were scanned with the heads tilted to the opposite side and neck slightly extended. The carotid intima medial thickness (CIMT) was defined as the distance between the leading edge of the luminal echo of the leading edge of the adventitia of the media. This measurement was taken at a site of 1.0 cm proximal to the carotid bulb.

3   Statistics

The data set were analysed using STATA 11.2, 2009 statistical software. The analysis of variance (ANOVA) was used to compare the dependent variables (right and left carotid intima media thickness with independent variables as follows: systolic blood pressure, diastolic blood pressure, fasting plasma glucose, 2 hour post-prandial plasma glucose, glycosylated haemoglobin, total cholesterol, high density lipoprotein cholesterol, uric acid, creatinine, left ventricular mass, body mass index and waist/hip ratio. Multivariate analysis was done for blood pressure (SBP and DBP) and fasting plasma glucose. The p values that were less than 0.05 were considered statistically significant.

4   Results

The 70 patients consisted of 36 females and 34 males. Their ages ranged from 30 to 71 years with a mean (SD) of 51.2 (10.63) years. The mean carotid intima thicknesses were largely equal on both sides. The mean (SD) values were 0.94 (0.12) mm and 0.94 (0.16) mm for the right and left sides respectively. Only 5 and 6 people smoked and drank significant amounts of alcohol respectively. These numbers were considered small and not further analysed. The cohort mean (SD) of the other measurements are shown in Table 1.

Risk Factor	Mean (SD)	Risk Factor	Mean (SD)	Risk Factor	Mean (SD)
FPG (mmol/l)	7.93 (4.74)	HDL – C (mmol/l)	1.71 (0.78)	BMI (kg/m2)	27.15 (4.36)
2hPPG (mmol/l)	12.4 (5.59)	UA (micromol /l)	256.63 (113.75)	WHR	0.94 (0.06)
HbA1c (%)	9.03(2.78)	Cr (micromol/l)	96.26 (35.11)	SBP (mmHg)	123.63 (11.07)
TC (mmol/l)	5.09(1.59)	LVM (g)	153.49 (47.26)	DBP (mmHg)	83.03 (5.00)

FPG– Fasting plasma glucose; 2hPPG – 2 hour post prandial plasma glucose; HbA1c – Glycosylated haemoglobin; TC – Total Cholesterol; HDL – C – High density lipoprotein cholesterol; UA – Serum uric acid; Cr – Serum Creatinine; LVM – Left ventricular mass; BMI – Body mass index; WHR – Waist to hip ratio; SBP – Systolic blood pressure; DBP – Diastolic blood pressure;

Table 1: Mean (SD) values of measured atherosclerotic vascular disease risk factors in the study population.

When subjected to analysis of variance, the following exhibited a statistically significant relationship with carotid intima media thickness on the right: SBP, DBP, FPG, 2hPPG, TC, HbA1c, HDL – C and UA. For the left carotid intima media thickness, there was statistically significant difference as follows: SBP, DBP, LVM, FBS, 2hPPG, TC, HbA1c, and UA. These are detailed in Table 2.

RF	Right CIMT			Left CIMT		
	RS	ARS	P	RS	ARS	P
SBP mmHg	0.9910	0.9838	< 0.0001	0.9913	0.9733	< 0.0001
DBP mmHg	0.9910	0.9838	< 0.0008	0.9913	0.9733	0.0115
FPG mmol/l	0.9995	0.9968	< 0.0001	0.9998	0.9985	< 0.0001
2hPPGmmol/l	0.9995	0.9968	< 0.0001	0.9998	0.9985	< 0.0001
TC mmol/l	0.9995	0.9968	< 0.0001	0.9998	0.9985	< 0.0001
HbA1c %	0.9995	0.9968	<0.0001	0.9998	0.9995	0.0005
UAmicmol/	0.9995	0.9968	<0.0001	0.9998	0.9985	< 0.0001

RF – Risk Factor, RS – R-Squared, ARS – Adjusted R-Squared, P – p value.

Table 2: Significant risk factors for atherosclerosis in Diabetes Mellitus.

It can be surmised from the above that the following are consistent significant risk factors for atherosclerotic vascular disease: SBP, DBP, FPG, 2hPPG, HbA1c, TC and UA.

Multivariate analysis was done for blood pressure indices and one parameter of glucose metabolism namely fasting plasma glucose. A significant positive association was found between SBP and FPG on the one hand (t=56.23, p<0.0001, 95% CI: 132.44 - 143.06); and DBP and FPG on the other (t=56.23, p< 0.0001, 95% CI: 90.64 - 97.23).

5   Discussion

Blood pressure when high is a risk factor for progressive atherosclerosis (Khan, 2006). The risk is linear with blood pressure, and starts as low as systolic blood pressure of 115 mmHg and diastolic blood pressure of 75 mmHg (Kozub, 2010). However some workers posit that there is no indication of a critical value (Kannel & Wilson, 2008). When hypertension co-exists with diabetes mellitus, microvascular and macrovascular complications leading to cardiovascular disease, stroke and end stage renal disease are accelerated (Sampanis & Zamboulis, 2008). As shown in this study even when within normal range, both systolic and diastolic blood pressures are associated significantly with carotid intima media thickness as well as measure of glucose metabolism namely fasting plasma glucose. Blacks have been found to manifest microvascular and macrovascular structural and functional abnormalities including even in the normotensive range of blood pressure (Din-Dziethan et al, 2004); including increased carotid intima media thickness (Heffernan et al 2008). As blood pressure rises the arterial walls respond to this stress by thickening its walls. The pulsatile force of blood flowing at high pressure damages the intima resulting in smooth muscle proliferation (Khan, 2006). For the carotids, these will result in increase in carotid intima media thickness. The implication of these is that in patients with diabetes mellitus, blood pressure should be as low as possible; provided there is no accompanying hypotensive or ischaemic features. As shown in the United Kingdom Prospective Diabetes Study, hypertensive-diabetic patients had less microvascular and macrovascular end points if blood pressure control was tight (UK Prospective Diabetic Study, 1998). This benefit needs persistent tight control to control as another study (Holman et al, 2008) showed that during a 10 year post-interventional follow up, if there was no attempt to maintain tight control the benefit was lost within two years.

Measures of glycaemic control be it fasting blood sugar, 2 hour post prandial blood sugar or glycosylated haemoglobin were associated significantly with carotid intima media thickness in this study. Most diabetes especially the type 2 variety has as the centerpiece insulin resistance and hyperinsulinaemia. This biochemical state results in impairment of the arterial wall irrespective of vessel size, the result of which is diabetes induced vasculopathy (Utsunomiya, 2012). This vasculopathy is critical to the development of cardiovascular disease risk factors (Reaven, 2011) which most of the time have atherosclerosis as the basis. Hyperglycaemia using a point test as in fasting blood sugar or one that assesses general control over a period like glycosylated haemoglobin are associated with atherosclerotic changes (Keen *et al*, 1999). In fact as shown in the Hoorn study of carotid artery stenosis which is related to carotid intima media thickness, the odds for developing atherosclerotic changes in the carotid artery is higher in hyperglycaemic states (Beks *et al*, 1997). Hyperglycaemia does this by inducing endothelial dysfunction, which has been shown to be less with lower glycosylated haemoglobin as a measure of glycaemic state (Jensen-Urstad *et al*, 1996). This relationship between insulin resistance and reduced function of vessels has also been reported more recently (Kubota *et al*, 2011), with cellular mechanisms resulting in reduction or elimination of endothelial nitric oxide synthase being culprit. 2 hour post prandial blood sugar even in the absence of abnormal baseline glucose metabolism could induce early atherosclerosis (Cerrielo, 1998). Infact recent perspectives see it as a greater independent cardiovascular disease risk factor than fasting hyperglycaemia (Hanefeld *et al*, 1996). Post prandial hyperglycaemia is said to predispose to atherosclerosis and cardiovascular disease by inducing endothelial dysfunction, low grade inflammation and oxidative stress; a phenomenon described as "vascular failure" (Node & Inoue, 2009). Specifically, 2 hour post prandial blood sugar has been shown in the Collaborative Analysis of Diagnostic Criteria in Europe (DECODE) study been shown to demonstrate a continuous graded and direct relationship with cardiovascular death (DECODE Study Group, 2003). Compared to either fasting blood sugar or glycosylated haemoglobin, it has been shown to be a better predictor of cardiovascular risk (Tominga *et al*, 1999). This risk is said to start from 80 mg/dl (4.4 mmol/l) and by 140 mg/dl (7.8 mmol/l), the risk for cardiovascular disease has already gone up by about 58% (Node & Inoue, 2009).

Cholesterol was another significant risk factor that emerged from this study. Total cholesterol was high and high density lipoprotein cholesterol low. In the process of atherosclerosis, the first step appears to be endothelial dysfunction. Once this injury is established, monocytes are attracted. They adhere and migrate into the intima where they get activated and form foam cells. If cholesterol (especially low density lipoprotein cholesterol) get into the sub-intimal space, they get oxidized with release of products of lipid oxidation, free radicals and toxic products. Inflammatory cells are attracted and a state of chronic low grade inflammation is established. With this comes attraction of smooth muscle cells which proliferate and get deposited in the intima resulting in atherosclerotic plaque (Khan, 2006; Gilles, 2001). Oxidation of lipoproteins is enhanced in the presence of hyperglycaemia and hypertriglyceridaemia (Dinneen &

Gestein, 1997). The latter is high in diabetes mellitus largely due to reduction in lipoprotein lipase activity (Gugliano *et al,* 1996). Low high density lipoprotein was also significantly associated with increased carotid intima media thickness in this study. Low high density lipoprotein cholesterol is typical of diabetic dyslipidaemia (Treatment Options for Type 2 Diaabetes Mellitus, 2000). This is because in the presence of hyperglycaemia, they are easily glycated increasing their clearance from circulation (Lyons, 1992).

Serum uric acid also had a significant association with carotid intima media thickness. Hyperuricaemia is an independent risk factor for cardiovascular disease (Lawrence Edwards, 2009). It could do this by its linkage with a wide variety of metabolic and vascular risk factors (Rich, 2000)as also shown in a study (Bo *et al,* 2001) where uric acid correlated with triglycerides, body mass index, systolic blood pressure, albumin excretion rate, C-peptide, creatinine clearance, high density lipoprotein cholesterol and glycosylated haemoglobin. Uric acid can stimulate vascular smooth muscle cell proliferation and endothelial dysfunction independent of hypertension (Beck, 1986). This in itself with increase in vascular intima media thickness will be further aggravated when hypertension, diabetes mellitus and dyslipidaemia are co-existing.

The association between carotid intima media thickness and left ventricular mass was significant only for one side; the left. There was however such tendency on the right, only that it did not attain statistical significance. Left ventricular mass is related to left ventricular hypertrophy which has been found to correlate positively with carotid intima media thickness (Sorof *et al,* 2003); leading the authors to suggest that the same adaptive process was operating in the myocardium and vascular media. All the factors that result in increased left ventricular mass, manifesting in the metabolic syndrome also initiate or worsen atherosclerosis. Hence it would be no surprise finding left ventricular mass as a significant association with atherosclerosis especially in diabetics.

In conclusion, when the skill and facilities are available, carotid intima media thickness can point to certain significant risk factors driving the process of athero-thrombosis. Targeting them by life style medicine and pharmacotherapy would then reduce the morbidity and mortality that would ordinarily accompany the disease in question. It is important to point out certain limitations in this work. Deliberate efforts were not made to exclude diabetics with pulmonary disease, obstructive sleep apnoea and systemic inflammatory diseases which could influence CIMT values. Pulmonary disease and systemic inflammatory diseases fuel atherosclerosis by background chronic inflammation and endothelial dysfunction. Obstructive sleep apnoea syndrome (Ciccone *et al,* 2012), gives rise to increased CIMT by a variety of mechanisms deriving from its pathophysiology namely hypoxia, hypercapnia, micro-arousals, sympathetic hyperactivity, oxidative stress, systemic inflammation and hypercoagulability.

References

Alberti KGMM,& Zimmet PZ.(1998). Definition, diagnosis and classification of diabetes mellitus and its complications. Part II. Diagnosis and Classification of diabetes mellitus. Provisional report of WHO Consultation. Diabetes Med,15, 539 – 643.

Alonge BA. (2007).Cardiovascular risk factors and carotid atherosclerosis in non hypertensive type 2 diabetes mellitus in Jos University Teaching Hospital, Jos. Dissertation submitted to the National Postgraduate Medical College of Nigeria for the award of Fellowship of the Medical College of Physicians (FMCP) in Cardiology

Beck L. (1986).Requiem for gouty nephropathy. Kidney Int. 30, 280 – 287

Beks PHJ, Mackay AJC, de Vries H, de Neeling JND, Bouten LM, & Heine RJ.(1997). Carotid artery stenosis is related to blood sugar level in an elderly Caucasian population: the Hoorn study. Diabetologia, 40, 290 – 298

Black HR. (1992).Cardiovascular risk factors. In: Zaret BL, Moser M, Calen LS (eds). Yale University School of Archive Heart Book. 24th edition.pp. 22 - 35. 48.Bo S, Cavallo- Perin P, Gentile L, Rapetti E, & Pagono G.(2001). Hypouri-caemia and hyperuricaemia in type 2 diabetes; two different phenotypes. Eur. J. Clin. Invest, 31(4), 318 – 321.

Bo S, Cavallo- Perin P, Gentile L, Rapetti E, & Pagono G.(2001). Hypouricaemia and hyperuricaemia in type 2 diabetes; two different phenotypes. Eur. J. Clin. Invest, 31(4), 318 – 321.

Bolinder G, Norin A, Defaire H,& Wahren J.(1997). Smokeless tobacco use and atherosclerosis. An ultrasonic investiga-tion of carotid intima medial thickness in healthy middle aged men. Atherosclerosis,132, 95 – 103

Bots ML, Launer LJ, Lindemans J, Hofman A, & Grobbee DE.(1997). Homocysteine, atherosclerosis and prevalent cardi-ovascular disease in the elderly. The Rottendam Study. J. Int. Med, 242(4), 339 – 347.

Caraway WT,& Watts NB. (1998).Determination of glucose in body fluids. In: Tiez NW (Ed). Fundamentals of Clinical Chemistry. 3rd edition. W.B. Saunders. Philadelphia. pp 426 – 430.

Ceriello A.(1998). The emerging role of post prandial hyperglycaemic spikes in the pathogenesis of diabetic complications. Diabet. Med, 15, 188 – 193.

Ciccone MM, Scicchitano P, Mitacchione G, Zito A, Gesualdo M, & Caputo P et al.(2012). Is there a correlation between OSAS duration/severity and carotid intima thickness? Respir Med,106(5), 740 - 746

DECODE Study Group. (2003). Is the current definition of diabetes relevant to mortality risk from all causes and Cardio-vascular and Non-cardiovascular disease? Diabetes Care, 26, 688 – 696.

Din-Dziethan R, Couper D, Evans G, Arnett DK, & Jones DW.(2004). Arterial stiffness is greater in African Americans than whites: evidence from the Forsyth County, North Carolina. ARIC Cohort. Am. J. Hypertens, 2004, 17. 304 – 313.

Dinneen SF, & Gestein HC.(1997). The association of microalbuminuria and mortality in non-insulin dependent diabetes mellitus. A systematic review of literature. Arch Intern. Med, 157, 1413 – 1418.

Dowse GK, & Zimmet P.(1992). A model protocol for diabetes and other non communicable diseases field study. Wld. Hlth. Stat. Quart, 45, 360 – 372.

Giles TD. (2001).Atherogenesis and coronary artery disease.In: CA Burtis, EA Ashwood (eds). Tietz Fundamentals of Clinical Chemistry. 5th edition. WB Saunders. Philadelphia, pp. 209 – 213.

Grobbee DE, & Bots ML.(1994) Carotid artery intima thickness as an indicator of generalized atherosclerosis. J. Int. Med, 235(5), 567 – 573.

Grundy SM, Pasternak R, Greenland PA, Smith S,& Valentin F. Statement for Healthcare Professionals from the American Heart Association and the American College of Cardiology. J. Am. Coll. Cardiol, 34, 134 - 159

Gugliano D, Ceriello A,& Paolisso G.(1996). Oxidative stress and diabetic complications. Diabetic Care, 19, 257 – 267.

Hanefeld M, Fischer S, Julius U, Schulze J, Schwanebeck V, Schmechel H, Ziegelasch HJ, & Lindner J.(1996). Risk factors for myocardial infarction and death in newly detected NIDDM: the Diabetes Intervention Study, 11 year follow – up. Diabetologia, 39, 1577 – 1583.

Heffernan KS, Joe SY, Wilend KR, Woods JA, & Fernahall B.(2008). Racial differences in central blood pressure and vas-cular function in young men. Am. J. Physiol. Heart Circ. Physiol. 295, H2380 – H2387.

Holman RR, Paul SK, Bethel MA, Neil HAW, & Matthews DR.(2008). Long term follow up after tight control of blood *pressure in type 2 diabetes. N. Eng. J. Med, 359, 1565 – 1576.*

Jensen – Urstad KJ, Reichard PG, Rosfoos JS, Lindblad LEL, & Jensen – Urstad MT.(1996). Early atherosclerosis is re-tarded by improved long term blood sugar control in patients with IDDM. Diabetes, 45, 1253 – 1257.

Kannel WB, & Wilson PWF.(2008). Cardiovascular risk factors and hypertension. In: JL Izzo, DA Sica, HR Black (eds). Hypertension Primer. The essentials of high blood pressure, Basic Science, Population Science and Clinical Man-agement. 4ᵗʰ edition. Lippincott, Williams and Wilkins. Philadelphia.pp. 244 – 248.

Keen H, Clark C, & Laakso M.(1999). Reducing cardiovascular burden of diabetes: Managing Cardiovascular Disease. Diabetes Metab. Res. Rev, 15, 186 – 196.

Keen H, Clark C, & Laakso M.(1999). Diabetes metabolism, research and review. Diabetes Metab. Res. Rev, 15, 186 – 196.

Khan MG. (2006). Arteriosclerosis. In MG Khan (ed). Encyclopaedia of Heart Diseases. Elsevier. 1ˢᵗ edition. Amsterdam. Boston. Heidelberg. London. New York. Oxford. Paris. San Diego. San Francisco. Singapore. Sydney. Tokyo. Pp. 101 – 103.

Khan MG. (2006).Atherosclerosis/Atheroma. Ibid 27. pp. 117 – 130.

Khan MG. (2006).Hypertension. Ibid 27, pp. 469 – 491.

Kozub E.(2010). Community Stroke Prevention Programme: An overview. J. Neuroscience Nursing, 42(3), 143 – 149.

Kubota T, Kubota N, Kumagai H, Yamagushi S, Kozono H, & Takahashi T et al.(2011). Impaired insulin signaling in en-dothelial cells reduces insulin induced glucose uptake by skeletal muscle. Cell Metab, 13, 294 – 307.

Lawrence Edwards N. ((2009).The role of hyperuricaemia in vascular disorders. Curr. Opin. Rheum, 21, 132 – 137.

Lazdan M, de la Horra A,& Pitcher A.(2010). Elevated blood pressure in offsprings born premature to hypertensive preg-nancy. Is endothelial dysfunction the underlying vascular mechanism? Hypertens,56, 159 – 165.

Lee AJ, Alowbray PI, Lowe GD, & Rumley A.(1998). Blood viscosity and elevated carotid intima media thickness in men and women. The Edinburgh Artery Study. Circulation, 15, 1467 – 1473.

Lyons T. (1992).Lipoprotein glycation and its metabolic consequences. Diabetes, 41(S2), 67.

Morrish NJ, Stevens LK, Head J, Fuller JH, Jarrett RJ & Keen H.(1990). A prospective study of morbidity among middle aged diabetic patients (The London cohort of WHO multinational study of vascular disease in diabetes)1: causes and death rates. Diabetologia,33, 538 – 540.

National Institute of Health. National Heart, Lung and Blood Institute.(1998). Clinical guidelines on identification, evalua-tion and treatment of overweight and obesity in adult. The evidence report. Obes. Res, 6, 51S – 209S

Newman DT, & Price CP.(2001). Non protein nitrogen metabolites. In: CA Burtis, ER Ashwood(eds). Tietz Fundamentals of Clinical Chemistry. 5ᵗʰ edition. W.B Saunders. Philadelphia.pp. 424 – 426.

Node K, & Inoue T.(2009). Post prandial hyperglycaemia as an aetiological risk factor in vascular failure. Cardiovascular Diabetology, 8, 23 doi: 10.1 186/1475 – 2840 – 8 – 23.

Reaven GM. (2011).Insulin resistance: the link between obesity and cardiovascular disease. Med. Clin North Am, 95, 875 – 892

Rich RW. (2000).Uric acid: Is it a risk factor for cardiovascular disease? Am. J. Cardiol, 85, 1018 – 1021.

Sampanis C,& Zamboulis C.(2008). Arterial hypertension in diabetes: from theory to clinical practice. Hippokratia, 12(2), 74 – 80.

Spencer K.(1986). Analytical reviews in Clinical Biochemistry. The estimation of creatinine. Ann. Clin. Biochem. 23, 1 –

25.

Sorof JM, Alexander V, Cardwell G, & Portman RJ.(2003). Carotid artery intima medial thickness and left ventricular hypertrophy in children with elevated blood pressure. Paediatrics, 111, 61 – 66.

Treatment options for type 2 Diabetes Mellitus. (2000). Am Fam. Phys. Momog, 1, 16 – 19.

Trinder P. (1981). Oxidase determination of cholesterol as cholesterol – 4 – en 3 – one using iso octane extraction Ann. Clin. Biochem. 18(pt 2), 64 – 70.

Tominga M, Eguchi H, Manaka H, Igarashi K, Kato T, & Sekikawa A.(1999). Impaired glucose tolerance is a risk factor for cardiovascular disease but not impaired fasting glucose. The Fungata Diabetes Study. Diabetes Care, 22, 920 – 924

UK Prospective Diabetes Study. (1998).Tight blood pressure control and risks of macrovascular and microvascular complications in type 2 diabetes. UKPDS 38. BMJ, 317, 703 – 713.

United Kingdom Prospective Diabetes Study. Implications of the UKPDS.(2002). Diabetes Care. 25(Suppl), S28 – S32.

Utsunomiya K. (2012).Treatment strategy for type 2 diabetes from the perspective of systemic vascular protection and insulin resistance. Vascular Health and Risk Management, 8, 429 – 436.

Yki Jarvinen H. (2000). Management of type 2 diabetes and cardiovascular risk: lessons from interventional trials. Drugs, 60, 975 – 983.

Diabetes Mellitus and Gastrointestinal Disorders

Mohamed Morsy
Department of Pharmaceutical Sciences
King Faisal University, Saudi Arabia

Promise Emeka
Department of Pharmaceutical Sciences
King Faisal University, Saudi Arabia

1   Introduction

Diabetes mellitus has been described as a metabolic disorder usually associated with hyperglycemia, which brings about complications, that affects multiple organs particularly if it persists for a long time either in type 1 or type 2 diabetes mellitus (Rodrigues & Motta, 2012). Although there are many differences in both types (Table 1), studies have shown that the gastrointestinal tract function is compromised, affecting the digestive processes, the motility and nervous control of the entire system (Bener *et al.*, 2012; Bernstein, 2000). These complications manifests in various forms and affecting about 75 % of long standing diabetics worldwide (Zhao *et al.*, 2006). The symptoms of this disorder seen in both the lower and upper gastrointestinal tract are caused by functional and/or structural changes. They may include gastroparesis, anorexia, vomiting, early satiety, intestinal enteropathy, diarrhea, constipation or fecal incontinence (Bytzer *et al.*, 2002; Bytzer *et al.*, 2001, Ko *et al.*, 1999; Feldman & Schiller, 1983). Hyperglycemia injures the nerves directly and also disrupts blood supply to the nerves in the gastrointestinal tract (Kashyap & Farrugia, 2010; Ordög *et al.*, 2009). The disruption of the nerve functions consequently affects the motility of the gut causing incomplete emptying of the different sections of the gastrointestinal tract. This could lead to gastroentropathy, a disorder of the esophagus, stomach and the colon. The effect of diabetes on digestive system can also cause malabsorption. Diabetics are reported to be at risk of developing gallstone due to decreased motility of the gallbladder as well (Yang *et al.*, 1984).

Characteristics	Type 1	Type 2
Etiology	Immune mediated with weak family influence (Vinik *et al.*, 2005)	Metabolic disorder with strong family influence (Kota *et al.*, 2012)
Pathogenesis	Loss of pancreatic β-cells leading to absolute insulin deficiency (Sparre *et al.*, 2005)	Complex but due to inadequate insulin secretion, insulin resistance or both (Sparre *et al.*, 2005)
Risk factors	Autoimmune diseases and environmental factors (Peng & Hagopian, 2006)	Obesity, familial and ethnic variations (Kota *et al.*, 2012)
Prevalence	5-10 % of diagnosed cases (Daneman, 2006)	Over 90 % of diagnosed cases (Kota *et al.*, 2012)
Onset	Abrupt. Symptoms usually start in childhood or adolescence	Slow. The disease is mostly discovered in adulthood, but an increasing number of children are being diagnosed with the disease
Clinical signs	Weight loss, and ketoacidosis (DiMeglio *et al.*, 2003)	Overweight (Kota *et al.*, 2012)
Management	Exogenous insulin	Exercise and diet plus medication e.g., oral hypoglycemics

Table 1: Differences between Type 1 and Type 2 Diabetes Mellitus.

Gastric mucosal damage has also been associated with diabetes (Morsy *et al.*, 2010). Diabetic patients are prone to acute gastric injury and impaired ulcer healing which could aggravate to acute stress-induced gastric lesion (Konturek *et al.*, 2010; Harsch *et al.*, 2003). It is reported that severe gastric inflammation or ulcer can affect gastric motility in diabetic patients (Boehme *et al.*, 2007). Healing impairment of chronic ulcers in diabetes mellitus has been attributed to release of proinflammatory cytokines such as tumor necrosis factor-α and the diminished activity of the mucosal antioxidative system (Brzozowska *et al.*, 2004). *Helicobacter pylori*, an organism implicated in ulcer has been noted to have a high prevalence amongst diabetics (Tseng, 2012).

2   Pathogenesis of Gastrointestinal Disorders in Diabetes Mellitus

It is well established that autonomic nervous supply to the gastrointestinal tract is affected in a chronic diabetic state (He *et al.*, 2001). The enteric system is the intrinsic nervous system of the gastrointestinal tract. This system, also termed "the brain of the gut", exerts a profound effect on the functions and activities of the gastrointestinal tract. It influences the digestive processes, whose actions include, motility, secretions, absorption, and gastrointestinal tract blood flow. The gastrointestinal tract function is mediated by both the extrinsic and intrinsic nerve fibers. The extrinsic neurons are controlled by the central nervous system and mediated via the parasympathetic and sympathetic nervous system (Figure 1), whereas the intrinsic nerves are found within the enteric nervous system where they originated from (Spångéus & El-Salhy, 2001; Spångéus *et al.*, 2000). The control of these systems and the balancing of their activities modulate gastrointestinal tract normal function (Kashyap & Farrugia, 2010). Embedded in the walls of the gastrointestinal tract are two nerve networks of the enteric nervous system called plexuses, which also run from the esophagus to the anus. The plexus comprises of three types of neurons namely sensory, motor and interneurons that elaborate an array of neurotransmitter substances. The major neurotransmitters are acetylcholine, norepinephrine, serotonin (5-HT) and vasoactive intestinal peptide. Current evidence indicates that there are various types of neurotransmitters involved in the nervous network of the gastrointestinal tract, while some are primary others are subsidiary neuromodulators. They include peptide and non-peptide neurotransmitters found within the enteric neurons. Studies have identified and located these neurotransmitters to specific neurons using specialized staining method. In the myenteric plexus, γ-aminobutyric acid is found to be involved in regulating muscle contraction, whereas 5-HT within the same location functions as interneuron transmitter. Adrenergic neurons are said to emanate from autonomic ganglia and are connected via synapses to enteric nervous system. Report indicates that neuropeptide Y secreted from adrenergic neurons is inhibitory in nature (Spångéus & El-Salhy, 2001).

The parasympathetic innervation produces excitatory effects, stimulating smooth muscle contraction as well as increasing blood flow, secretions and release of enteric hormones (Frøkjaer *et al.*, 2007). On the other hand the sympathetic nerve stimulation provides inhibition of gastrointestinal tract secretions, motor activities and decrease of blood flow. The submucosal plexus, an integral part of the enteric nervous system, is stimulated by the release of acetylcholine and inhibited by vasoactive intestinal peptide via the cholinergic neurons (Spångéus & El-Salhy, 2001; Tonini *et al.*, 2000). Also, the sympathetic neurons by the release of norepinephrine modulate the secretory responses and blood flow (Lomax *et al.*, 2010). The myenteric plexus neurons mediate contractile responses via the cholinergic system and these responses are inhibited by vasoactive intestinal peptide and nitric oxide by provoking relaxation responses (Iwasaki *et al.*, 2006). On the other hand, epinephrine/norepinephrine mediates vasoconstriction, reduces gastrointestinal tract secretions and relaxation in addition to the contraction of sphincters (Lomax *et al.*, 2010; Sarna, 2006). There is evidence that combined effect of the sympathetic system and activities of the dopaminergic inhibitory system is geared to reduce acetylcholine elaboration which consequently reduces gastrointestinal tract contractility (Eshraghian & Eshraghian, 2011).

There are abnormalities of neurotransmitters in the neurons of enteric nerve fibers in diabetic animal model. These abnormalities are seen from the esophagus to the anal region of the gastrointestinal tract (Spångéus & El-Salhy, 2001). Studies have shown that reduced vagal activity in acute hyperglycemic state decreases release of nitric oxide from the myenteric plexus and results in impaired gastric relaxation and delayed gastric emptying (Ishiguchi *et al.*, 2001). The enzyme responsible for the elaboration of nitric oxide, nitric oxide synthase, is found to be reduced in diabetic patients and experimental diabetic animal models. This is said to be critical in development of gastric dysmotility because the expression of neuronal nitric oxide synthase is found to be decreased in diabetic gastroparesis. The damaging effects of hyperglycemia on gastric motility stress the importance of rigorous metabolic control in the management of diabetic patients. There are indications that changes in the excitatory and inhibitory neurons or contents of the neurotransmitter in diabetes will lead to gastrointestinal tract dysfunction and these have been demonstrated in diabetic patients (Chandrasekharan & Srinivasan, 2007). This is seen as a significant decrease in the density of these inhibitory neurons. Since diabetes produces a state of oxidative stress precipitating conditions of advanced glycosylation end products, there is evidence that inhibitory neurons such as vasoactive intestinal peptide, nitric oxide and neuropeptide are mostly affected when compared to excitatory neurons (Iwasaki *et al.*, 2006; Sheetz & King, 2002). The decrease and/or increase in the density of these neurons is believed to be responsible for altered gastrointestinal tract motility and gastric emptying observed in diabetic patients, while the loss of neurons could be due to apoptosis or necrosis in hyperglycemic state (Guo *et al.*, 2004; Wautier & Guillausseau, 2001). Thus the diabetic state affects the innervation of gastrointestinal tract in both animal model and diabetic patients.

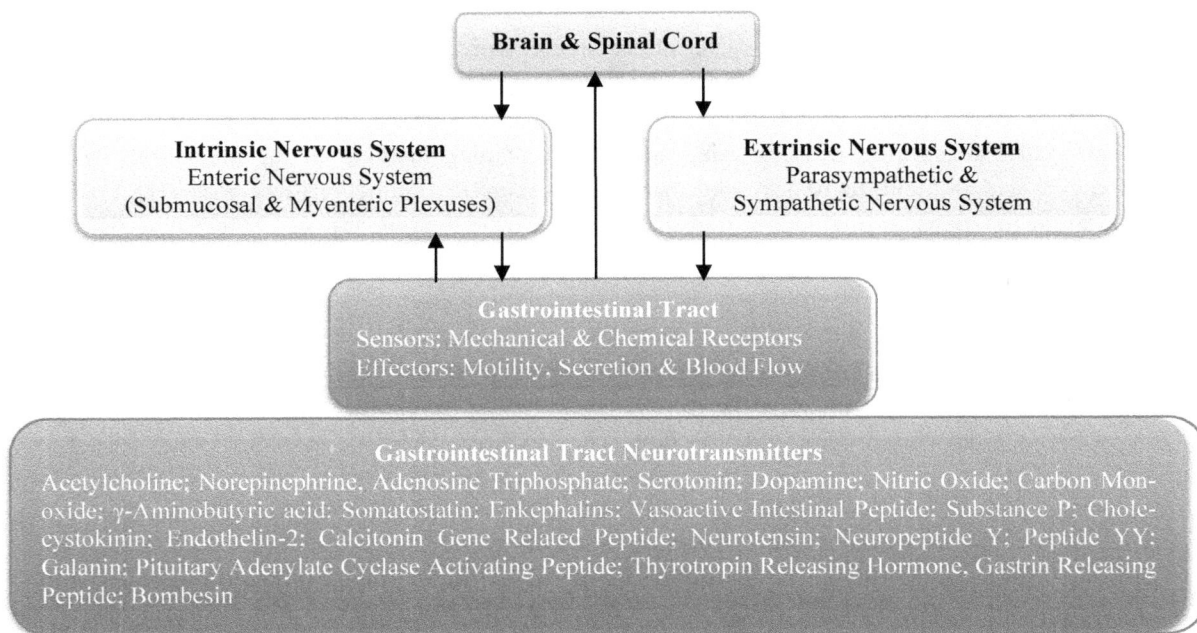

Figure 1: Gastrointestinal Tract Innervations and Neurotransmitters

The key to the pathogenesis of gastrointestinal tract disorders in diabetic patients is reported to be related to autonomic neuropathy (Shakil *et al.*, 2008). The pathogenic mechanism of this abnormality appears to be multifactorial, manifesting in one or more of the gastrointestinal tract segments as form of demyelination of enteric neurons, decreased neuronal size, reduction in hormonal secretions and degeneration of axons in the submucous plexus (Bernstein, 2000). The theories proposed by scientists in the pathology of diabetic gastric dysfunction include, oxidative stress within the cells, impaired fatty acid metabolism, synthesis of advanced glycosylation end products in hyperglycemic state, increased sorbitol production by aldose reductase enzyme and reduction of blood flow in the gastrointestinal tract (Chandrasekharan *et al.*, 2011).

3 Affected Signaling Pathways in Diabetic Gastrointestinal Tract Disorders

The pathophysiology of gastrointestinal tract disorders in diabetes involves signaling pathways and disruption to any one of these could lead to autonomic neuropathy. In the presence of persistent high blood glucose, non enzymic glycosylation occurs resulting in excess glycosylation of proteins, particularly hemoglobin and cellular structures (Brownlee *et al.*, 1988). Advanced glycosylation end products are protein and lipids that have been converted to glycated products upon exposure to sugars. They are predominant in diabetics and affect cellular structure and functions. The development of advanced glycosylation end products in diabetes, will affect the cell function, especially membrane cells (Bernstein, 2000). Advanced glycosylation end products impair nitric oxide production by reducing the half-life of neuronal nitric oxide synthase (Xu *et al.*, 2003; Rojas *et al.*, 2000). Polyol signaling pathway activity is also enhanced in a high blood glucose level condition where glucose is converted to sorbitol by the enzyme aldose reductase and is involved in autonomic neuropathy (Bernstein, 2000). Sorbitol may also glycate protein thus producing advanced glycosylation end products. Because this compromises the cell integrity, cellular information is disrupted and hence, nerve transmission is affected and morphological changes occur, altering nerve fibers within the enteric nervous system. Also excess sorbitol is known to decrease nitric oxide concentration in diabetic condition. This decrease in concentration of nitric oxide is reported to reduce gastrointestinal tract relaxation responses to non-adrenergic non-cholinergic nerves (Jenkinson & Reid, 1995).

4 Morphological and Functional Changes in Gastrointestinal Tract of Diabetic Patients

Impairment of nervous system function by diabetic neuropathy can occur anywhere in the body. Along the gastrointestinal tract, it produces conditions that are akin to vagotomy (Vittal *et al.*, 2007; Kong & Horowitz, 2005). In diabetic conditions, advanced glycosylation end products are produced and this brings about morphological changes which occur in the presence of hyperglycemia. These changes, lead to biomechanical remodeling of the gastrointestinal tract (Zhao *et al.*, 2010; Zhao *et al.*, 2006). It is the accumulation of advanced glycosylation end products in the diabetic cells that causes the modification of structure and function of protein matrix. This has been demonstrated in animal models of diabetes mellitus and found to be one of the key mechanisms involved in gastrointestinal tract alterations in diabetes mellitus (Suzuki *et al.*, 2012). A significant number of long standing diabetics exhibit different forms of symptoms due to disruption of function or changes in the gastrointestinal tract structure (He *et al.*, 2001). Mandelstam and Lieber (1967) was the first to satisfactorily describe the relationship between esophageal dysfunction and diabetes mellitus. Several studies have since shown that esophageal motor dysfunction is common in patients with associated diabetic neuropathy (Kim *et al.* 2012; la Roca-Chiapas & Cordova-Fraga, 2011; Shakil *et al.*, 2008; Frøkjaer *et al.*, 2007; Chandran *et al.* 2003). Findings have now revealed swelling, irregularity of caliber and disruption of parasympathetic fibers both within the myenteric plexus and in the extrinsic trunks in the walls of the esophagus (Ordög *et al.*, 2009; Bernstein, 2000). In the esophagus, distress may be described as dysphagia, chest pain and odynophagia (Kotler & Hsu, 2010). It is postulated that hyperglycemia which affects the vagal control of the esophagus, increases the relaxation of the esophageal sphincter (Ordög *et al.*, 2009). It usually results in the delay of esophageal transit and seen in about 50% of the chronic diabetic cases (Kotler & Hsu, 2010). This effect is attributed to either peristaltic failure or development of focal low amplitude waves which consequently leads to gastroesophageal reflux (Holloway *et al.*, 1999). Studies have shown that esophageal motor dysfunction in diabetes is more prevalent in the presence of neuropathy (Ordög *et al.*, 2009; Shakil *et al.*, 2008). Therefore changes are seen in both the structure and function of part or whole of the gastrointestinal tract. The structural changes are described as demyelination of the enteric nerves and loss of Schwann cells in the parasympathetic fibers, both in the wall and extrinsic nerves. The observed loss of function is as a result of reduced cholinergic stimulation. The parasympathetic innervation controls the peristalsis and relaxation of the esophagus and hence this loss will lead to distinctive alteration of both morphology and function. It is convenient to describe the clinical picture as loss of contraction amplitude, or reduced velocity in peristaltic movement and/or delay in esophageal emptying time (Zhao *et al.*, 2006).

The stomach has two parts namely proximal and distal segments with two ends, cardiac and pylorus. The movement of food out of the stomach into duodenum is controlled by two processes, peristaltic and gastric emptying process (la Roca-Chiapas & Cordova-Fraga, 2011). Morphologically, the stomach is well suited in receiving and grinding food particle and stretching. The myenteric plexus is said to be responsible for gastric motility and in maintaining muscular tone of the stomach. In the presence of hyperglycemia, the stomach experiences cellular anatomic disruption in form of swelling of nerve cells with a consequent loss of myelin fibers, and smooth muscle are observed to be rounded and hyalinized (Bernstein, 2000). The diabetic stomach is reported to have a reduced ability to distend in response to food due to morphological structural changes in the musculature. Ordög *et al.* (2009) reported the presence of eosinophilic bodies and smooth muscle atrophy with accumulation of collagen in diabetic affected cells. While other workers reported diffuse smooth muscle atrophy and fibrosis of the stomach in diabetes mellitus (Pasricha *et al.*, 2008). Abnormalities of gastric motility is said to occur in 20-30% of diabetic patients and, like esophageal motor dysfunction, they are often without clinical symptoms or manifestations (Shakil *et al.*, 2008).

From human studies, disorders of gastric emptying is said to occur frequently in diabetes and acknowledged as disordered gastric contractile activity (Chandrasekharan *et al.*, 2011; Bernstein, 2000). This motility dysfunction is said to manifest in amplitude and frequency of contractions and pyloric dysfunction (Zhao *et al.*, 2006). Kassander in 1958 first recognized gastroparesis which he termed "gastroparesis diabeticorum" signifying delayed gastric emptying seen in diabetic patients. Delayed gastric emptying or gastric retention may present as nondescript abdominal discomfort. The cause of delayed gastric emptying is suggested to be because of vagal neuropathy, since the vagi are responsible for regulating gastric motility and transit. Support for this hypothesis is that there is a constant intragastric pressure within the normal stomach, despite receiving large volumes of food. This receptive relaxation, which the vagal nerves mediate has been shown to be impaired after vagotomy and is similar as seen in patients with diabetes mellitus (Vittal *et al.*, 2007). In all, there is motor dysfunction of the stomach resulting in irregularity and uncoordinated motor activity as a consequence of diabetic neuropathy. Therefore in diabetic patients with gastric dysfunction, the activities of the stomach are grossly hampered. Studies have shown a decrease in the density of myenteric neurons caused by prolonged hyperglycemia in diabetic patients (Spångéus & El-Salhy, 2001). Evidence suggests that the condition of a hyperglycemic state will cause autonomic neuropathy, which is a causal factor that precipitates disturbances of gastric motility (Ordög et al., 2009; Tieppo et al., 2009). This phenomenon has been reported in both animal and human studies (Kashyap & Farrugia, 2010). It can be argued that loss of myenteric neurons whether sensory or motor will mean a decreased innervation and motility of the stomach. Studies have provided evidence that increased production of fructose in hyperglycemic conditions will result in edema and rupture of nerve sheath, ultimately reducing nerve impulse conduction (De Freitas et al., 2008). The proposed mechanism is described as decrease in inositol metabolism, which reduces the activation of protein kinase C. The resultant excess intracellular sodium causes edema and rupture of myelin sheath, affecting transmission of nerve impulses (De Freitas et al., 2008). This will in turn affect the functions of the stomach as evidenced by the slowing of gastric emptying seen in diabetic patients and has also been demonstrated in animal models (Liu et al., 2004; Mehta et al., 2002). The slowing of gastric emptying is observed as slowing transit with food retention and loss of motility of the gastric wall (Smith & Ferris, 2003). The abnormalities of the fundus and pylorus were demonstrated also in diabetic animals by James et al. (2004) as seen frequently in patients with diabetes mellitus of either type 1 or 2 or both. Interestingly, studies that show the link with diabetes, also demonstrated that induced hyperglycemia in healthy subjects lead to slowing of gastric transit and food retention (Samsom et al., 1997; Abrahamsson, 1995).

Small intestinal dysfunction appears to be more common in diabetes when compared with esophageal or gastric dysfunction and with more severe symptoms. Like in the esophagus and stomach, the small intestine may be extensively affected in conditions of diabetes mellitus. The diabetic effect on the small intestine usually manifests with many symptoms when compared with the disorders involving the esophagus and stomach which may go on unnoticed. A decrease in the intestinal tone of diabetic patients has been attributed to an increase in cholinergic activities and a decrease in adrenergic receptor activation (Anjaneyulu & Ramarao, 2002). The effect is seen as both slowing and rapid transit of the small intestine and is well documented also in animal studies (De Freitas et al., 2008). The small intestine of diabetic patients undergoes structural and functional changes. These changes are responsible for the impairments of motility, slowing of transit time, and affecting both secretory as well as absorptive functions. Evidence show that increase in the sorbitol production causes changes in the intracellular osmolality, which leads to neuronal death (Zanoni et al., 2002). This effect will deplete the small intestine of neurons and thereby decrease its neuronal stimulatory actions. From animal studies, diabetes induced rats will present with hyperplasia and hypertrophy of the mucosa and submucosa of the layers of the small intestine (De Freitas et al., 2008). Clinical examinations have revealed a number of histological changes due to angiopathy in the intestinal mucosa of diabetic patients and are therefore associated with autonomic neuropathy. These changes which are strongly associated with reduced mesenteric perfusion are atrophic in nature with thick walls, reduced villi and possibly change in permeability (De Las Casas & Finley, 1999; Kandemir et al., 1995). The disruption of the intestinal mucosal cell integrity will compromise its functional ability as a surface barrier to prevent the passage of possible harmful agents. The observed increase in permeability of the small intestine to potentially dangerous substances in diabetic patients has also been documented in human studies and is related to its functional abnormality as well (de Kort et al., 2011).

The diabetic colon is more susceptible to damage when exposed to hyperglycemia (Rodrigues & Motta, 2012; Chandrasekharan et al., 2011). This damage can manifest as apoptosis of the enteric neurons and reduction in the size of the ganglionic neurons in the colon. The consequent development of this disorder is due to the creation of an oxidative state (Kashyap & Farrugia, 2011). Functional disorders will follow when there is a profound structural disruption in tissues. Evidence abound that show a delayed transit in the diabetic colon (Unal et al., 2008; Jung et al., 2003). As with the small intestine, these changes have been demonstrated in both human and animal models of diabetes mellitus in form of neu-ronal necrosis and hyperplasia resulting in increased thickness of the epithelial layers with reduced cell density (Unal *et al.*, 2008). The development of morphological changes due to diabetes has been shown to bring about functional changes also in the colon. These functional changes could significantly affect the total colonic transit time due to a marked alteration in motility as a result of the loss and injury to in-terstitial cells of Cajal in the colonic submucosal cells (Forrest *et al.*, 2008). Evidence from studies in humans show that the dysfunctional diabetic colon is related to the development of diabetic neuropathy, with absent postprandial response (Mirakhur & Walshaw, 2003). Also the prolonged diabetic conditions will blunt receptor-mediated responses and reduce contractions. This is said to be attributable to de-creased ganglion size and increased enteric neuron apoptosis in a diabetic colon (Chandrasekharan *et al.*, 2011).

The functions of anorectal region of the gastrointestinal tract are also affected in long standing dia-betes mellitus. Changes are seen as alterations in evacuation and continence mechanisms (Tieppo *et al.*, 2009). Fecal incontinence is the main sign seen in patients with anorectal dysfunction in patients with diabetes mellitus (Weiss & Sumpio, 2006). It is characterized by involuntary release of flatus's and/or liquid or solid feces, causing both hygienic and social problems. These social problems could lead to stigmatization and can cause serious psychological depression. This anorectal dysfunction is attributable to conditions of hyperglycemia which cause the impairment of the sphincter muscle function, altering the anal pressure (Tieppo *et al.*, 2009). There is clinical evidence from diabetic neuropathy studies to show that the dysfunction of the anal sphincter in long standing diabetes mellitus is common (Ricci, *et al.*, 2000). Diarrhea is usually accompanied by accidental passage of feces which is described as fecal incon-tinence. In these patients, the diarrhea is protracted with the presence of diabetic neuropathy occasioned by abnormal anal sphincter motor function (Bjelaković *et al.*, 2005). This is said to be as a result of a de-fective autonomic nervous system regulation of the internal sphincter and/or abnormal intrinsic sphincter smooth muscle (Yang *et al.*, 1984). Evidence from animal studies show that this is brought about by de-crease in sphincter pressure and contraction of anorectal muscle (Tieppo *et al.*, 2009). The alteration in function and structure of this region of gastrointestinal tract has been attributed to hyperglycemia. The state of hyperglycemia is known to induce an increase in apoptosis and causes the reduction of phospha-tidyl inositol-3-kinase signaling in the enteric neurons (Chandrasekharan *et al.*, 2011).

5   Consequences of Diabetic Neuropathy on the Gastrointestinal Tract

Poor glycemic control in diabetes mellitus has been suggested to be responsible for the many complica-tions observed in gastrointestinal tract disorders (Ordög *et al.*, 2009). Demonstrations of this disorder in both human and animals show that it is evident in type 1 as well as type 2 diabetes mellitus and that they are equally affected (Mishima *et al.*, 2009). Previous studies show that diabetic neuropathy has an enor-mous influence on the sensory and motor functions from the esophagus to the terminal portion of the gas-trointestinal tract (Chandrasekharan *et al.*, 2011). It is believed that chronic hyperglycemic state in diabet-ic patients will create a condition of oxidative stress which is known to play a critical role in cellular inju-ry. This condition is said to stimulate the generation of free radicals which are very reactive chemically and can impose a damaging effect on tissues causing injury to cell membrane and DNA (Kim *et al.*, 2012). Both animal and human have shown the attenuation of vascular dysfunction seen in diabetes with antioxidant (Zhao *et al.*, 2010). Increased oxidative stress is related to loss of hemeoxygenase-1 which in turn leads to loss of the interstitial cells of Cajal and reduced expression of neuronal nitric oxide synthase and initiation of apoptotic process within the cells (Suzuki *et al.*, 2012; Forrest *et al.*, 2008). Oxidative stress in diabetes mellitus is reported to be activated by hyperglycemia (Rösen *et al.*, 2001). In diabetes mellitus, the production of reactive oxygen species causes the activation of several metabolic reactions within the cells. In high glucose concentration, the enzyme aldose reductase converts glucose to sorbitol which is the first step in the polyol pathway, eventually converting it to fructose. The continuous activation of this pathway is reported to affect other oxidative reactions within the cells such as reduced levels of glutathione due to shunting of glucose through the polyol pathway critically reducing NADPH (King & Loeken, 2004). There is the likelihood of reduction of antioxidant potentials, which will critically expose cells to oxidation and damage compromising their function and integrity. In these conditions the activities of other stress sensitive intracellular signaling pathways are altered. There is an increase in the mitochondrial superoxide and hydroxyl radical formation precipitated also by these reactions. Again this is responsible for the high oxidative state in which protein cellular structures and membrane lipids are modified. Kasznicki *et al.* (2012) reported that hyperglycemia decreased plasma nitric oxide content in diabetic subjects because superoxide anion can inhibit endothelial nitric oxide synthase by reacting with nitric oxide. The decrease of nitric oxide by hyperglycemia is suggested to be the major cause of endothelial dysfunction seen in diabetic conditions. The development of oxidative stress leads to diabetic neuropathy and has been documented in animal models of diabetes mellitus and reported also in diabetic patients (Chandrasekharan *et al.*, 2011). Due to overproduction of reactive oxy and hydroxyl radicals in the presence of hyperglycemia in diabetic conditions, the created high oxidative state causes endothelial injury (Kim *et al.*, 2012). The non enzymic reaction of glucose with protein forms advanced glycosylation end products in which various reports have shown to promote other complications of gastrointestinal tract disorders (Chandrasekharan *et al.*, 2011; Kashyap & Farrugia, 2010; De Freitas *et al.*, 2008).

6   Symptoms of Gastrointestinal Disorders in Diabetes Mellitus

Symptoms of gastrointestinal tract disorders in diabetic patients are diverse and can be related. These have also been reported to be observed in various sections of the gastrointestinal tract, from the esophagus to the anorectal region either in part or as whole (Hasler, 2007; Bjelaković *et al.*, 2005; Kong and Horowitz, 2005). The role of hyperglycemia in the disorders of gastrointestinal tract is well documented (Onitilo *et al.*, 2012; Marmuthu *et al.*, 2011; Stacher, 2001). These effects are either acute or chronic, however both conditions produce similar outcome. According to reports, acute glycemia decreases the tone of the fundus and contractile activities of the stomach and intestine (Rodrigues & Motta, 2012). The decrease in gastric motility and impaired emptying by hyperglycemia has been demonstrated in animal experiments. In the colon, it affects muscular contractility and alters emptying time with attendant hypotonia of the sphincter muscle of the anus. These are clinically described as esophageal enteropathy and gastroentropathy which are associated with autonomic neuropathy. The main disorders of the esophagus are described as peristalsis abnormality and dysfunction of the lower esophageal sphincter (Ebert, 2005). These disorders are said to be due to dysfunctional vagus nerve. The resultant consequences of this in both type 1 and type 2 diabetes are impaired esophagus transit and abnormal gastric acid reflux (Bjelaković *et al.*, 2005). Symptoms experienced by diabetics are heartburn, dysphagia and sometimes regurgitation. From animal studies it is revealed that gastroesophageal reflux could lead to the development of oxidative stress which is capable of causing epithelial mucosal damage (Kim *et al.*, 2012; Zhao *et al.*,

2010). However these symptoms observed in the esophagus might be also a direct effect of a developed dysfunctionality in the gastric section of the gastrointestinal tract.

In the diabetic stomach, symptoms of dysfunction are commonly seen in both types of diabetes (Hasler, 2007). It is dynamic in development particularly with the presence of prolonged hyperglycemia and described as gastroparesis. Gastroparesis is increasingly becoming a significant health issue as the problem of diabetes mellitus increases across nations. Gastroparesis is reported to be the outcome of a variety of potentially disabling upper gastrointestinal tract. Some diabetic patients with impaired gastric motility do not show any symptoms of gastroparesis (Shakil et al., 2008; Zochodne, 2007; Carnethon et al., 2006). The impairment of gastrointestinal tract function as in delayed gastric emptying seems to be closely related to parasympathetic insufficiency (Jørgensen et al., 1991). Delayed gastric emptying is a common feature of gastroparesis. About 90 % of ingested food in healthy subjects and non-diabetic patients are emptied after 4 hours from the stomach which allows for gastric accommodation (Tougas et al., 2000). This is a form of physiological response that permits the stomach to stretch and accommodate the ingested food without increasing intragastric pressure or cause discomfort. However, long standing diabetic patients with gastroparesis, have delayed gastric emptying, which is attributed to antral hypomotility and recognized as a major pathophysiological mechanism underlying the symptoms of gastroparesis with impaired gastric accommodation. Because the accommodation reflex is mediated by the vagal pathway, therefore this results from impaired autonomic nervous system. This impaired gastric accommodation plays a critical role in the generation of certain symptoms seen in patients with gastroparesis (Yin et al., 2010). Gastroparesis may enhance bezoar formation and acute gastric dilatation, intestinal obstruction, vomiting, respiratory aspiration, and affect the glycemic control in diabetes mellitus by impeding the absorption of oral medications (Kashyap & Farrugia, 2010; Bernstein, 2000). This may lead to inconsistent blood glucose readings and will further aggravate the hyperglycemic situation and worsens the gastroparesis condition. Gastroparesis symptoms are nonspecific and because of this the diagnosis is often missed and so the degree of diabetic neuropathy does not show any relationship with the symptoms no matter how severe the presentation (Grover et al., 2011). In the condition of gastroparesis, gastric emptying could be fast, due to impaired relaxation and autopyloroduodenal coordination or slow emptying due to reduced motility. In some patients with type 2 diabetes, both accelerated and retarded gastric emptying has been reported (Intagliata & Koch, 2007). The activity of gastric emptying is dependent on the function of the vagus nerve which has been said to be affected in a persistent hyperglycemic state. It is established that hyperglycemia can have a profound effect on sensory and motor functions of the gastrointestinal tract (Kim et al., 2011).

The relationship between hyperglycemia and gastric dysfunction is unequivocal in that it causes the relaxation of the fundus and abolishes impulse propagation. This situation is capable of precipitating ketoacidosis and a condition of acute gastroparesis (Kotler & Hsu, 2010). Other factors which may be secondary can include damage to cells of interstitial cells of Cajal and lack of nitric oxide inhibitory actions due to oxidative stress. The interstitial cells of Cajal are known to serve a variety of functions within the gastrointestinal tract. The slow wave generated by interstitial cells of Cajal is transmitted to the smooth muscles initiating membrane depolarization (Ordög et al., 2009). Therefore loss of interstitial cells of Cajal as seen in gastroparesis will affect slow wave generation and transmission causing gastric dysmotility (Horváth et al., 2006). The consequence of disrupted gastric motility is the development of delayed gastric emptying. Studies in animals show that high oxidative state in diabetes ultimately leads to the emergence of diabetic gastroparesis which procures the loss of interstitial cells of Cajal (Forrest et al., 2008; Choi et al., 2007; Forster et al., 2005). The interstitial cells of Cajal are known to mediate neuronal activities within the gastrointestinal tract and therefore play crucial role in its motility (Kim *et al.*, 2011). There is an abundance of evidence showing that in diabetic state, interstitial cells of Cajal network is depleted causing a condition of neuropathy and this has been demonstrated in both human and animal experiments (Forrest *et al.*, 2008). Therefore, delayed gastric emptying in diabetes is suggested to be a feature of gastroparesis caused by poor glycemic control. Clinically, gastroparesis is said to be difficult to diagnose, however, features like anorexia, bloating, epigastric discomfort/pain, early satiety, distention, nausea and vomiting are common (Aljarallah, 2011). Gastroparesis is reported to be common amongst diabetes and leads to gastric stasis affecting other sections of the gastrointestinal tract and causing the deterioration of gastroesophageal reflux with all the associated symptoms. Koch and Uwaifo (2008) described gastroparesis as the dysfunction of the enteric nervous system as well as muscular and hormonal activities of the gastrointestinal tract. The presence of gastroparesis is common amongst diabetes suffering patients affecting their intestinal functions (Camilleri *et al.*, 2012). Manifestations can be described as diarrhea and constipation due to impaired motility and secretory activities related to development of diabetic neuropathy (Camilleri *et al.*, 2011, Ma *et al.*, 2009).

Intestinal and colonic motility disorders in both types of diabetes mellitus can lead to diarrhea. Diabetic diarrhea can be described as the presence of chronic diarrhea which usually is brown, watery, profuse stool and might be associated with tenesmus. The diarrhea is long lasting, typically episodic, and consistent with hyperglycemia and the presence of diabetic neuropathy. Diabetic diarrhea has been described as a worrying debilitating gastrointestinal tract complication seen in about 10-22 % of diabetic patients (Wolosin & Edelman, 2000; Ogbonnaya & Arem, 1990). It is seen in patients with long standing history of diabetes mellitus and accompanied with abnormal rapid transit of fluids, increased frequency and urgency (Wolosin & Edelman, 2000). Due to altered absorptive process, volume of stool may also increase. It appears to be episodic and can last for several days to weeks or months. The pathogenesis of diabetic diarrhea is difficult to predict. However, the proposed mechanism is thought to be as a result of autonomic neuropathy (Murao & Hosokawa, 2010). A body of evidence has shown that disordered gastrointestinal tract motility coupled with abnormal intestinal secretions, reduced fluid absorption and sometimes bacterial overgrowth are among causative factors (Rodrigues & Motta, 2012; Ebert, 2005; Lysy *et al.*, 1999; Virally-Monod *et al.*, 1998; Keshavarzian & Iber, 1986). Particularly, studies have revealed the association between *Clostridium difficile* infection and its role in diabetic diarrhea (Shakov *et al.*, 2011). These conditions are also said to exacerbate fecal incontinence (Rodrigues & Motta, 2012). Rayner *et al.* (2001) reported that stasis syndrome, a condition of altered motility, is also associated with diarrhea. These episodes are often followed by an occasional constipation with intervals of weeks to months of normal movements. The pathogenic mechanism is said to be related to decrease adrenergic receptor activity, abnormal gastrointestinal tract motility and delayed transit time.

The enteric neurons in concert with autonomic nervous system regulate the gastrointestinal tract motility. Excitatory neurons like cholinergic and serotonergic nerves are known to stimulate the gastrointestinal tract, whereas the sympathetic, nitrergic and vasoactive intestinal peptide nerves mediate relaxation response (Chandrasekharan & Srinivasan, 2007). Therefore neuronal changes either morphological or functional due to diabetes mellitus will affect the excitatory and inhibitory responses. Studies in both human and animal models of diabetes have shown loss of inhibitory neurons (Murao & Hosokawa, 2010). The reported loss of inhibitory responses to sympathetic relaxation and loss of nitric oxide neurons in diabetic patients is said to be responsible for the intestinal hypermotility. Also implicated in diabetic diarrhea is the loss of interstitial cells of Cajal (He *et al.*, 2001). They are identified as enteric neuron pacemaker cells, involved in the regulation of intestinal motility (Sanders *et al.*, 2000). Their role in this regard has been demonstrated in patients with diabetes mellitus (Iwasaki *et al.*, 2006). Therefore the balance between excitatory and inhibitory stimulation in the enteric neurons hold the key to the control of this complex motor function. Critically the disturbance of this balance regulation in diabetic state is said to cause dysmotility function. This phenomenon has been described in experimental diabetic models as lack of inhibitory responses (Chandrasekharan & Srinivasan, 2007).

The intestinal symptoms in experimentally-induced diabetes in rats are very similar to those observed in human diabetes, thus the results of experimental models might be applied to the study of the illness in humans, in order to gain a better knowledge of the alterations caused on the nerves of the enteric system by this illness. Recent studies on experimental diabetes have shown alterations in the adrenergic, cholinergic and peptidergic innervation in the gastrointestinal tract of streptozotocin-induced diabetic rat (Belai *et al.*, 1988; Schmidt *et al.*, 1988; Lincoln *et al.*, 1984) suggesting autonomic dysfunction (Cuervas-Mons *et al.*, 1990). About 17 % of diabetic patients were associated with ischemic colitis (Cubiella Fernández *et al.*, 2010; Longstreth & Yao, 2010; Longo *et al.*, 1992). This condition is said to affect all segments of the colon where it is transitorily deprived of blood supply. Persistent hyperglycemia affects arteries supplying the bowel which could cause hardening and narrowing, effectively precipitating ischemic colitis in which mesenteric microcirculation deteriorates considerably (Karayiannakis *et al.*, 2011; Nagai *et al.*, 1998; Sharieff *et al.*, 1997; Spotnitz *et al.*, 1984).

Constipation is seen as a major gastrointestinal tract complaint in patients with diabetes than in non-diabetics. It is estimated that 44 % of diabetic patients are affected by constipation and is the most common gastrointestinal complication resulting from diabetic neuropathy (Kotler & Hsu, 2010; Shakil *et al.*, 2008). Gastrocolic reflex is altered with a diffuse disorder of colonic motility. The pathophysiology of colonic dysmotility in diabetes is believed to be due to delay or absent postprandial motility caused by dysfunction of autonomic nervous system. Clinical examination usually reveals occasional massive amount of fecal material found in the large atonic and dilated colon of diabetic patients (Taub *et al.*, 1979). This condition may present as intestinal obstruction or fecal impaction capable of causing stercoral ulcerations associated with colonic distension and consequent mucosal erosion in patients (Taub *et al.*, 1979). It might be due to loss of intestinal nervous control attributed to dysfunction of intrinsic and extrinsic intestinal neurons and decreased or absent of postprandial gastrocolic reflex (Vinik *et al.*, 2003). It is the most definable symptom of the gastrointestinal tract disorders in both type 1 and type 2 diabetes mellitus.

Diabetic patients may present with several different symptoms of gastrointestinal tract motor dysfunctions whose clinical features may differ from patient to patient (Nowak *et al.*, 1995). Clinical features are suggestive of gastroparesis and enteropathy as mentioned earlier which is termed gastroenteropathy because it reflects a similar wide range of symptomatologic spectrum (Quigley, 1999). Different evaluation methods are currently been used by clinicians to assess gastric emptying, antral contractility, colonic segmental transit time, sphincter tone and the rectal anal inhibitory reflex (Vinik *et al.*, 2003; Quigley, 1999). These evaluations employ different investigative tools for the detection of gastrointestinal tract dysfunction in diabetics like breath test based on 13C-octanoic acid, electrogastrography, ultrasonography, magnetic resonance imaging and manometry for effective management (Vinik *et al.*, 2003; Quigley, 1999).

6.1   Treatment of Diabetic Gastroparesis

Gastroparesis has the potential to cause a wide range of health problems among diabetics that is often times very difficult to assess and treat. By the time symptoms of diabetic autonomic neuropathy begin to appear, nerve damage would have been evident, irreversible and most likely to be advanced with poor prognosis. Hence, the best form of treatment would be to aim at preventing the progression of diabetes mellitus. This will limit the progression to autonomic neuropathies seen in chronic diabetes. Therefore adequate glycemic control, diet monitoring and prompt medication needs will decrease the development of gastroparesis and its debilitating consequences. For this reason, management of gastroparesis, is often a challenge and mostly dependent upon patients glycemic control and frequency and severity of symptoms presented (Forgacs & Patel, 2011). However, the early recognition of gastrointestinal motility disorders may be important for the better long-term management of patients. Sometimes the patient's nutritional status becomes a factor in considering mode of treatment. Despite the fact that glycemic control and dieting are important aspect of treatment, they cannot suffice particularly where symptoms are debilitating. Definitive and individualized management of patients is likely to improve functionality, quality of life and ensure glycemic control. Therefore, a better understanding of the nature and pathophysiology of the diseased condition in animal models and human as well as a confirmed symptom evaluation, will help to guide management decisions. Drugs acting on central and peripheral satiety centres may possibly improve nutrition and prevent excessive weight loss. However, agents that are prokinetic are useful in the control of symptoms and treatment of gastroparesis. Therefore, several drugs used in the management of gastroparesis has prokinetic activity. The dopamine receptor antagonists and 5-HT receptor antagonist like metoclopramide, domperidone and cisapride are currently been used as form of management which act locally to increase released acetylcholine at the myenteric plexus (Table 2).

Drug	Mechanism of action	Effects	Adverse reactions	References
Metoclopramide	Antagonist of dopamine (D_2) and 5-HT_3 receptors	Improves gastrointestinal tract contractions	Extrapyramidal symptoms and hyperprolactinemia	Parkman et al., 2004
Domperidone	Dopamine antagonist	Increases antral contractions and decrease receptive relaxation of the proximal stomach	Hyperprolactinemia such as gynecomastia	Talley, 2003
Cisapride	Partial agonist on 5-HT_4 and 5-HT_3 receptors	Beneficial effects on small bowel motility	Arrhythmia and diarrhea	Chandran et al., 2003
Erythromycin	Motilin agonist	Improves symptoms and gastric emptying	Abdominal pain and antibiotic resistance	Maganti et al., 2003
Bethanechol	Nonspecific cholinergic muscarinic receptor agonist	Increases amplitude of contractions	Abdominal cramps, salivation, blurred vision and bladder spasm	Parkman et al., 2004
Botulinum toxin	A potent inhibitor of neuromuscular transmission	Improves both symptoms and gastric emptying	Swallowing difficulties and muscle weakness	Miller et al., 2002

Table 2: Pharmacological Treatment of Diabetic Gastroparesis.

Metoclopramide is a derivative of benzamide which has been used for years in the treatment of gastroparesis as a prokinetic agent. It releases acetylcholine from intrinsic myenteric cholinergic neurons by activating 5-HT_4 receptors as well as acting as a dopamine receptor antagonist in the stomach with a weak 5-HT_3 receptor antagonism (Parkman et al., 2004). Metoclopramide increases lower esophageal sphincter pressure and it improves symptoms of postprandial fullness and nausea. The prokinetic properties of metoclopramide are felt more in esophageal and fundus. However, it crosses the blood-brain barrier to cause extrapyramidal symptom, drowsiness and irritability. These adverse effects are dose-related and may be irreversible (Parkman *et al.*, 2004).

Domperidone is a substituted prokinetic benzimidazole derivative and a specific dopamine (D_2) receptor antagonist that is similar to metoclopramide in action. However, it does not readily cross the blood-brain barrier and less likely to cause extrapyramidal side effects like metoclopramide. Apart from its prokinetic effects on the stomach, domperidone possesses centrally mediated antiemetic properties by its action on the area postrema. Because of reduced side effects, dose increases can be employed although tachyphylaxis has been reported in patients (Horowitz *et al.*, 1985). Other side effects noted from using domperidone include hyperprolactinemia, menstrual disturbance and galactorrhea due to its antidopaminergic activity.

Cisapride is among prokinetic agents used by practitioners to treat patients with gastroparesis. It is an agonist of 5-HT_4 receptor and through this facilitates the release of acetylcholine in the gut. Cisapride is said to stimulate contractile responses to acetylcholine and improves antroduodenal coordination, and accelerates gastric emptying (Braden *et al.*, 2002). It increases the rate of gastric emptying time and decreases symptoms associated with gastroparesis. However, it causes cardiac arrhythmias which could lead to sudden death (Rabine & Barnett, 2001). Therefore, its use is contraindicated in individuals with underlying cardiac disease.

Erythromycin, a macrolide antibiotic, is a motilin receptor agonist which has a powerful prokinetic action and stimulates the contractility of the antrum and gastric emptying. In the process, smooth muscle and enteric nerves are also stimulated (Galligan & Vanner, 2005). Erythromycin has been shown to stimulate gastric emptying in diabetic gastroparesis and idiopathic gastroparesis. It is used to relieve symptoms associated with gastroparesis with a good safety profile. It has been reported that hyperglycemia attenuates the stimulation of antral contractility and gastric emptying by erythromycin (Parkman *et al.*, 2004).

The effect of erythromycin is said to diminish with time due to tachyphylaxis caused by downregulation of motilin receptors (Frazee & Mauro, 1994). The most common side effects exhibited by erythromycin are abdominal pain, nausea and skin rashes.

Bethanechol is a nonspecific cholinergic muscarinic receptor agonist which has been shown to enhance the amplitude of contractions throughout the gut. It lacks coordinated contractions and therefore gastric emptying is not demonstrable. It is however used as an adjunct with other agents. It exhibits cholinergic side effects.

For patients who are refractory to pharmacotherapy, botulinum toxin type A injection into the pylorus, or surgery can be considered. Botulinum toxin A is a bacterial toxin that causes muscle paralysis by inhibiting acetylcholine release. It has been shown to improve both symptoms and gastric emptying (Lacy & Zayat, 2002). Pylorospasm has been reported to occur in diabetic patients with gastroparesis.

6.2   Treatment of Diabetic Diarrhea

The treatment of diabetic diarrhea begins with non-pharmacological measures of fluid and electrolyte replacement, glycemic control and then symptomatic treatment. Octreotide a somatostatin analogue has been used in both normal and diabetic subjects to treat several types of refractory diarrhea (Table 3). It delays gastric emptying by prolonging intestinal transit, improves fluid and electrolyte absorption and directly suppresses gastrointestinal motility together with splanchnic vasoconstriction (Mourad *et al.*, 1992; Dudl *et al.*, 1987).

Drug	Mechanism of action	Effects	Adverse reactions	References
Octreotide	Somatostatin analogue	Reduce intestinal mucosal secretions and enhance absorption	Gallstones, allergic skin reactions, hair loss and inflammation	Dudl et al., 1987
Ramosetron	Selective 5-HT$_3$ receptor antagonist	Prolongs colonic transit time, inhibit intestinal bowel secretion and ameliorates fecal incontinence	Hard stools	Murao & Hosokawa, 2010
Clonidine	α_2 receptor agonist	Inhibits intestinal secretions	Hypotension, dry mouth, dizziness and constipation	Chang et al., 1986
Loperamide	Opioid-receptor agonist	Slows intestinal transit time and increases the internal anal sphincter tone	Toxic megacolon, bloating, nausea, vomiting and constipation	Vinik & Erbas, 2001
Antibiotics (metronidazole & tetracycline)	Decreases ability of bacteria to make protein	Inhibit and kill intestinal bacteria growth	Nausea and diarrhea	Dukowicz et al., 2007

Table 3: Pharmacological Treatment of Diabetic Diarrhea.

Ramosetron a 5-HT$_3$ serotonin receptor antagonist has also been employed in the treatment of diabetic diarrhea. It enhances absorption, prolongs colonic transit time, inhibits intestinal bowel secretion and ameliorates fecal incontinence (Murao & Hosokawa, 2010). However, because of the risk for constipation its use is reserved for severe cases. Studies have shown that loss of adrenergic innervation may play a role in autonomic neuropathy-induced intestinal fluid and electrolyte malabsorption in diabetic patients. Stimulation of α_2-adrenergic receptors on enterocytes promotes fluid and electrolyte absorption and inhibits anion secretion (Ogbonnaya & Arem, 1990). Clonidine, an α_2-adrenergic agonist, has been used to treat patients with diabetic diarrhea when other treatments had failed. It exhibits antisecretory and antimotility effect (Chang *et al.*, 1986). Loperamide, a drug used for symptomatic treatment of diabetic diarrhea, is known to slow intestinal transit time and increases the internal anal sphincter tone. However, it can be associated with abdominal pain and bloating, nausea, vomiting and constipation (Vinik & Erbas, 2001). In healthy subjects, there are usually normal intestinal flora in the small intestine. Diabetic conditions change the nature of these bacteria leading to overgrowth causing bloating and diarrhea. Sometimes the use of antibiotic therapy like tetracyclines and metronidazole is employed in such patients (Dukowicz *et al.*, 2007).

6.3   Treatment of Diabetic Constipation

Management of constipation in diabetic patients is similar to non-diabetic patients. Constipation may alternate with diabetic diarrhea and is one of the most common complications of diabetes mellitus. However, apart from conventional treatment methods of employing the use of laxatives, treatment might include good hydration, regular physical activity, and increased fiber intake. Sorbitol or lactulose can also be used to treat constipation (Shakil *et al.*, 2008). Lactulose and sorbitol are poorly absorbed sugars in the intestine and work by increasing the amount of water that is secreted within the intestines. Lactulose is effective in increasing stool frequency, volume and weight in chronic constipated patients. Also sorbitol has been shown to be equally effective as lactulose in increasing bowel movements and good stool consistency with similar side effects like abdominal bloating and flatulence (Foxx-Orenstein *et al.*, 2008; Rayner *et al.*, 2001). Acarbose is another useful agent that has been found to be valuable in the treatment of constipating diabetics (Hücking *et al.*, 2005). It reduces prolonged colonic transit times in addition to its beneficial effect in controlling diabetes (Ron *et al.*, 2002). Prucalopride, a 5-HT$_4$ agonist, has been shown to increase small bowel and colonic transit time and thereby improving the symptoms of constipation (Lacy & Weiser, 2006; Bouras *et al.*, 2001). It also accelerates orocecal transit and increases stool frequency in patients with chronic constipation (Coremans *et al.*, 2003) (Table 4).

Drug	Mechanism of Action	Effects	Adverse Reactions	References
Sorbitol/lactulose	Osmotic laxatives	Increase intestinal bulk	Abdominal bloating and flatulence	Rayner et al., 2001f
Acarbose	α-Glucosidase inhibitor	Impairing carbohydrate absorption	Abdominal pain, diarrhea and flatulence	Hücking et al., 2005
Prucalopride	Selective 5-HT$_4$ agonist	Increases stool frequency and colonic transit time	Abdominal pain, nausea and diarrhea	Lacy & Weiser, 2006

Table 4: Pharmacological Treatment of Diabetic Constipation.

7   Symptoms of End Stage Disease of the Gastrointestinal Tract in Diabetes Mellitus

There have been speculations in the past linking diabetes mellitus to several cancers of the gastrointestinal tract. Risk factors associated with diabetes mellitus and gastrointestinal tract cancers are shared by many other cancers linked with it. Evidence is emerging from assessments conducted studies by various workers, who have demonstrated a possible association between diabetes and gastrointestinal malignancy of the esophagus, stomach, colon and rectal (Onitilo *et al.*, 2012; Marimuthu *et al.*, 2011; Omran & Ismail, 2010; Larsson *et al.*, 2005). Epidemiological evidence has shown that the development of hypomotility in the stomach could lead to Barrett's esophagus and eventually adenocarcinoma (Sun & Yu, 2012). It is estimated that significant numbers of diabetics have increased risks of developing colorectal cancer and esophageal cancer compared with non-diabetic patients (Huang *et al.*, 2012; Sun & Yu, 2012). These associations were observed more in type 2 than that in type 1 and in both sexes. A state of hyperglycemia and increased oxidative stress may act together to contribute to the increase in cancer risk among diabetics. Similar mechanisms have been postulated for the etiology of diabetes induced cancers (Giovannucci *et al.*, 2010). This may be due to common fundamental pathophysiological mechanisms which include hyperinsulinemia, poor glycemic control, presence of advanced glycosylation end products and oxidative stress (Onitilo *et al.* 2012). Reports from studies have shown that hyperglycemia in diabetes is implicated with increased incidence and mortality for a range of cancers of the gastrointestinal tract (Deng *et al.*, 2012; Onitilo *et al.*, 2012; Jee *et al.,* 2005). This is associated with systemic inflammation, which could explain the role of oxidative stress. Because glycolysis is essential for cancer cells energy metabolism, hypergylcemia can promote carcinogenesis via the generation of reactive oxygen species within the cells (Sun & Yu, 2012). Oxidative radicals can damage the DNA directly or inhibit DNA repair mechanism (Onitilo *et al.*, 2012). It is reported that oxidative stress can influence the expression of gene signaling molecules (Reuter *et al.*, 2010). Anitha *et al.* (2006) demonstrated that hyperglycemia caused a dose-dependent increase in enteric neuronal apoptosis by inhibiting the glial-derived neurotrophic factor which promotes enteric neuron survival (Srinivasan *et al.*, 2005). Glial-derived neurotrophic factor mediates its activity by the expression of phosphatidylinositol-3-kinase signaling (Kashyap & Farrugia, 2011). There is strong evidence that hyperglycemia decreases phosphatidylinositol-3-kinase signaling by its inhibitory action on derived neurotrophic factor (Anitha *et al.*, 2006). It is believed that alteration in the phosphatidylinositol-3-kinase pathway can contribute to loss of gastrointestinal motility in both acute and chronic hyperglycemia. The regulations of the phosphatidylinositol-3-kinase pathway may be altered in a hyperglycemic state therefore suggesting that the expression of phosphatidylinositol-3-kinase plays a critical role in development of cancer associated with diabetes.

Clear understanding of the various mechanisms of hyperglycemia-induced enteric neuronal damage may provide a better management option of gastrointestinal disorders. It will also help in identifying potential therapeutic targets that will aid the development of new agents which will improve the disease burden of diabetic neuropathy in long standing diabetic patients.

Acknowledgement

This work was supported in part by Deanship of Scientific Research, King Faisal University, Saudi Arabia.

References

Abrahamsson, H. (1995). Gastrointestinal motility disorders in patients with diabetes mellitus. *Journal of Internal Medicine, 237(4), 403–409.*

Aljarallah, B. M. (2011). Management of diabetic gastroparesis. *Saudi Journal of Gastroenterology, 17(2), 97–104.*

Anitha, M., Gondha, C., Sutliff, R., Parsadanian, A., Mwangi, S., Sitaraman, S. V., & Srinivasan, S. (2006). GDNF rescues hyperglycemia-induced diabetic enteric neuropathy through activation of the PI3K/Akt pathway. *The Journal of Clinical Investigation, 116(2), 344–356.*

Anjaneyulu, M. & Ramarao, P. (2002). Studies on gastrointestinal tract functional changes in diabetic animals. *Methods and Findings in Experimental and Clinical Pharmacology, 24(2), 71–75.*

Belai, A., Lincoln, J., Milner, P., & Burnstock, G. (1988). Progressive changes in adrenergic, serotonergic, and peptidergic nerves in proximal colon of streptozotocin-diabetic rats. *Gastroenterology, 95(5), 1234–1241.*

Bener, A., Ghuloum, S., Al-Hamaq, A. O., & Dafeeah, E. E. (2012). Association between psychological distress and gastrointestinal symptoms in diabetes mellitus. *World Journal of Diabetes, 3(6), 123–129.*

Bernstein, G. (2000). The diabetic stomach: management strategies for clinicians and patients. *Diabetes Spectrum, 13, 11.*

Bjelaković, G., Nagorni, A., Stamenković, I., Benedeto-Stojanov, D., Bjelaković, M., Petrović, B., & Antić, S. (2005). Diabetes mellitus and digestive disorders. *ACTA Facultatis Medicae Naissensis, 22(1), 43–50.*

Boehme, M. W., Autschbach, F., Ell, C., & Raeth, U. (2007). Prevalence of silent gastric ulcer, erosions or severe acute gastritis in patients with type 2 diabetes mellitus--a cross-sectional study. *Hepato-gastroenterology, 54(74), 643–648.*

Bouras, E. P., Camilleri, M., Burton, D. D., Thomforde, G., McKinzie, S., & Zinsmeister, A. R. (2001). Prucalopride accelerates gastrointestinal and colonic transit in patients with constipation without a rectal evacuation disorder. *Gastroenterology, 120(2), 354–360.*

Braden, B., Enghofer, M., Schaub, M., Usadel, K. H., Caspary, W. F., & Lembcke, B. (2002). Long-term cisapride treatment improves diabetic gastroparesis but not glycaemic control. *Alimentary Pharmacology & Therapeutics, 16(7), 1341–1346.*

Brownlee, M., Cerami, A., & Vlassara, H. (1988). *Advanced glycosylation end products in tissue and the biochemical basis of diabetic complications. The New England Journal of Medicine, 318(20), 1315–1321.*

Brzozowska, I., Targosz, A., Sliwowski, Z., Kwiecien, S., Drozdowicz, D., Pajdo, R., Konturek, P. C., Brzozowski, T., Pawlik, M., Konturek, S. J., Pawlik, W. W., & Hahn, E. G. (2004). *Healing of chronic gastric ulcers in diabetic rats treated with native aspirin, nitric oxide (NO)-derivative of aspirin and cyclooxygenase (COX)-2 inhibitor. Journal of Physiology and Pharmacology, 55(4), 773–790.*

Bytzer, P., Talley, N. J., Hammer, J., Young, L. J., Jones, M. P., & Horowitz, M. (2002). *GI symptoms in diabetes mellitus are associated with both poor glycemic control and diabetic complications. The American Journal of Gastroenterology, 97(3), 604–611.*

Bytzer, P., Talley, N. J., Leemon, M., Young, L. J., Jones, M. P., & Horowitz, M. (2001). *Prevalence of gastrointestinal symptoms associated with diabetes mellitus: a population-based survey of 15,000 adults. Archives of Internal Medicine, 161(16), 1989–1996.*

Camilleri, M., Bharucha, A. E., & Farrugia, G. (2011). *Epidemiology, mechanisms, and management of diabetic gastroparesis. Clinical Gastroenterology and Hepatology, 9(1), 5–12; e7.*

Camilleri, M., Grover, M., & Farrugia, G. (2012). *What are the important subsets of gastroparesis? Neurogastroenterology and Motility, 24(7), 597–603.*

Carnethon, M. R., Prineas, R. J., Temprosa, M., Zhang, Z. M., Uwaifo, G., & Molitch, M. E.; Diabetes Prevention Program Research Group. (2006). *The association among autonomic nervous system function, incident diabetes, and intervention arm in the Diabetes Prevention Program. Diabetes Care, 2006 29(4), 914–919.*

Chandran, M., Chu, N. V., & Edelman, S. V. (2003). *Gastrointestinal disturbances in diabetes. Current Diabetes Reports, 3(1), 43–48.*

Chandrasekharan, B., Anitha, M., Blatt, R., Shahnavaz, N., Kooby, D., Staley, C., Mwangi, S., Jones, D. P., Sitaraman, S. V., & Srinivasan. S. (2011). *Colonic motor dysfunction in human diabetes is associated with enteric neuronal loss and increased oxidative stress. Neurogastroenterology and Motility, 23(2), 131–8.*

Chandrasekharan, B. & Srinivasan S. (2007). *Diabetes and the enteric nervous system. Neurogastroenterology & Motility, 19(12), 951–960.*

Chang, E. B., Fedorak, R. N., & Field, M. (1986). *Experimental diabetic diarrhea in rats. Intestinal mucosal denervation hypersensitivity and treatment with clonidine. Gastroenterology, 91(3), 564–569.*

Choi, K. M., Gibbons, S. J., Roeder, J. L., Lurken, M. S., Zhu, J., Wouters, M. M., Miller, S. M., Szurszewski, J. H., & Farrugia, G. (2007). *Regulation of interstitial cells of Cajal in the mouse gastric body by neuronal nitric oxide. Neurogastroenterology and Motility, 19(7), 585–595.*

Coremans, G., Kerstens, R., De Pauw, M., & Stevens M. (2003). *Prucalopride is effective in patients with severe chronic constipation in whom laxatives fail to provide adequate relief. Results of a double-blind, placebo-controlled clinical trial. Digestion, 67(1-2), 82–89.*

Cubiella Fernández, J., Núñez Calvo, L., González Vázquez, E., García García, M. J., Alves Pérez, M. T., Martínez Silva, I., & Fernández Seara, J. (2010). *Risk factors associated with the development of ischemic colitis. World Journal of Gastroenterology, 16(36), 4564–4569.*

Cuervas-Mons, M., Morte, L., Junquera, C., & Ramón y Cajal, S. (1990). *Effects of experimental diabetes in the noradrenergic and cholinergic nerves of the rat small intestine. Histology and Histopathology, 5(2), 193–198.*

Daneman, D. (2006). *Type 1 diabetes. Lancet, 367(9513), 847–858.*

De Freitas, P., Natali, M. R., Pereira, R. V., Miranda Neto, M. H., & Zanoni, J. N. (2008). *Myenteric neurons and intestinal mucosa of diabetic rats after ascorbic acid supplementation. World Journal of Gastroenterology, 14(42), 6518–6524.*

de Kort, S., Keszthelyi, D., & Masclee, A. A. (2011). *Leaky gut and diabetes mellitus: what is the link? Obesity Reviews, 12(6), 449–458.*

De Las Casas, L. E. & Finley, J. L. (1999). Diabetic microangiopathy in the small bowel. Histopathology, 35(3), 267–270.

Deng, L., Gui, Z., Zhao, L., Wang, J., & Shen, L. (2012). Diabetes mellitus and the incidence of colorectal cancer: an updated systematic review and meta-analysis. Digestive Diseases and Sciences, 57(6), 1576–1585.

DiMeglio, L. A., Chaet, M. S., Quigley, C. A., & Grosfeld, J. L. (2003). Massive ischemic intestinal necrosis at the onset of diabetes mellitus with ketoacidosis in a three-year-old girl. Journal of Pediatric Surgery, 38(10), 1537–1539.

Dudl, R. J., Anderson, D. S., Forsythe, A. B., Ziegler, M. G., & O'Dorisio, T. M. (1987). Treatment of diabetic diarrhea and orthostatic hypotension with somatostatin analogue SMS 201–995. The American Journal of Medicine, 83(3), 584–588.

Dukowicz, A. C., Lacy, B. E., & Levine, G. M. (2007). Small intestinal bacterial overgrowth: a comprehensive review. Gastroenterology & Hepatology (N Y), 3(2), 112–122.

Ebert, E. C. (2005). Gastrointestinal complications of diabetes mellitus. Disease-a-Month, 51(12), 620–663.

Eshraghian, A. & Eshraghian, H. (2011). Interstitial cells of Cajal: a novel hypothesis for the pathophysiology of irritable bowel syndrome. Canadian Journal of Gastroenterology, 25(5), 277–279.

Feldman, M. & Schiller, L. R. (1983). Disorders of gastrointestinal motility associated with diabetes mellitus. Annals of Internal Medicine, 98(3), 378–384.

Forgacs, I. & Patel, V. (2011). Diabetes and the gastrointestinal tract. Medicine, 39(5), 288–292.

Forrest, A., Huizinga, J. D., Wang, X. Y., Liu, L. W., & Parsons, M. (2008). Increase in stretch-induced rhythmic motor activity in the diabetic rat colon is associated with loss of ICC of the submuscular plexus. American Journal of Physiology, Gastrointestinal and Liver Physiology, 294(1), G315–G326.

Forster, J., Damjanov, I., Lin, Z., Sarosiek, I., Wetzel, P., & McCallum, R. W. (2005). Absence of the interstitial cells of Cajal in patients with gastroparesis and correlation with clinical findings. Journal of Gastrointestinal Surgery, 9(1), 102–108.

Foxx-Orenstein, A. E., McNally, M. A., & Odunsi, S. T. (2008). Update on constipation: one treatment does not fit all. Cleveland Clinic Journal of Medicine, 75(11), 813–824.

Frazee, L. A. & Mauro, L. S. (1994). Erythromycin in the Treatment of Diabetic Gastroparesis. American Journal of Therapeutics, 1(4), 287–295.

Frøkjaer, J. B., Andersen, S. D., Ejskaer, N., Funch-Jensen, P., Arendt-Nielsen, L., Gregersen, H., & Drewes, A. M. (2007). Gut sensations in diabetic autonomic neuropathy. Pain, 131(3), 320–329.

Galligan, J. J. & Vanner, S. (2005). Basic and clinical pharmacology of new motility promoting agents. Neurogastroenterology and Motility, 17(5), 643–653.

Giovannucci, E., Harlan, D. M., Archer, M. C., Bergenstal, R. M., Gapstur, S. M., Habel, L. A., Pollak, M., Regensteiner, J. G., & Yee, D. (2010). Diabetes and cancer: a consensus report. CA: a Cancer Journal for Clinicians, 60(4), 207–221.

Grover, M., Farrugia, G., Lurken, M. S., Bernard, C. E., Faussone-Pellegrini, M. S., Smyrk, T. C., Parkman, H. P., Abell, T. L., Snape, W. J., Hasler, W. L., Ünalp-Arida, A., Nguyen, L., Koch, K. L., Calles, J., Lee, L., Tonascia, J., Hamilton, F. A. & Pasricha, P. J.; NIDDK Gastroparesis Clinical Research Consortium. (2011). Cellular changes in diabetic and idiopathic gastroparesis. Gastroenterology, 140(5), 1575–1585.e8.

Guo, C., Quobatari, A., Shangguan, Y., Hong, S., & Wiley, J. W. (2004). Diabetic autonomic neuropathy: evidence for apoptosis in situ in the rat. Neurogastroenterology and Motility, 16(3), 335–345.

Harsch, I. A., Brzozowski, T., Bazela, K., Konturek, S. J., Kukharsky, V., Pawlik, T., Pawlowski, E., Hahn, E. G., & Konturek, P. C. (2003). Impaired gastric ulcer healing in diabetic rats: role of heat shock protein, growth factors, prostaglandins and proinflammatory cytokines. European Journal of Pharmacology, 481(2-3), 249–260.

Hasler, W. L. (2007). Type 1 diabetes and gastroparesis: diagnosis and treatment. Current Gastroenterology Reports, 9(4), 261–269.

He, C. L., Soffer, E. E., Ferris, C. D., Walsh, R. M., Szurszewski, J. H., & Farrugia, G. (2001). Loss of interstitial cells of cajal and inhibitory innervation in insulin-dependent diabetes. Gastroenterology, 121(2), 427–434.

Holloway, R. H., Tippett, M. D., Horowitz, M., Maddox, A. F., Moten, J., & Russo, A. (1999). Relationship between esophageal motility and transit in patients with type I diabetes mellitus. The American Journal of Gastroenterology, 94(11), 3150–3157.

Horowitz, M., Harding, P. E., Chatterton, B. E., Collins, P. J., & Shearman, D. J. (1985). Acute and chronic effects of domperidone on gastric emptying in diabetic autonomic neuropathy. Digestive Diseases and Sciences, 30(1), 1–9.

Horváth, V. J., Vittal, H., Lörincz, A., Chen, H., Almeida-Porada, G., Redelman, D., & Ordög, T. (2006). Reduced stem cell factor links smooth myopathy and loss of interstitial cells of cajal in murine diabetic gastroparesis. Gastroenterology, 130(3), 759–770.

Huang, W., Ren, H., Ben, Q., Cai, Q., Zhu, W., & Li, Z. (2012). Risk of esophageal cancer in diabetes mellitus: a meta-analysis of observational studies. Cancer Causes & Control, 23(2), 263–272.

Hücking, K., Kostic, Z., Pox, C., Ritzel, R., Holst, J. J., Schmiegel, W., & Nauck, M. A. (2005). alpha-Glucosidase inhibition (acarbose) fails to enhance secretion of glucagon-like peptide 1 (7-36 amide) and to delay gastric emptying in Type 2 diabetic patients. Diabetic Medicine, 22(4), 470–476.

Intagliata, N. & Koch, K. L. (2007). Gastroparesis in type 2 diabetes mellitus: prevalence, etiology, diagnosis, and treatment. Current Gastroenterology Reports, 9(4), 270–279.

Ishiguchi, T., Nakajima, M., Sone, H., Tada, H., Kumagai, A. K., & Takahashi, T. (2001). Gastric distension-induced pyloric relaxation: central nervous system regulation and effects of acute hyperglycaemia in the rat. The Journal of Physiology, 533(Pt 3), 801–813.

Iwasaki, H., Kajimura, M., Osawa, S., Kanaoka, S., Furuta, T., Ikuma, M., & Hishida, A. (2006). A deficiency of gastric interstitial cells of Cajal accompanied by decreased expression of neuronal nitric oxide synthase and substance P in patients with type 2 diabetes mellitus. Journal of Gastroenterology, 41(11), 1076–1087.

James, A. N., Ryan, J. P., Crowell, M. D., & Parkman, H. P. (2004). Regional gastric contractility alterations in a diabetic gastroparesis mouse model: effects of cholinergic and serotoninergic stimulation. American Journal of Physiology. Gastrointestinal and Liver Physiology, 287(3), G612–G619.

Jee, S. H., Ohrr, H., Sull, J. W., Yun, J. E., Ji, M., & Samet, J. M. (2005). Fasting serum glucose level and cancer risk in Korean men and women. JAMA: the Journal of American Medical Association, 293(2), 194–202.

Jenkinson, K. M. & Reid, J. J. (1995). Effect of diabetes on relaxations to non-adrenergic, non-cholinergic nerve stimulation in longitudinal muscle of the rat gastric fundus. British Journal of Pharmacology, 116(1), 1551–1556.

Jørgensen, F., Boesen, F., Andersen, E. B., & Hesse, B. (1991). Oesophageal transit in patients with autonomic dysfunction. The effect of treatment with fludrocortisone. Clinical Physiology, 11(1), 83–92.

Jung, H. K., Kim, D. Y., Moon, I. H., & Hong, Y. S. (2003). Colonic transit time in diabetic patients--comparison with healthy subjects and the effect of autonomic neuropathy. Yonsei Medical Journal, 44(2), 265–272.

Kandemir, O., Utas, C., Gönen, O., Patiroglu, T. E., Ozbakir, O., Kelestimur, F., & Yücesoy, M. (1995). Colonic subepithelial collagenous thickening in diabetic patients. Diseases of the Colon and Rectum, 38(10), 1097–1100.

Karayiannakis, A. J., Bolanaki, H., Kouklakis, G., Dimakis, K., Memet, I., & Simopoulos, C. (2011). Ischemic colitis of the left colon in a diabetic patient. Case Reports in Gastroenterology, 5(1), 239–245.

Kashyap, P. & Farrugia, G. (2010). Diabetic gastroparesis: what we have learned and had to unlearn in the past 5 years. Gut, 59(12), 1716–1726.

Kashyap, P. & Farrugia, G. (2011). Oxidative stress: key player in gastrointestinal complications of diabetes. Neurogastroenterology and Motility, 23(2), 111–114.

Kassander, P. (1958). Asymptomatic gastric retention in diabetics (gastroparesis diabeticorum). Annals of Internal Medicine, 48(4), 797–812.

Kasznicki, J., Kosmalski, M., Sliwinska, A., Mrowicka, M., Stanczyk, M., Majsterek, I., & Drzewoski, J. (2012). Evaluation of oxidative stress markers in pathogenesis of diabetic neuropathy. Molecular Biology Report, 39(9), 8669–8678.

Keshavarzian, A. & Iber, F. L. (1986). Intestinal transit in insulin-requiring diabetics. The American Journal of Gastroenterology, 81(4), 257–260.

Kim, S. J., Park, J. H., Song, D. K., Park, K. S., Lee, J. E., Kim, E. S., Cho, K. B., Jang, B. K., Chung, W. J., Hwang, J. S., Kwon, J. G., & Kim, T. W. (2011). Alterations of colonic contractility in long-term diabetic rat model. Journal of Neurogastroenterology and Motility, 17(4), 372–380.

Kim, Y. J., Kim, E. H., & Hahm, K. B. (2012). Oxidative stress in inflammation-based gastrointestinal tract diseases: challenges and opportunities. Journal of Gastroenterology and Hepatology, 27(6), 1004–1010.

King, G. L, & Loeken, M. R. (2004). Hyperglycemia-induced oxidative stress in diabetic complications. Histochemistry and Cell Biology, 122(4), 333–338.

Ko, G. T., Chan, W. B., Chan, J. C., Tsang, L. W., & Cockram, C. S. (1999). Gastrointestinal symptoms in Chinese patients with Type 2 diabetes mellitus. Diabetic Medicine, 16(8), 670–674.

Koch, C. A. & Uwaifo, G. I. (2008). Are gastrointestinal symptoms related to diabetes mellitus and glycemic control? European Journal of Gastroenterology & Hepatology, 20(9), 822–825.

Kong, M. F. & Horowitz, M. (2005). Diabetic gastroparesis. Diabetic Medicine, 22(Suppl 4), 13–18.

Konturek, P. C., Brzozowski, T., Burnat, G., Szlachcic, A., Koziel, J., Kwiecien, S., Konturek, S. J., & Harsch, I. A. (2010). Gastric ulcer healing and stress-lesion preventive properties of pioglitazone are attenuated in diabetic rats. Journal of Physiology and Pharmacology, 61(4), 429–436.

Kota, S. K., Meher, L. K., Jammula, S., Kota, S. K., & Modi, K. D. (2012). Genetics of type 2 diabetes mellitus and other specific types of diabetes; its role in treatment modalities. Diabetes & Metabolic Syndrome, 6(1), 54–58.

Kotler, D. P. & Hsu, S. (2010). Gastrointestinal Manifestations of Diabetes. In: Poretsky, L. (ed.), Principles of Diabetes Mellitus, (2nd edition), Springer Science+Business Media, LLC, DOI 10.1007/978-0-387-09841-8_27, (pp. 419–434).

Lacy, B. E. & Weiser, K. (2006). Gastrointestinal motility disorders: an update. Digestive Diseases, 24(3-4), 228–242.

Lacy, B. E., Zayat, E. N., Crowell, M. D., & Schuster, M. M. (2002). Botulinum toxin for the treatment of gastroparesis: a preliminary report. The American Journal of Gastroenterology, 97(6), 1548–1552.

la Roca-Chiapas, J. M. & Cordova-Fraga, T. (2011). Biomagnetic techniques for evaluating gastric emptying, peristaltic contraction and transit time. World Journal of Gastrointestinal Pathophysiology, 2(5), 65–71.

Larsson, S. C., Orsini, N., & Wolk, A. (2005). Diabetes mellitus and risk of colorectal cancer: a meta-analysis. Journal of the National Cancer Institute, 97(22), 1679–1687.

Lincoln, J., Bokor, J. T., Crowe, R., Griffith, S. G., Haven, A. J., & Burnstock, G. (1984). Myenteric plexus in streptozotocin-treated rats. Neurochemical and histochemical evidence for diabetic neuropathy in the gut. Gastroenterology, 86(4), 654–661.

Liu, J., Qiao, X., Micci, M. A., Pasricha, P. J., & Chen, J. D. (2004). Improvement of gastric motility with gastric electrical stimulation in STZ-induced diabetic rats. Digestion, 70(3), 159–166.

Lomax, A. E., Sharkey, K. A., & Furness, J. B. (2010). The participation of the sympathetic innervation of the gastrointestinal tract in disease states. Neurogastroenterology and Motility, 22(1), 7–18.

Longo, W. E., Ballantyne, G. H., & Gusberg, R. J. (1992). Ischemic colitis: patterns and prognosis. Diseases of the Colon and Rectum, 35(8), 726–730.

Longstreth, G. F. & Yao, J. F. (2010). Diseases and drugs that increase risk of acute large bowel ischemia. Clinical Gastroenterology and Hepatology, 8(1), 49–54.

Lysy, J., Israeli, E., & Goldin, E. (1999). The prevalence of chronic diarrhea among diabetic patients. The American Journal of Gastroenterology, 94(8), 2165–2170.

Ma, J., Rayner, C. K., Jones, K. L., & Horowitz, M. (2009). Diabetic gastroparesis: diagnosis and management. Drugs, 69(8), 971–986.

Maganti, K., Onyemere, K., & Jones, M. P. (2003). Oral erythromycin and symptomatic relief of gastroparesis: a systematic review. The American Journal of Gastroenterology, 98(2), 259–263.

Mandelstam, P. & Lieber, A. (1967). Esophageal dysfunction in diabetic neuropathy-gastroenteropathy. Clinical and roentgenological manifestations. JAMA: the Journal of American Medical Association, 201(8), 582–586.

Marimuthu, S. P., Vijayaragavan, P., Moysich, K. B., & Jayaprakash, V. (2011). Diabetes mellitus and gastric carcinoma: Is there an association? Journal of Carcinogenesis, 10, 30.

Mehta, N., Veliath, S., & Thombre, D. P. (2002). Effect of experimental diabetes and vagotomy on gastric emptying in rats. Indian Journal of Physiology and Pharmacology, 46(4), 441–448.

Miller, L. S., Szych, G. A., Kantor, S. B., Bromer, M. Q., Knight, L. C., Maurer, A. H., Fisher, R. S., & Parkman, H. P. (2002). Treatment of idiopathic gastroparesis with injection of botulinum toxin into the pyloric sphincter muscle. The American Journal of Gastroenterology, 97(7), 1653–1660.

Mirakhur, A. & Walshaw, M. J. (2003). Autonomic dysfunction in cystic fibrosis. Journal of the Royal Society of Medicine, 96(Suppl 43), 11–7.

Mishima, Y., Amano, Y., Takahashi, Y., Mishima, Y., Moriyama, N., Miyake, T., Ishimura, N., Ishihara, S., & Kinoshita, Y. (2009). Gastric emptying of liquid and solid meals at various temperatures: effect of meal temperature for gastric emptying. Journal of Gastroenterology, 44(5), 412–418.

Morsy, M. A., Ashour, O. M., Fouad, A. A., & Abdel-Gaber, S. A. (2010). Gastroprotective effects of the insulin sensitizers rosiglitazone and metformin against indomethacin-induced gastric ulcers in Type 2 diabetic rats. Clinical and Experimental Pharmacology & Physiology, 37(2), 173–177.

Mourad, F. H., Gorard, D., Thillainayagam, A. V., Colin-Jones, D., & Farthing, M. J. (1992). Effective treatment of diabetic diarrhoea with somatostatin analogue, octreotide. Gut, 33(11), 1578–1580.

Murao, S. & Hosokawa, H. (2010). Serotonin 5-HT3 receptor antagonist for treatment of severe diabetic diarrhea. Diabetes Care, 33(3), e38.

Nagai, T., Tomizawa, T., Monden, T., & Mori, M. (1998). Diabetes mellitus accompanied by nonocclusive colonic ischemia. Internnal Medicine, 37(5), 454–456.

Nowak, T. V., Johnson, C. P., Kalbfleisch, J. H., Roza, A. M., Wood, C. M., Weisbruch, J. P., & Soergel, K. H. (1995). Highly variable gastric emptying in patients with insulin dependent diabetes mellitus. Gut, 37(1), 23–29.

Ogbonnaya, K. I. & Arem, R. (1990). Diabetic diarrhea. Pathophysiology, diagnosis, and management. Archives of Internal Medicine, 150(2), 262–267.

Omran, S. & Ismail, A. A. (2010). Knowledge and beliefs of Jordanians toward colorectal cancer screening. Cancer Nursing, 33(2), 141–8.

Onitilo, A. A., Engel, J. M., Glurich, I., Stankowski, R. V., Williams, G. M., & Doi, S. A. (2012). Diabetes and cancer II: role of diabetes medications and influence of shared risk factors. Cancer Causes & Control, 23(7), 991–1008.

Ordög, T., Hayashi, Y., & Gibbons, S. J. (2009). Cellular pathogenesis of diabetic gastroenteropathy. Minerva Gastroenterologica e Dietologica, 55(3), 315–343.

Parkman, H. P., Hasler, W. L., Fisher, R. S.; & American Gastroenterological Association. (2004). American Gastroenterological Association technical review on the diagnosis and treatment of gastroparesis. Gastroenterology, 127(5), 1592–1622.

Pasricha, P. J., Pehlivanov, N. D., Gomez, G., Vittal, H., Lurken, M. S., & Farrugia, G. (2008). Changes in the gastric enteric nervous system and muscle: a case report on two patients with diabetic gastroparesis. BMC Gastroenterology, 8, 21.

Peng, H. & Hagopian, W. (2006). Environmental factors in the development of Type 1 diabetes. Reviews in Endocrine & Metabolic Disorders, 7(3), 149–162.

Quigley, E. M. (1999). The evaluation of gastrointestinal function in diabetic patients. World Journal of Gastroenterology, 5(4), 277–282.

Rabine, J. C. & Barnett, J. L. (2001). Management of the patient with gastroparesis. Journal of Clinical Gastroenterology, 32(1), 11–18.

Rayner, C. K., Samsom, M., Jones, K. L., & Horowitz, M. (2001). Relationships of upper gastrointestinal motor and sensory function with glycemic control. Diabetes Care, 24(2), 371–381.

Reuter, S., Gupta, S. C., Chaturvedi, M. M., & Aggarwal, B. B. (2010). Oxidative stress, inflammation, and cancer: how are they linked? Free Radical Biology & Medicine, 49(11), 1603–1616.

Ricci, J. A., Siddique, R., Stewart, W. F., Sandler, R. S., Sloan, S., & Farup, C. E. (2000). Upper gastrointestinal symptoms in a U.S. national sample of adults with diabetes. Scandinavian Journal of Gastroenterology, 35(2), 152–159.

Rodrigues, M. L. & Motta, M. E. (2012). Mechanisms and factors associated with gastrointestinal symptoms in patients with diabetes mellitus. Jornal de Pediatria (Rio J), 88(1), 17–24.

Rojas, A., Romay, S., González, D., Herrera, B., Delgado, R., & Otero, K. (2000). Regulation of endothelial nitric oxide synthase expression by albumin-derived advanced glycosylation end products. Circulation Research, 86(3), E50–E54.

Ron, Y., Wainstein, J., Leibovitz, A., Monastirsky, N., Habot, B., Avni, Y., & Segal, R. (2002). The effect of acarbose on the colonic transit time of elderly long-term care patients with type 2 diabetes mellitus. The Journals of Gerontology. Series A, Biological Sciences and Medical Sciences, 57(2), M111–M114.

Rösen, P., Nawroth, P. P., King, G., Möller, W., Tritschler, H. J., & Packer, L. (2001). The role of oxidative stress in the onset and progression of diabetes and its complications: a summary of a Congress Series sponsored by UNESCO-MCBN, the American Diabetes Association and the German Diabetes Society. Diabetes/Metabolism Research and Reviews, 17(3), 189–212.

Samsom, M., Akkermans, L. M., Jebbink, R. J., van Isselt, H., vanBerge-Henegouwen, G. P., & Smout, A. J. (1997). Gastrointestinal motor mechanisms in hyperglycaemia induced delayed gastric emptying in type I diabetes mellitus. Gut, 40(5), 641–646.

Sanders, K. M., Ördög, T., Koh, S. D., & Ward, S. M. (2000). A novel pacemaker mechanism drives gastrointestinal rhythmicity. News in Physiological Sciences, 15(6), 291–298.

Sarna, S. K. (2006). Molecular, functional, and pharmacological targets for the development of gut promotility drugs. American Journal of Physiology. Gastrointestinal and Liver Physiology, 291(4), G545–G555.

Schmidt, R. E., Plurad, D. A., & Roth, K. A. (1988). Effects of chronic experimental streptozotocin-induced diabetes on the noradrenergic and peptidergic innervation of the rat alimentary tract. Brain Research, 458(2), 353–360.

Shakil, A., Church, R. J., & Rao, S. S. (2008). Gastrointestinal complications of diabetes. American Family Physician, 77(12), 1697–1702.

Shakov, R., Salazar, R. S., Kagunye, S. K., Baddoura, W. J., & DeBari, V. A. (2011). Diabetes mellitus as a risk factor for recurrence of Clostridium difficile infection in the acute care hospital setting. American Journal of Infection Control, 39(3), 194–198.

Sharieff, G. Q., Shad, J. A., & Garmel, G. (1997). An unusual case of mesenteric ischemia in a patient with new-onset diabetes mellitus. The American Journal of Emergency Medicine, 15(3), 282–284.

Sheetz, M. J. & King, G. L. (2002). Molecular understanding of hyperglycemia's adverse effects for diabetic complications. The Journal of the American Medical Association, 288(20), 2579–2588.

Smith, D. S. & Ferris, C. D. (2003). Current concepts in diabetic gastroparesis. Drugs, 63(13), 1339–1358.

Spångéus, A. & El-Salhy, M. (2001). Myenteric plexus of obese diabetic mice (an animal model of human type 2 diabetes). Histology and Histopathology, 16(1), 159–165.

Spångéus, A., Suhr, O., & El-Salhy, M. (2000). Diabetic state affects the innervation of gut in an animal model of human type 1 diabetes. Histology and Histopathology, 15(3), 739–744.

Sparre, T., Larsen, M. R., Heding, P. E., Karlsen, A. E., Jensen, O. N., & Pociot, F. (2005). Unraveling the pathogenesis of type 1 diabetes with proteomics: present and future directions. Molecular & Cellular Proteomics, 4(4), 441–457.

Spotnitz, W. D., Van Natta, F. C., Bashist, B., Wolff, M., Green, P., & Weber, C. J. (1984). Localized ischemic colitis in a young woman with diabetes. Diseases of the Colon and Rectum, 27(7), 481–484.

Srinivasan, S., Anitha, M., Mwangi, S., & Heuckeroth, R. O. (2005). Enteric neuroblasts require the phosphatidylinositol 3-kinase/Akt/Forkhead pathway for GDNF-stimulated survival. Molecular and Cellular Neurosciences, 29(1), 107–119.

Stacher, G. (2001). Diabetes mellitus and the stomach. Diabetologia, 44(9), 1080–1093.

Sun, L. & Yu, S. (2012). Diabetes mellitus is an independent risk factor for colorectal cancer. Digestive Diseases and Sciences, 57(6), 1586–1597.

Suzuki, H., Nishizawa, T., Tsugawa, H., Mogami, S., & Hibi, T. (2012). Roles of oxidative stress in stomach disorders. Journal of Clinical Biochemistry and Nutrition, 50(1), 35–39.

Talley, N. J. (2003). Diabetic gastropathy and prokinetics. The American Journal of Gastroenterology, 98(2), 264–271.

Taub, S., Mariani, A., & Barkin, J. S. (1979). Gastrointestinal manifestations of diabetes mellitus. Diabetes Care, 2(6), 437–447.

Tieppo, J., Kretzmann Filho, N. A., Seleme, M., Fillmann, H. S., Berghmans, B., & Possa Marroni, N. (2009). Anal pressure in experimental diabetes. International Journal of Colorectal Disease, 24(12), 1395–1399.

Tonini, M., De Giorgio, R., De Ponti, F., Sternini, C., Spelta, V., Dionigi, P., Barbara, G., Stanghellini, V., & Corinaldesi R. (2000). Role of nitric oxide- and vasoactive intestinal polypeptide-containing neurones in human gastric fundus strip relaxations. British Journal of Pharmacology, 129(1), 12–20.

Tougas, G., Eaker, E. Y., Abell, T. L., Abrahamsson, H., Boivin, M., Chen, J., Hocking, M. P., Quigley, E. M., Koch, K. L., Tokayer, A. Z., Stanghellini, V., Chen, Y., Huizinga, J. D., Rydén, J., Bourgeois, I., & McCallum, R. W. (2000). Assessment of gastric emptying using a low fat meal: establishment of international control values. The American Journal of Gastroenterology, 95(6), 1456–1462.

Tseng, C. H. (2012). Diabetes, insulin use and Helicobacter pylori eradication: a retrospective cohort study. BMC Gastroenterology, 12, 46.

Unal, A., Guven, K., Yurci, A., Torun, E., Gursoy, S., Baskol, M., Ozturk, F., & Arsav, V. (2008). Is increased colon subepithelial collagen layer thickness in diabetic patients related to collagenous colitis? An immunohistochemical study. Pathology, Research and Practice, 204(8), 537–544.

Vinik, A. I., Anandacoomaraswamy, D., & Ullal, J. (2005). Antibodies to neuronal structures: innocent bystanders or neurotoxins? Diabetes Care, 28(8), 2067–2072.

Vinik, A.I. & Erbas, T. (2001). Recognizing and treating diabetic autonomic neuropathy. Cleveland Clinic Journal of Medicine, 68(11), 928-930, 932, 934–944.

Vinik, A. I., Maser, R. E., Mitchell, B. D., & Freeman, R,. (2003). Diabetic autonomic neuropathy. Diabetes Care, 26(5), 1553–1579.

Virally-Monod, M., Tielmans, D., Kevorkian, J. P., Bouhnik Y., Flourie, B., Porokhov, B., Ajzenberg, C., Warnet, A., & Guillausseau, P. J. (1998). Chronic diarrhoea and diabetes mellitus: prevalence of small intestinal bacterial overgrowth. Diabetes & Metabolism, 24(6), 530–536.

Vittal, H., Farrugia, G., Gomez, G., & Pasricha, P. J. (2007). Mechanisms of disease: the pathological basis of gastroparesis--a review of experimental and clinical studies. Nature Clinical Practice. Gastroenterology & Hepatology, 4(6), 336–346.

Wautier, J. L. & Guillausseau, P. J. (2001). Advanced glycation end products, their receptors and diabetic angiopathy. Diabetes & Metabolism, 27(5 Pt 1), 535–542.

Weiss, J. S. & Sumpio, B. E. (2006). Review of prevalence and outcome of vascular disease in patients with diabetes mellitus. European Journal of Vascular and Endovascular Surgery, 31(2), 143–150.

Wolosin, J. D. & Edelman, S. V. (2000). Diabetes and the Gastrointestinal Tract. Clinical Diabetes, 18(4), 148–151.

Xu, B., Chibber, R., Ruggiero, D., Kohner, E., Ritter, J., & Ferro, A. (2003). Impairment of vascular endothelial nitric oxide synthase activity by advanced glycation end products. FASEB Journal, 17(10), 1289–1291.

Yang, R., Arem, R., & Chan, L. (1984). Gastrointestinal tract complications of diabetes mellitus. Pathophysiology and management. Archives of Internal Medicine, 144(6), 1251–1256.

Yin, J., Chen, J., & Chen, J. D. (2010). Ameliorating effects and mechanisms of electroacupuncture on gastric dysrhythmia, delayed emptying, and impaired accommodation in diabetic rats. American Journal of Physiology. Gastrointestinal and Liver Physiology, 298(4), G563–570.

Zanoni, J. N., Hernandes, L., Bazotte, R. B., & Miranda Neto, M. H. (2002). Terminal ileum submucous plexus: Study of the VIP-ergic neurons of diabetic rats treated with ascorbic acid. Arquivos de Neuro-psiquiatria, 60(1), 32–37.

Zhao, J., Frøkjaer, J. B., Drewes, A. M., & Ejskjaer, N. (2006). Upper gastrointestinal sensory-motor dysfunction in diabetes mellitus. World Journal of Gastroenterology, 12(18), 2846–2857.

Zhao, J., Liao, D., Yang, J., & Gregersen, H. (2010). Biomechanical Remodeling of the Diabetic Gastrointestinal Tract. In: Levy, J. H. (ed.), Biomechanics: Principles, Trends and Applications, Nova Science Publishers, ISBN: 978-1-61761-865-9, (pp.137–162).

Zochodne, D. W. (2007). Diabetes mellitus and the peripheral nervous system: manifestations and mechanisms. Muscle & Nerve, 36(2), 144–166.

Anthropometric Detection of Macrosomia in Nigerian Fetuses

Emmanuel Stephen Mador
Department of Anatomy
University of Jos, Nigeria

John Oluwole Ogunranti
Department of Anatomy
University of Jos, Nigeria

Ishaya Chuwang Pam
Department of Obstetrics & Gynaecology
University of Jos, Nigeria

1   Introduction

It has been suggested long ago that there should be clinical anthropologists in developing countries whose main responsibility would be the making available of anthropological information for the diagnosis of diseases and their treatment. In nearly all cases this would be the physician working in a particular community, who would need all the anthropometric data of that community for making a diagnosis. For instance, serial measurements of fetal growth by ultrasonography and measurements of biparietal diameter and trunk circumference have been reported to allow some assessment of normal fetal size during intrauterine life but the use of these fetal parameters together with their ratios in the detection of abnormal fetal growth have not been reported in Jos, Nigeria. Only when the values of these parameters are available then can the physician arrive at a meaningful diagnosis of abnormal fetal growth in this setting. The development of macrosomia, just like that of macrocephaly, can be identified by ultrasonography. Macrosomic fetal growth can be discovered sonographically when estimated fetal weight is greater than the 90th percentile of the general population or when the abdominal circumference is found to be above the 95th percentile. The ratio of femur length to abdominal circumference can be used for early detection of accelerated fetal growth. The biparietal diameter, head circumference, occipitofrontal diameter, abdominal circumference and femur length of 13,740 healthy Nigerian fetuses drawn from a population of healthy pregnant women were studied in a cross-sectional fashion from 12 – 42 weeks and the 3rd, 5th, 10th, 50th, 90th, 95th and 97th centiles derived for all the measured parameters. The predictive formulae of the 95th centiles were also derived so also the 90th centile for estimated fetal weight. The importance of the 90th and the 95th percentiles in the diagnosis of macrosomia is discussed.

Macrosomia refers to a fetus weighing 4kg or more at birth. Severe macrosomia refers to birth weight of 4.5g or more. Closely related to macrosomia is the term macrocephaly which is said to be present when the fetal head dimensions are above the 95th percentile (Mador *et al.*, 2012a). Macrosomia is associated with increased perinatal morbidity and mortality (Ballard *et al* 1984; Boyd *et al.*, 1983; Hansmann & Hinckers, 1974; Stevenson *et al.*, 1982). When Modanlou and his co-workers (1980) studied the maternal, fetal and neonatal implications of macrosomia they found that the mortality in infants with birth weight greater than 4500g was twice as high as in infants with normal size. During labour, a large fetal head and trunk can cause dystocic complications. If a relative disproportion is already present, a cesarean delivery is inevitable. In some cases a cesarean section can be avoided by detecting accelerated fetal growth at an early stage and scheduling preterm induction at approximately 38 weeks. The development of macrosomia, like that of macrocephaly, can be detected sonographically. Macrosomic growth can be detected sonographically either by intrauterine weight estimation (Farmer *et al.*, 1992; Mador *et al.*, 2012b), fetal weight greater than 90th centile or by determining the abdominal circumference (Deter *et al.*, 1985; Hadlock *et al.*, 1985; Tamura *et al.*, 1986, Mador *et al.*, 2012c; Pam *et al.*, 2012a). Hadlock *et al* (1985) recommend using the ratio of FL/AC for early detection of accelerated fetal growth which was also confirmed by Pam and his co-workers (Pam *et al.*, 2012b). One disadvantage of weight estimation is that there is tendency to overestimate weight due to excessive fat deposition in macrosomic fetuses (Bernstein & Catalano, 1992). While fat markedly increases the abdominal girth, it is less dense than muscle tissue. Macrosomia is assumed to be present when abdominal measurements yield dimensions that are above 95th percentile. If only the head dimensions are above the 95th percentile, macrocephaly is diagnosed (Mador *et al.*, 2012a). Macrosomic growth is described as proportional when head and trunk dimensions are above the normal range by an equal degree. If the measurements are at or slightly above the upper limit of normal, the differential diagnosis should include a genetically large offspring of large parents. If only trunk growth is accelerated, the macrosomia is described as disproportional. Increased abdominal growth with a relatively normal head circumference is seen in diabetic macrosomia, for example. The degree of disproportionality in these cases can be evaluated by calculating the head/trunk ratio (Mador, 2012). If only the trunk is enlarged, the head/trunk ratio will be low. With proportional macrosomia, the head/trunk ratio will be unchanged. In macrocephaly or macrocephalic head growth due to advanced hydrocephalus, both the biparietal diameter and head circumference are too large (Mador, 2012). Because the abdominal dimensions are within normal limits, the head/trunk ratio is correspondingly high. The causes of fetal macrosomia are largely unknown. Empirical factors that can alert the physician to the development of macrosomia include maternal birth weight, multiparity, the previous delivery of a macrosomic infant, maternal obesity, an extreme weight gain during pregnancy and large parents (Timofeev *et al.*, 2012; Dyer & Rosenfeld, 2011; Udall *et al.*, 1978; Larkin *et al.*, 2011; Tarim & Cok, 2011; Baptiste-Roberts *et al.*, 2012; Stallone & Ziel 1974; Alberico *et al.*, 2010; Mulder *et al.*, 2010; Klebanoff *et al.*, 1985; Parks & Ziel, 1978; Wiedemann *et al.*, 1983). In some cases, fetal macrosomia can be related to specific syndromes such as wiedemann-Beckwith syndrome, satos syndrome or weaver syndrome (Wiedemann *et al.*, 1983). An established cause of macrosomia is maternal diabetes mellitus, though this disease is implicated in fewer than 10% of large for gestational age cases.

2   Control of Fetal Growth

Every individual spends the first nine months of its life within the womb (uterus) of its mother (Welin, 2004; Simonstein, 2006; Wheeler *et al.*, 2007). During this period it develops from a small one-celled structure to an organism having billions of cells. During the first two months the developing individual is called an embryo. After that it is called a fetus. Intrauterine growth of the fetus is influenced by maternal factors (Le Clair *et al.*, 2009; Fall, 2009; Yajnik & Deshmukh, 2008; Kanaka-Gantenbein, 2010), placental factors and fetal factors (Koukoura *et al.*, 2012; Sandovici *et al.*, 2012; Jansson & Powell, 2007; Robinson *et al.*, 1995; Angiolini *et al.*, 2006; Wilhelm-Benartzi *et al.*, 2012). Adequate availability of nutrition in maternal blood, and its transfer across the placenta, is essential for normal growth of the fetus. Malnutrition in the mother affects fetal growth and can possibly cause fetal malformation. As a rule maternal hormones do not pass through the placenta and hence they cannot affect fetal growth. However, they can influence the fetus indirectly by controlling maternal metabolic processes. Hormones secreted by the placenta can influence the fetus indirectly by influencing maternal metabolism. For example, somatomammotropin secreted by the placenta has an anti-insulin effect leading to increased plasma levels of glucose and amino acids in maternal blood. The availability of these to the fetus is, thereby, increased. Placental hormones also have a direct influence on fetal growth. Somatomammotropin increases fetal growth. Human chorionic gonadotropin (hCG) stimulates growth of the fetal testis. Fetal factors that influence fetal growth are genetic. However, genetic factors that determine the height of the individual operate mainly in postnatal life through the action of the growth hormone and thyroid hormones. When the growth of a fetus is less than that seen in 90 per cent of fetuses (i.e. it is below the 90th percentile) the phenomenon is described as intrauterine growth retardation. Such infants are described as small for gestational age. Apart from genetic factors like chromosomal abnormalities, growth retardation can be caused by infections, poor nutrition, and use of harmful drugs, by the mother.

3   Diabetes in Pregnancy

Several investigators (Pöyhönen-Alho *et al.*, 2012; Saxena *et al.*, 2012; Ozanne *et al.*, 2011; Salbaum & Kappen, 2011) have reported that pregnancy affects maternal diabetes and produces an increase in insulin requirements, at the same time; diabetes has a significant effect on the pregnancy (Retnakaran *et al.*, 2012; Colatrella *et al.*, 2012; Kwak *et al.*, 2012). With appropriate management and careful regulation of blood glucose levels, perinatal losses can be minimized and will approach levels in the normal population. This management is best undertaken by a combined team of physicians and obstetricians and delivery should always be effected in a major obstetric hospital which has first class neonatal services.

All forms of diabetes are associated with increased perinatal loss unless properly managed. The degree of risk is related to the severity of the diabetes. According to the British Diabetic Association, potential diabetes refers to patients with no evidence of clinical diabetes but who have a family history of diabetes, a previous history of delivering an infant in excess of 4kg, or a history of an unexplained fetal death. Glycosuria is not a reliable sign, but should be investigated if it is persistent. Latent or gestational diabetes on the other had refer to women who develop overt diabetes in later life develop chemical or clinical diabetes during pregnancy. Apart from these two, there is chemical diabetes. Women with chemical diabetes have an abnormal glucose tolerance test, but no symptoms of diabetes. Perinatal morbidity is significantly increased in this category of patients. The fourth variant is clinical diabetes which can either be insulin dependent or independent. Insulin dependent diabetes requires careful control throughout pregnancy and should preferably be regulated before pregnancy is commenced.

The American Classification introduced by White in 1965 also linked management and prognosis to further sub classification of diabetes as follows:

a)   class A – chemical diabetes only

b)   class B – diabetes of adults; onset after 20 years of age

c)   Class C – diabetes of long duration (between 10 and 19 years) with no evidence of vascular disease

d)   Class D – diabetes present since before the age of 10 years and present for 20 years or more with vascular disease, calcification of vessels or benign retinopathy

e)   Class E – diabetes associated with calcification of the limb vessels

f)   Class F – diabetes-associated nephropathy

g)   Class G – the presence of proliferating diabetic retinopathy.

In women with suspected abnormalities of glucose tolerance, a glucose tolerance test should be performed. This test involves the oral administration of 50g of glucose. An abnormal test is defined by the following criteria:

a)   A fasting value of blood glucose in excess of 5.5mmol/l

b)   A 1 hour value over 9mmol/l

c)   A 2 hour value over 7mmol/l

3.1   Maternal Complications

1. Pregnancy is diabetogenic and diabetic control therefore becomes difficult. Hyperglycaemia is common and if uncontrolled leads to the development of ketoacidosis with the risk of both fetal and maternal death. Hyperglycaemia may result in fetal death only if it is severe and prolonged, and it is more likely to occur in early pregnancy which is complicated by excessive vomiting.

2. Hydramnios is a common complication of diabetic pregnancy and may result in an unstable lie and premature rupture of the membranes

3. Pre-eclampsia is common in diabetics and is made worse by poor control of the diabetes. Both fetal and maternal prognosis are significantly worse where the pregnancy is complicated by diabetic nephropathy

4. Dystocia and operative delivery – the fetus may be abnormally large and an obstructed and difficult labour (dystocia) is a recognized complication. The problem may occur after the head has been delivered because of shoulder obstruction. If there is evidence of potential cephalo-pelvic disproportion, the fetus should be delivered by caesarean section.

3.2   Fetal Complication

Babies born to diabetic mothers tend to be larger than normal. There is generalized macrosomia and body fat is commonly increased. Fetal distress associated with intra-uterine asphyxia and acidosis is a complication of labour.

3.3   Neonatal Complications

1. Hypoglycaemia – there is hyperplasia and hyperplasia and hypertrophy of the islets of Langerhans and, as a result, the newborn infant is particularly likely to develop hypoglycaemia. It is therefore important to perform frequent examinations of blood glucose levels in the first 48 hours of life.

2. Respiratory distress syndrome – there is higher incidence of respiratory distress syndrome in diabetic infants than in normal infants born at comparable gestational ages

3. Congenital abnormalities – there is a slightly higher incidence of fetal abnormalities in infants born to mothers with diabetes

4   Management of Diabetes

All grades of diabetes carry a significant risk to the fetus. It may be possible to control gestational diabetes with dietary control, but all other forms of diabetes should be controlled with insulin. In general, it should be the aim to keep the blood glucose levels below 7 mmol/l at all times by appropriate regulation of diet and insulin administration. Hospital admission is not essential unless there is an additional complication of the pregnancy or it is possible to control the diabetes at home. It is the policy in some hospitals to train women to measure their own blood glucose levels and to perform profiles every 2 weeks in the first two trimesters, and weekly in the last 12 weeks. Joint management is undertaken by the physicians and obstetricians and by a diabetic clinic sister who visits patients at home and keeps a close check on the glucose profile.

4.1   Antenatal Assessment

Serial measurement of placental function and fetal growth are performed throughout pregnancy. Placental function tests are of limited value because oestrol and placental lactogen measurements tend to be abnormally high. However, low values are particularly significant and the tests are therefore worth performing. Cardiotocography is also of value in assessment of feto-placental function. Serial measurements of fetal growth by ultrasonography and the measurement of biparietal diameter and trunk circumference allow some assessment of fetal size.

4.2   Method of Delivery

If good diabetic control is achieved and there are no other complications, it should be possible to allow the pregnancy to proceed to full term, although delivery is usually effected between 38 weeks and term. Induction of labour and vaginal delivery can be achieved with careful regulation of blood glucose levels during labour and continuous intrapartum fetal monitoring. If there is any evidence of fetal distress or delay in labour, caesarean section should be performed. Amniocentesis performed before induction or elective caesarean section to measure the lecithin/sphingomyelin ratio or lecithin concentration will enable the prediction of fetal lung maturity.

4.3   Neonatal Management

The two major hazards that affect the neonate born to a diabetic mother are respiratory distress syndrome and neonatal hypoglycaemia. These infants should therefore be admitted to the special care neonatal unit to monitor blood glucose levels and to administer oral glucose until feeding is satisfactorily established. *Perinatal mortality:* It should be possible to achieve perinatal loss rates that are comparable to the overall perinatal mortality figures. Fetal anomalies occur in 5 to 6% and are frequently associated with polyhydramnios.

5   The Place of Ultrasound in Obstetrics

To ascertain the size and to observe the growth of the fetus *in utero* are matters of great importance to the obstetrician, yet the methods previously available have been either imprecise or of limited application. Practically the only part of the fetus which can be measured is the head; this measurement has been made by x-ray with varying reliability. The use of the ultrasonic echo-sounding has been shown to have advantages over radiography.

The cardinal importance of knowledge of the size and shape of the fetal head in order to understand the mechanism of labour was recognized by Smellie (1752), who also pointed out that it is the biparietal diameter which passes through the narrowest part of the brim of the pelvis. Denman (1795), in advocating the induction of premature labour in cases of contracted pelvis, regretted that it was impossible to make accurate measurement on which to base the indications for operation. "it would be highly satisfactory", he wrote, "if I were able to state with precision the exact dimensions of the cavity of the pelvis ……. to enable us by them to form an unerring guide to practice: and as the head of a child before it is born can never be accurately measured, of course the exact relation between them must be unknown, and the determination must be therefore left to opinion." After the times of Smellie and Denman, numerous methods of x-ray cephalometry were developed. Cephalometry has been used for two main reasons: to assess disproportion andto assess the growth and maturity of the fetus. Scammon & Calkins (1922, 1929) and Recce (1935) were among the earliest workers to use cephalometry as an index of fetal growth and maturity. They stated that the biparietal diameter increase by 2.5mm, a week. Despite the work which has been done on the subject, many obstetricians remain unconvinced of the value of x-ray cephalometry. Savage (1951) was of the opinion that the head could not be measured accurately in utero. Mengert & Korkmans (1957), with an experience of obstetric radiology, gave up measuring the head altogether and contented themselves with a clinical impression as to whether the head was a large, medium or small.

Crichton (1962) in his William Blair Bell Memorial lecture on "the Accuracy and Value of Cephalo-pelvimetry" reviewed the work of 9 years, first at Oxford, then at Durban, assessing over 3,000 cases. He stressed the value of the biparietal diameter as the most important measurement of the fetal head and, in particular, he showed that its significance is superior to that of the average cranial circumference – the method advocated by Ball (1935, 1936). Crichton prefers intra-partum to antenatal cephalo-pelvimetry because in labour the head is usually fixed. "Unfortunately", he says, "the biparietal diameter of any high head – which one associates with brim disproportion – has a tendency to present unfavourably in this (i.e. the lateral) radiograph. Thus only 33 percent of unmoulded biparietal diameter presented, or could be deduced fairly accurately from antenatal radiography in the present series." This statement shows the severe limitations of the radiological method.

To know the size of the fetal head in cases of suspected disproportion and in malpresentations, and to observe by repeated measurements the growth of the fetal head in normal and abnormal pregnancy would be more than worth while. In cases complicated by placental degeneration due to pre-eclampsia, chronic nephritis or hypertension, in case of ante-partum haemorrhage, in diabetes, or in any other condition where it may be desirable in the interests of the fetus to terminate the pregnancy prematurely, knowledge of the size of the child, of which the size of the head is an indirect index, would be of great value, and any indication of reduced rate of growth would be even more important. A small fetus may be starving from placental failure; similarly, the presence of a well-grown fetus in a case of, say, hypertension, might lead the obstetrician to conclude that "placental insufficiency" was not a feature of the case. Butler (1962) stated that one-third of all "premature" babies weighing 2.5kg or less were born at 39 weeks or more of gestation, and that these babies had a mortality rate 2½ times the average. Sjostedt *et al.* (1958) used the term "dysmature" to describe such infants. The cause of death in cases of "placental insufficiency" has often been ascribed to anoxia, but evidence is accumulating to suggest that lack of oxygen is only part of the picture. It seems likely that these babies starve to death in the same way as an adult does when deprived of food, and it is possible that they may actually begin to lose weight *in utero.* All that the obstetrician can do is to observe all cases in which (whether due to toxaemia or other factors) there appears to be failure of fetal growth and hope to intervene at the right time. The purpose of ultrasonic cephalometry in these cases is to demonstrate whether or not adequate fetal growth is taking place and whether the growth rate is altering. Clinical estimation of the size of a baby is little more than guesswork. The thickness of the abdominal wall, the tension of the uterus, the amount of liquor amnii and the presentation and attitude of the fetus are liable to influence judgment. A method of measuring the biparietal diameter of the fetus in utero by ultrasound has been evolved by Donald & Brown, 1961; Willocks, 1962

6   Ultrasound Studies of Nigerian Fetuses

This was a prospective cross-sectional study (Mador, 2012) carried out in Jos, the capital of Plateau state of Nigerian. The study involved a population of pregnant women with fetuses from 12 – 42 weeks of gestation undergoing ultrasound examination. The sample used in the research consisted of all women with uncomplicated pregnancy who presented for routine ultrasound at Centre for Reproductive Health Research Jos, a division of Tadam limited. The study was approved by the Ethics Committee of Jos University Teaching Hospital and before inclusion of the patients, informed consent was obtained. In seeking the informed consent, the following information was provided to each subject: a description of the procedure to be followed, a description of any reasonably foreseeable risks or discomfort, a description of benefits to the subjects or to others which may reasonably be expected from the research, a disclosure of appropriate procedure that might be advantageous to the subject, a statement describing the extent to which confidentiality of records identifying the subject will be maintained, an explanation of whom to contact for answers to pertinent questions about the research and research subjects' rights, and whom to contact in the event of a research related injury to the subject; and refusal to participate will involve no penalty or loss of benefits to which the subject is otherwise entitled, and that the subject may discontinue participation at any time without penalty or loss of benefits to which the subject is otherwise entitled.

Only singleton pregnancies were included. Pregnant women with concomitant disease possibly affecting fetal growth (e.g. diabetes mellitus, asthma, hypertension, renal disease, thyroid disease) were not included as were those with complications of pregnancy known at the moment of the ultrasound scan (e.g. bleeding, pre-eclampsia). If a fetal malformation was detected during the examination the patient was excluded. Patients with a history of obstetric complications, intrauterine growth retardation or macrosomia were also excluded. The investigator did not take into account complications or diagnosis that occurred later in the pregnancy, after the ultrasound measurements were performed. Every fetus was measured and included only once so that a pure cross-sectional set of data was constructed. For each patient the gestational age was recorded, as were last menstrual period, maternal age and parity. Maternal age was calculated in completed years at the moment of the ultrasound.

The area of study was Jos. Jos is a city in the middle belt of Nigeria and the capital of Plateau State. It is located near the center of the Jos Plateau on the Dilimi River and it is about 1250 meters (about 4100 ft) above sea level. Plateau State derives its name from the geographical landscape that predominates in this part of the country. It has a population of 3,178,712 (2006 estimate). The state lies between latitude 7 and 11 degrees north of the Equator and longitude 7 degrees east. Although located in the tropical zone, the climate of plateau state is the nearest equivalent of a temperate climate in Europe and United States of America. The state has over 50 ethnic groups each with a proud cultural heritage with no single group large enough to claim majority position. Nature has richly endowed this State with scenic beauty making it a tourist haven. Coupled with the invigorating climate, people from all over the country love staying in Jos that is why the state has been rightly described as a miniature Nigeria because it contains within itself almost, if not all the various ethnic groups of Nigeria. The sample size in this study was estimated from pilot study findings. From simple statistics, it is known that the standard error of the mean is equal to the standard deviation of the characteristic divided by the square root of the number in the sample i.e. $SE = SD/\sqrt{n}$ where SE is standard error of mean, SD is standard deviation and n is sample size. From the pilot study that was carried out, the standard deviation of fetal biparietal diameter at 23 weeks was 2.1. Since the size of the sample is the denominator of the fraction in the equation above, the standard error of mean in the study was set at 0.1 so as to get a larger random sample. So, the sample size for each week of gestation from 12 – 42 weeks was found to be approximately 441 fetuses. When 441 is multiplied by 31 (12 – 42 weeks), that will give the approximate number of fetuses to form the sample size which is roughly 13,671 fetuses. Although this figure served as a guide during the course of study, the actual number of singleton fetuses that were scanned was 13,740 and their biometric parameters documented for analysis. The patient to be scanned had to lie on the examination couch such that she is able to see the screen easily. Most scans were performed with the patient supine. However, in later pregnancy many patients feel dizzy in this position and it was necessary for such patients to be tilted to one side. This is easily achieved by placing a pillow under one of the buttocks. The patient had to be uncovered just sufficiently to allow the examination to be performed. This will include the first inch of the area covered by the pubic hairs and will extend far enough upwards to allow the fundus of the uterus to be visualized. A full bladder was the only prerequisite for an ultrasound examination.

Fetal biometric measurements were performed by using Philips Real time ultrasound machine equipped with 3.5MHz transducer and an electronic caliper system set at a velocity of 1540m/s (Mador, 2012). Fetal head measurements were made in an axial plane at the level where the continuous midline echo is broken by the cavum septum pellucidum in the anterior third and that includes the thalamus. This transverse section should demonstrate an oval symmetrical shape. Measurement of BPD was from the outer edge of the closest temporomandibular bone to the outer edge of the opposite temporomandibular bone. Measurement of OFD was from the outer edge of the frontal bone to the outer edge of the occipital bone. The HC was measured around the calvarium from the same axial image as for the BPD. The abdominal circumference was measured through the transverse section of the fetal abdomen at the level of the stomach and bifurcation of the main portal vein into its right and left branches. The femur length was measured from the greater trochanter to the lateral condyle, with both ends clearly visible and at a horizontal angle $< 45^0$. All measurements were expressed in millimeters. Estimated fetal weight was calculated in grams by the formulae described by Shepard and by Hadlock, as these are included in the software of most commercially available ultrasound scanners (Shepard *et al*., 1982). To enable appropriate statistical comparison of data, only studies with the number of examined fetuses indicated were included since many studies do not indicate the number of fetuses and are reported in graphic rather than tabular forms. Statistical analyses were performed using Number cruncher statistical system (NCSS/PASS 2006 Dawson Edition, USA). The normality of measurements at each week of gestation was assessed using Shapiro-Wilk test, Anderson-Darling test, Martinex-Iglewicz test, Kolmogorov-Sminov test, D'Agostino Skewness test, D'Agostino Kurtosis test and D'Agostino Omnibus test. Given the large sample size, statistically significant nonnormality was accepted unless the normal plot showed clear deviation from a straight line (Altman & Chitty, 1994). For each measurement, a regression analysis was applied, examining linear, logarithmic, polynomial, power, exponential models for association with gestational age in weeks. The best model was selected based on visual inspection of the regression line that best fitted the data scattergram.

Over a period of five years, the biparietal diameter (Mador *et al*., 2011a), head circumference (Mador *et al*., 2011b), occipitofrontal diameter (Mador, 2012), abdominal circumference (Pam *et al*., 2012a) and femur length (Mador *et al*., 2012d) of a total of 13,740 Nigerian fetuses in Jos were measured in a cross-sectional fashion. Fetal weight of 12,080 fetuses from 17 – 42 weeks was also estimated by the ultrasound machine (Mador *et al*., 2012b). The measurements of the fetal parameters were classified into thirty one groups (i.e. from 12 – 42 weeks) and the set of data in each group arranged in order of magnitude and divided into one hundred equal parts in order to obtain percentiles for the respective parameters (Mador, 2012). Tables 1, 2, 3, 4 and 5 give the centile values for fetal biparietal diameter, head circum-

GA (wks, days)	Biparietal diameter (mm)						
	3rd	5th	10th	50th	90th	95th	97th
12 to 12+6	19.0	19.0	19.0	20.0	24.0	25.5	26.0
13 to 13+6	20.0	22.0	22.5	25.0	27.0	27.0	27.0
14 to 14+6	26.2	27.0	28.0	29.0	31.0	31.0	32.0
15 to 15+6	31.0	31.0	32.0	34.0	35.0	35.0	35.4
16 to 16+6	33.0	34.0	35.0	37.0	39.0	39.0	39.0
17 to 17+6	37.0	38.0	38.8	41.0	42.0	42.0	43.2
18 to 18+6	41.0	41.0	42.0	44.0	45.0	46.0	47.0
19 to 19+6	44.0	44.2	45.0	46.0	47.0	49.0	50.0
20 to 20+6	46.0	47.0	48.0	49.0	51.0	52.0	53.4
21 to 21+6	49.0	50.0	51.0	53.0	54.0	55.0	56.0
22 to 22+6	53.0	53.0	54.0	56.0	57.0	59.0	60.0
23 to 23+6	55.0	56.0	57.0	59.0	61.0	61.0	62.0
24 to 24+6	56.6	58.0	60.0	63.0	64.0	65.0	67.0
25 to 25+6	62.0	63.0	64.0	66.0	68.0	69.0	70.0
26 to 26+6	63.0	64.0	66.0	69.0	70.0	72.0	74.0
27 to 27+6	64.0	66.0	68.0	71.0	72.7	74.0	75.0
28 to 28+6	69.0	71.0	72.0	74.0	75.1	77.0	78.0
29 to 29+6	70.7	73.0	74.0	76.0	78.0	78.8	79.0
30 to 30+6	71.0	72.0	74.0	79.0	81.0	84.0	85.0
31 to 31+6	74.7	76.0	78.0	81.0	83.0	84.0	84.3
32 to 32+6	77.0	78.0	80.0	83.0	85.0	87.0	87.0
33 to 33+6	80.0	82.0	82.0	85.0	87.0	88.0	88.0
34 to 34+6	80.4	82.0	83.5	87.0	89.0	91.0	92.0
35 to 35+6	82.0	83.0	85.0	89.0	91.0	92.0	93.0
36 to 36+6	84.0	85.0	87.0	90.0	92.0	93.0	94.0
37 to 37+6	87.0	87.0	89.0	92.0	94.0	94.0	95.0
38 to 38+6	88.0	89.0	90.0	93.0	96.0	97.0	98.0
39 to 39+6	90.0	91.0	92.0	94.0	98.0	99.0	99.0
40 to 40+6	91.0	91.0	93.0	95.0	98.7	100.0	100.0
41 to 41+6	91.2	92.0	93.0	96.0	100.0	101.0	101.0
42 to 42+6	91.0	91.0	91.0	98.0	99.0	99.0	99.0

Table 1: Fetal biparietal diameter centiles from 12 – 42 weeks.

ference, occipitofrontal diameter, abdominal circumference and estimated fetal weight. From Table 1, it can be seen the 10th percentile of biparietal diameter at 20 to 20 + 6 weeks gestation is 48 millimeters. This means that 10% of the fetuses at 20 to 20 + 6 had a mean biparietal diameter less than 48 millimeters, while 90% had a mean biparietal diameter greater than 48 millimeters. Similarly, the 97th percentile of biparietal diameter at 36 to 36 + 6 is 94 millimeters. Hence 97% of fetuses at 36 to 36 + 6 had a mean biparietal diameter less than 94 millimeters while 3% had a mean biparietal diameter greater than 94 millimeters. When the 95th percentiles of biparietal diameter of fetuses in Jos were plotted against gestational age in weeks, the best-fitted regression model to describe the relationship between 95th biparietal diameter percentile and gestational age is as shown in Figure 1. There is a positive polynomial correlation

Gestational age	Head circumference centiles (mm)						
	3rd	5th	10th	50th	90th	95th	97th
12 to 12+6	56.0	61.5	69.0	79.0	96.0	98.5	101.0
13 to 13+6	75.0	78.0	82.0	94.0	106.0	108.0	109.0
14 to 14+6	92.2	94.0	96.0	108.0	118.8	122.0	126.0
15 to 15+6	104.6	110.0	111.0	120.0	134.0	141.0	155.4
16 to 16+6	116.0	119.0	121.0	133.0	145.0	149.0	151.0
17 to 17+6	122.7	130.0	135.0	146.0	159.0	163.0	170.0
18 to 18+6	131.0	134.0	146.0	159.0	172.2	196.2	203.0
19 to 19+6	140.0	150.0	156.3	168.0	183.0	191.9	200.5
20 to 20+6	160.0	164.0	169.0	180.0	195.0	201.0	210.0
21 to 21+6	171.0	175.0	181.0	193.0	206.9	214.0	222.0
22 to 22+6	181.0	186.0	190.0	201.0	215.0	220.1	223.0
23 to 23+6	183.0	191.0	199.0	212.0	227.0	233.0	239.6
24 to 24+6	200.0	205.0	214.0	225.0	239.9	247.0	250.0
25 to 25+6	206.4	216.5	225.9	238.0	253.0	261.7	265.0
26 to 26+6	220.0	226.0	232.2	249.0	265.0	272.0	279.0
27 to 27+6	230.0	232.7	240.3	260.0	278.0	287.0	292.0
28 to 28+6	243.0	247.0	255.0	270.0	284.0	289.0	292.0
29 to 29+6	229.2	246.3	260.0	277.0	290.0	294.0	302.0
30 to 30+6	250.0	262.3	269.0	286.0	300.0	309.0	315.4
31 to 31+6	253.0	267.0	276.0	293.0	309.0	311.0	314.3
32 to 32+6	274.1	279.2	284.4	300.0	316.0	320.0	322.0
33 to 33+6	280.0	286.0	293.0	308.0	321.0	324.0	328.0
34 to 34+6	286.0	290.5	300.0	315.0	330.5	335.0	340.0
35 to 35+6	291.2	297.0	301.0	320.0	333.0	338.0	340.8
36 to 36+6	301.0	303.0	306.0	326.0	339.0	346.0	351.0
37 to 37+6	300.0	302.7	312.3	333.0	344.7	351.0	358.0
38 to 38+6	310.9	315.0	320.0	337.0	352.0	359.0	364.0
39 to 39+6	318.0	320.3	326.2	342.0	359.0	372.0	378.0
40 to 40+6	323.0	324.3	330.0	344.0	360.0	373.5	382.5
41 to 41+6	316.0	329.0	335.0	348.5	366.0	366.0	367.6
42 to 42+6	306.0	306.0	306.0	353.0	387.0	387.0	387.0

Table 2: Centiles of fetal head circumference measurements

between gestational age and 95th biparietal diameter percentile with a correlation of determination of $R^2 = 0.9985$ ($P < 0.0001$) in Nigerian fetuses in Jos. The relationship is best described by the second order polynomial regression equation:

$$y = -0.0486x^2 + 5.2729x - 33.052 \qquad (1)$$

where y is the biparietal diameter 95th percentile and x is the gestational age in weeks. This means that fetal gestational age could predict the 95th percentile of biparietal diameter by 99.85 percent ($R^2 = 0.9985$) in 13,740 fetuses in this study. Again, plotting the 95th percentiles of head circumference alongside gestational age in weeks, a positive polynomial correlation between gestational age and 95th head circumference percentile with a correlation of determination of $R^2 = 0.9964$ ($P < 0.0001$) was found.

Gestational age	Occipitofrontal diameter centiles (mm)						
	3rd	5th	10th	50th	90th	95th	97th
12 to 12+6	19.0	21.0	24.0	27.0	33.0	34.0	35.0
13 to 13+6	26.0	27.0	28.0	33.0	37.0	38.0	38.0
14 to 14+6	32.0	33.0	33.0	38.0	41.0	42.0	44.0
15 to 15+6	36.0	38.0	39.0	42.0	47.0	49.0	54.0
16 to 16+6	40.0	41.0	42.0	46.0	50.0	52.0	52.0
17 to 17+6	42.8	45.0	47.0	51.0	55.0	57.0	59.0
18 to 18+6	45.0	47.0	51.0	55.0	59.6	68.0	70.0
19 to 19+6	49.0	52.0	54.3	58.0	64.0	66.9	69.5
20 to 20+6	56.0	57.0	59.0	63.0	68.0	70.0	73.0
21 to 21+6	59.0	61.0	63.0	67.0	72.0	74.0	77.0
22 to 22+6	63.0	65.0	66.0	70.0	75.0	76.1	77.0
23 to 23+6	64.0	66.0	69.0	74.0	79.0	81.0	83.0
24 to 24+6	69.0	71.0	74.0	78.0	83.0	86.0	87.0
25 to 25+6	72.1	75.0	78.0	83.0	88.0	90.6	92.0
26 to 26+6	76.0	78.0	81.0	86.0	92.0	94.0	97.0
27 to 27+6	79.9	81.0	83.3	90.0	97.0	100.0	101.0
28 to 28+6	84.0	86.0	89.0	94.0	99.0	100.0	101.0
29 to 29+6	79.8	85.3	90.0	96.0	101.0	102.0	105.0
30 to 30+6	87.0	91.0	93.0	99.0	104.0	107.0	109.2
31 to 31+6	88.0	93.0	96.0	102.0	107.0	108.0	109.0
32 to 32+6	95.0	97.0	99.0	104.0	110.0	111.0	112.0
33 to 33+6	97.0	99.0	102.0	107.0	111.0	113.0	114.0
34 to 34+6	99.0	101.0	104.0	109.0	115.0	116.0	118.0
35 to 35+6	101.0	103.0	105.0	111.0	116.0	117.0	118.0
36 to 36+6	105.0	105.0	106.0	113.0	118.0	120.0	122.0
37 to 37+6	104.0	105.0	108.3	116.0	119.7	122.0	124.0
38 to 38+6	108.0	109.0	111.0	117.0	122.0	125.0	126.0
39 to 39+6	110.0	111.0	113.6	119.0	125.0	129.0	131.0
40 to 40+6	112.0	112.7	115.0	119.0	125.0	129.4	132.8
41 to 41+6	110.0	114.0	116.0	121.0	127.0	127.0	127.8
42 to 42+6	106.0	106.0	106.0	123.0	134.0	134.0	134.0

Table 3: Fetal occipitofrontal diameter centiles from 12 – 42 weeks

The correlation is best described by the second order polynomial regression equation

$$y = -0.1789x^2 + 19.048x - 106.64 \qquad (2)$$

where y is the head circumference 95th percentile and x is the gestational age in weeks (Figure 2). This means that fetal gestational age could predict the 95th percentile of head circumference by 99.85 percent ($R^2 = 0.9964$) in 13,740 fetuses in this study. Once more, when the 95th percentiles of occipitofrontal diameter of fetuses in Jos were plotted against gestational age in weeks, the best-fitted regression model to illustrate the relationship between 95th occipitofrontal diameter percentile and gestational age is as made known in Figure 3. There is a positive polynomial correlation linking gestational age and 95th occipitofrontal diameter percentile with a correlation of determination of $R^2 = 0.9966$ ($P < 0.0001$) in Nigerian fetuses in Jos.

Gestational age	Abdominal circumference centiles (cm)						
	3rd	5th	10th	50th	90th	95th	97th
12 to 12+6	53	54	54	65	95	101	101
13 to 13+6	58	59	62	79	95	99	101
14 to 14+6	71	75	80	92	107	112	118
15 to 15+6	87	91	93	103	118	124	133
16 to 16+6	99	100	102	113	131	135	143
17 to 17+6	104	107	113	124	145	158	168
18 to 18+6	116	120	126	138	158	179	191
19 to 19+6	124	129	137	149	169	178	182
20 to 20+6	134	136	143	159	180	190	194
21 to 21+6	149	149	153	170	191	200	208
22 to 22+6	159	162	165	179	200	208	214
23 to 23+6	159	166	172	190	213	218	228
24 to 24+6	170	176	185	200	221	230	237
25 to 25+6	187	192	194	214	237	245	251
26 to 26+6	200	207	210	226	251	261	268
27 to 27+6	204	209	216	235	262	273	282
28 to 28+6	218	226	230	246	267	279	285
29 to 29+6	225	226	233	254	278	283	285
30 to 30+6	239	241	247	267	291	298	302
31 to 31+6	229	241	255	276	297	300	305
32 to 32+6	259	263	268	286	305	311	319
33 to 33+6	261	264	274	296	316	320	329
34 to 34+6	273	278	284	305	326	332	339
35 to 35+6	281	283	290	313	334	342	355
36 to 36+6	291	294	299	320	340	350	354
37 to 37+6	295	302	310	332	351	359	366
38 to 38+6	309	312	318	336	359	364	369
39 to 39+6	305	310	323	347	369	382	388
40 to 40+6	305	314	331	346	378	384	385
41 to 41+6	323	329	337	351	370	373	373
42 to 42+6	309	309	315	349	387	387	387

Table 4: Fetal abdominal circumference centiles from 12 – 42 weeks

The relationship is preeminently portrayed by the second order polynomial regression equation

$$y = -0.0621x^2 + 6.6146x - 36.814 \qquad (3)$$

where y is the occipitofrontal diameter 95th percentile and x is the gestational age in weeks. This means that fetal gestational age could predict the 95th percentile of occipitofrontal diameter by 99.66 percent (R^2 = 0.9966) in 13,740 fetuses in this study. Yet again, whilst the 95th percentiles of abdominal circumference of fetuses in Jos were plotted against gestational age in weeks, the best-fitted regression model to describe the relationship between 95th abdominal circumference percentile and gestational age is as shown in Figure 4. There is a positive polynomial correlation between gestational age and 95th abdominal circumference percentile with a correlation of determination of $R^2 = 0.9962$ ($P < 0.0001$) in Nigerian fetuses in Jos.

Gestational age	Weight centiles (grams)						
	3rd	5th	10th	50th	90th	95th	97th
17 to 17+6	300	300	300	300	400	400	400
18 to 18+6	300	300	300	400	1900	2400	2400
19 to 19+6	300	300	400	400	400	500	860
20 to 20+6	400	400	400	400	500	600	700
21 to 21+6	400	400	400	500	600	600	700
22 to 22+6	500	500	500	600	600	700	700
23 to 23+6	500	500	600	600	800	800	800
24 to 24+6	600	600	700	800	900	900	1073
25 to 25+6	643	700	800	900	1100	1100	1157
26 to 26+6	800	900	900	1100	1300	1400	1500
27 to 27+6	800	900	1000	1200	1400	1600	1700
28 to 28+6	1000	1100	1200	1400	1500	1690	1874
29 to 29+6	1100	1200	1300	1500	1800	1800	1900
30 to 30+6	1300	1300	1500	1700	2000	2100	2440
31 to 31+6	1260	1300	1600	1900	2100	2200	2400
32 to 32+6	1600	1700	1800	2100	2400	2500	2600
33 to 33+6	1700	1800	1900	2300	2600	2700	2900
34 to 34+6	2000	2100	2200	2500	2900	3065	3200
35 to 35+6	2000	2180	2300	2700	3100	3300	3400
36 to 36+6	2200	2300	2500	2900	3200	3400	3400
37 to 37+6	2500	2600	2700	3100	3400	3600	3600
38 to 38+6	2600	2700	2900	3300	3700	3800	3900
39 to 39+6	2800	3000	3000	3500	4000	4100	4200
40 to 40+6	2900	3100	3200	3600	4200	4435	4600
41 to 41+6	3100	3155	3210	3800	4190	4545	4600
42 to 42+6	2900	2900	2960	3900	4600	4600	4600

Table 5: Frequency distribution table of fetal weight measurements showing the 3rd, 5th, 10th, 50th, 90th, 95th and 97th centile values from 17 – 42 weeks.

The relationship is best described by the second order polynomial regression equation

$$y = -0.01127x^2 + 16.162x - 87.966 \qquad (4)$$

where y is the abdominal circumference 95th percentile and x is the gestational age in weeks. This means that fetal gestational age could predict the 95th percentile of abdominal circumference by 99.62 percent ($R^2 = 0.9962$) in 13,740 fetuses in this study. Finally, by plotting the 90th percentiles of estimated fetal weight alongside gestational age in weeks, a positive polynomial correlation between gestational age and 95th estimated fetal weight percentile with a correlation of determination of $R^2 = 0.9965$ ($P < 0.0001$) was found. The correlation is best described by the second order polynomial regression equation

$$y = 2.7792x^2 + 20.277x - 1122.1 \qquad (5)$$

where y is the estimated fetal weight 90th percentile and x is the gestational age in weeks (Figure 5). This means that fetal gestational age could predict the 95th percentile of estimated fetal weight by 99.65 percent ($R^2 = 0.9965$) in 13,740 fetuses in this study.

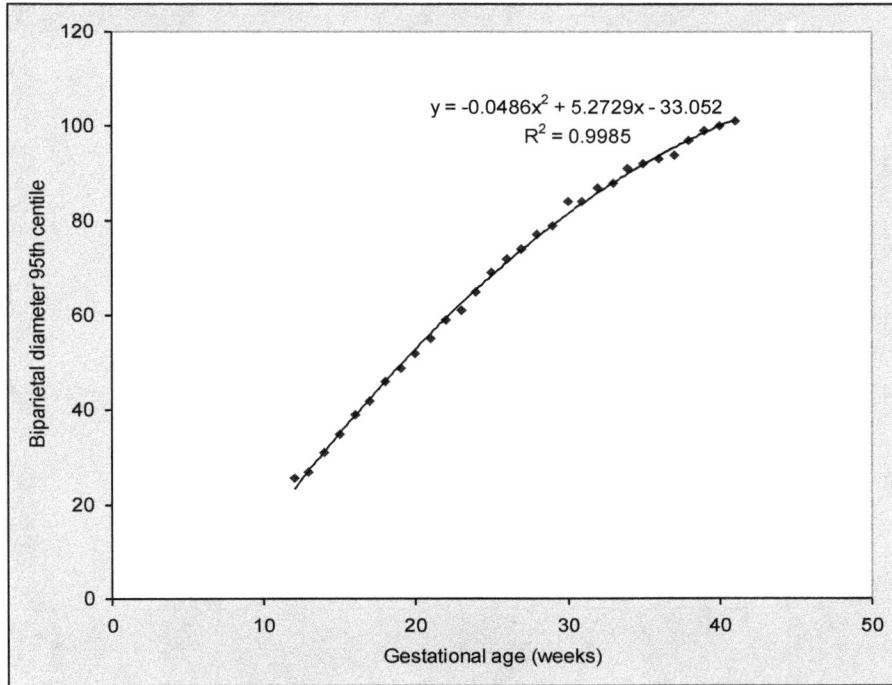

Figure 1: Graph Showing Correlation and Regression Equation of biparietal iameter 95th centile Plotted against Gestational Age in Weeks.

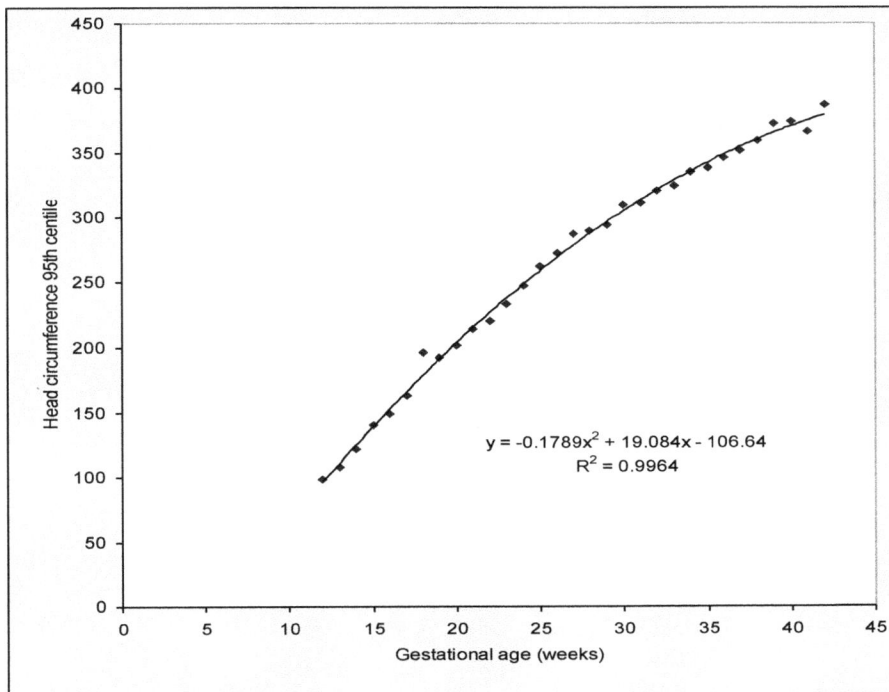

Figure 2: Graph Showing Correlation and Regression Equation of head ircumference 95th centile Plotted against Gestational Age in Weeks

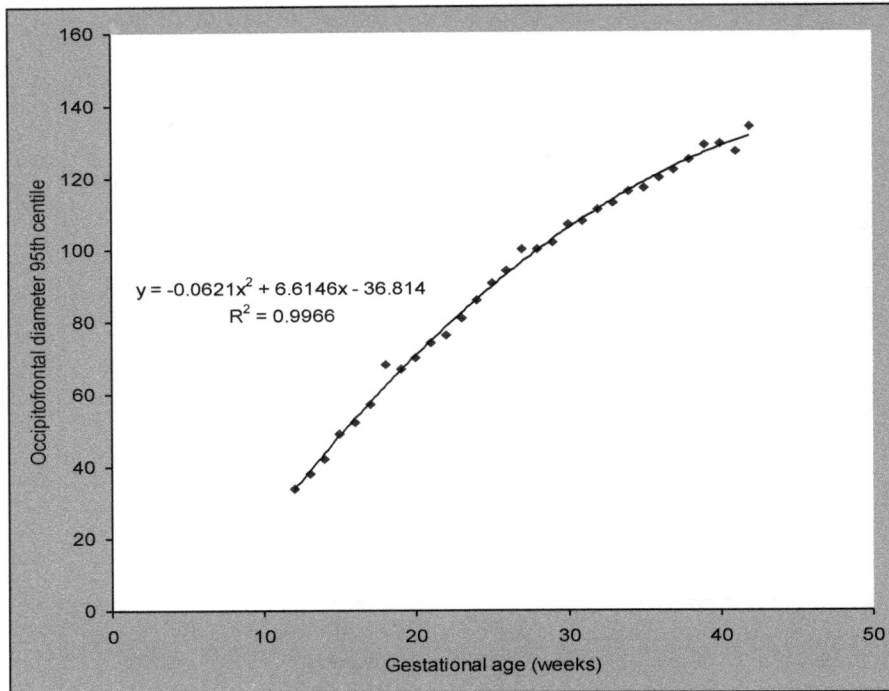

Figure 3: Graph Showing Correlation and Regression Equation of occipitofrontal diameter 95th centile Plotted against Gestational Age in Weeks

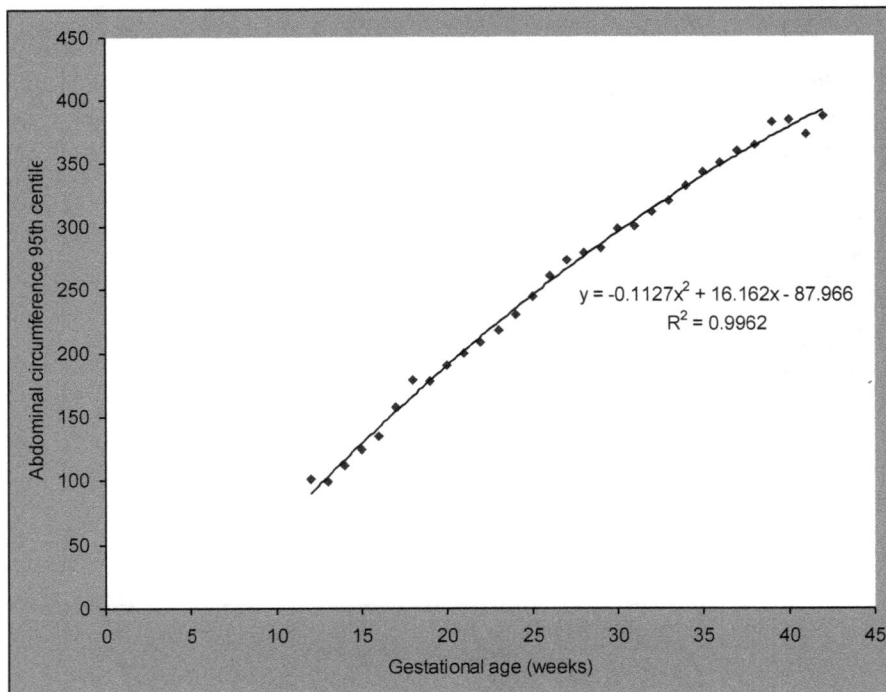

Figure 4: Graph Showing Correlation and Regression Equation of abdominal ircumference 95th centile Plotted against Gestational Age in Weeks.

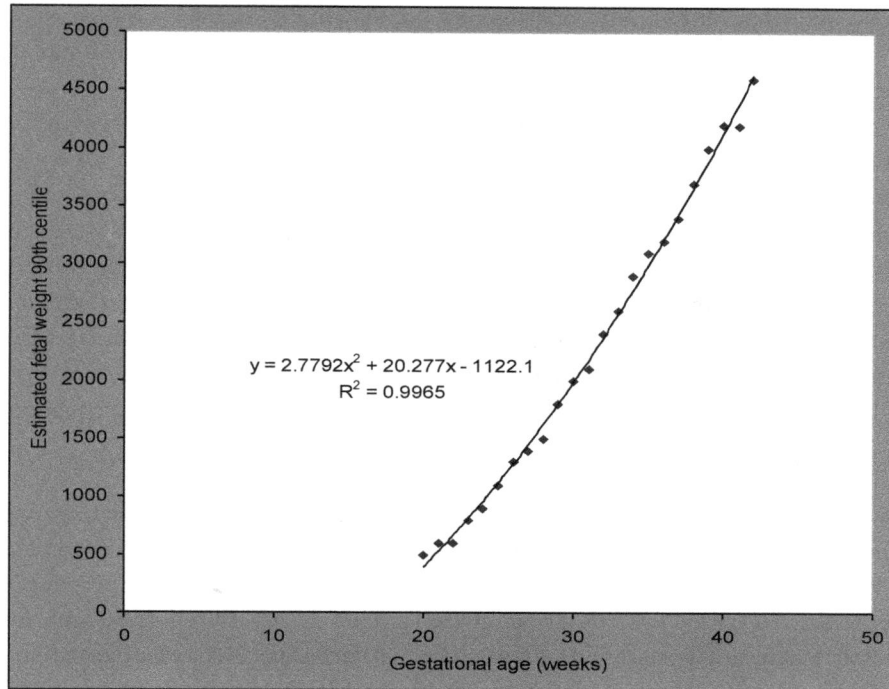

Figure 5: Graph Showing Correlation and Regression Equation of estimated fetal weight Plotted against Gestational Age in Weeks.

7 Ratio of Femur Length to Abdominal Circumference in Nigerian Fetuses

Fetal femur length to abdominal circumference ratio is an important proportion for the assessment of fetal growth. The proportional relationship between these two fetal parameters has been studied thoroughly on western population by many researchers but there is nothing in the literature to show that a similar work has been done in our environment. This is why this study was designed to establish chart of fetal femur length to abdominal circumference ratio in Nigeria. A proportional relationship between two different fetal femur parameters is a tool which illustrates whether the fetal parameters in question are growing size for size or not. The most useful parameters are those that remain constant through some period. DuBose (1996) in his elegant study on size/age analysis reported that ratios of fetal cranium are constant throughout the second and third trimesters. Several investigators (Deter *et al.*, 1983; Divon *et al.*, 1986; Lockwood *et al.*, 1987; Hadlock *et al.*, 1983; Ott, 1985; Fescina & Ucieda 1980) have reported fetal ratios on western population. The ratio of fetal femur length to abdominal circumference is an important ratio for the assessment of fetal growth. It is constant in the normally growing fetus from 21 weeks of gestation to term being independent of menstrual age. An increase in the ratio above normal can be seen in fetuses that are small for gestational age. Fetuses that are small for gestational age (Divon *et al.*, 1986) have a ratio that is greater or equal to 23.5. Fetuses that show appropriate development for gestational age have a ratio less than 23.5 with values around 22. Large for gestational age infants have a ratio around 21. So far no study has been conducted on this ratio on Nigerian population. This is why this prospective cross-sectional study was carried out to produce a table with mean, standard deviation and standard error of mean of this ratio based on our Nigerian population.

The mean values of FL/AC at each week of gestation from 12 – 42 are as shown in Table 6. This table gives the mean values of fetal femur lengths to abdominal circumference ratio for each gestational age in weeks from 12 – 42 weeks together with their corresponding standard deviations and standard errors of mean. The group with the highest number of observations was from 34 weeks 0 days to 34 weeks 6 days while 42 weeks 0 days to 42 weeks 6 days group had the lowest number of observations. When the mean values of femur length to abdominal circumference ratio were plotted against gestational age, a positive polynomial correlation between gestational age and femur length to abdominal circumference ratio with a coefficient of determination of $R^2 = 0.9545$ ($P < 0.0001$) in Nigerian fetuses in Jos was found (Figure 6). The relationship is best described by the sixth order polynomial regression equation:

$$y = 7\text{E-}09x^6 - 7\text{E-}07x^5 + 2\text{E-}5x^4 - 0.005x^3 - 0.0039x^2 - 0.0098x + 0.1892 \qquad (6)$$

where y is the femur length to abdominal circumference ratio and x is the gestational age weeks. Mean values of fetal femur length to abdominal circumference ratio of fetuses of Nigerian women have been established. The findings are consistent with those reported from other parts of the world (Divon et al., 1986; Lockwood et al., 1987; Ott, 1985; Sabrina, 2009; Hadlock et al., 1985). The femur length to abdominal circumference ratio in this study was found to be constant from 21 week of gestation up to term. The ratio of the femur to abdominal circumference is constant in the normally growing fetus from 21 weeks of gestation to term being independent of menstrual age. An increase in the ratio above normal can be seen in fetuses that are small for gestational age. Infants who are small for gestational age have a ratio that is greater or equal to 23.5 (or 0.235); however due to the low prevalence of growth retardation in a general population only 25% of infants with a ratio greater or equal to 23.5 will be growth retarded (Divon et al., 1986). Divon and his co-workers (1986) further reported that fetuses that show appropriate development for gestational age have a ratio less than 23.5 with values around 22 (or 0.22). Large for gestational age infants have a ratio around 21 (or 0.21). From Table 1, it can be seen that before 21 weeks of gestation the fetuses were large for gestational age while after the 39th week of gestation, they become small for gestational age. Once an infant has been identified as being at risk for growth retardation by the femur length to abdominal circumference ratio then other criteria for growth should be monitored rather than the ratio as the ratio can return to normal in infants who are growth retarded (Divon et al., 1986; Hadlock et al., 1983; Ott, 1985). From the result obtained from the investigation into the relationship between fetal femur length to abdominal circumference ratio and gestational age, it is concluded that femur length to abdominal circumference ratio correlate positively with gestational age. Correlation and regression analysis have shown that a fetus's femur length to abdominal circumference ratio could be predicted using gestational age. Gestational age could explain the prediction of a fetus' femur length to abdominal circumference ratio by 95.45 percent ($r^2 = 0.9545$) in the 13,740 fetuses scanned during this study.

8   Sonographic Detection of Macrosomia in Nigerian Fetuses

The development of macrosomia in Nigerian fetuses can be detected by using either intrauterine weight estimation in view of the fact that the 90th percentile of estimated fetal weight of Nigerian fetuses 17 – 42

Gestational Age (wks)	Number of fetuses	Mean FL/AC	SD	SE
12	49	0.18	0.05	0.007
13	384	0.19	0.12	0.006
14	371	0.18	0.06	0.003
15	351	0.18	0.03	0.001
16	505	0.20	0.06	0.003
17	427	0.20	0.03	0.001
18	446	0.20	0.02	0.001
19	282	0.21	0.03	0.002
20	553	0.21	0.03	0.001
21	400	0.22	0.04	0.002
22	398	0.21	0.02	0.001
23	478	0.22	0.03	0.001
24	520	0.22	0.02	0.001
25	388	0.22	0.02	0.001
26	511	0.22	0.02	0.001
27	432	0.22	0.02	0.001
28	548	0.22	0.02	0.001
29	484	0.22	0.02	0.001
30	625	0.22	0.02	0.001
31	523	0.22	0.02	0.001
32	583	0.22	0.01	0.001
33	516	0.22	0.02	0.001
34	744	0.22	0.01	0.001
35	739	0.22	0.01	0.001
36	599	0.22	0.01	0.001
37	532	0.22	0.02	0.001
38	481	0.22	0.02	0.001
39	525	0.22	0.02	0.001
40	252	0.22	0.01	0.001
41	72	0.24	0.03	0.006
42	22	0.24	0.03	0.006
Total	13740			

Table 6: Frequency Distribution Table of Fetal Mean Femur Length to abdominal Circumference Ratio Together With Standard Deviation (SD) and Standard Error of Mean of from 12 – 42 Weeks.

weeks has already been derived using large sample size or by means of the 95th centiles of biparietal diameter (Mador *et al.*, 2011a), head circumference (Mador *et al.*, 2011b), occipitofrontal diameter (Mador, 2012), and abdominal circumference (Mador *et al.*, 2012c; Pam *et al.*, 2012a). Otherwise, ratio of FL/AC can be used for early detection of accelerated fetal growth (Pam *et al.*, 2012b). In situations where the 90th percentile of estimated fetal weight is unknown (this is often the case in some rural communities), weight may be recorded using ultrasound machine and 90th centile predicted from the propounded prediction formula (Mador *et al.*, 2012b). When the estimated fetal weight is above the 90th percentile of the Nigerian fetuses, it implies that that particular fetus is macrosomic. Similarly, in circumstances where the

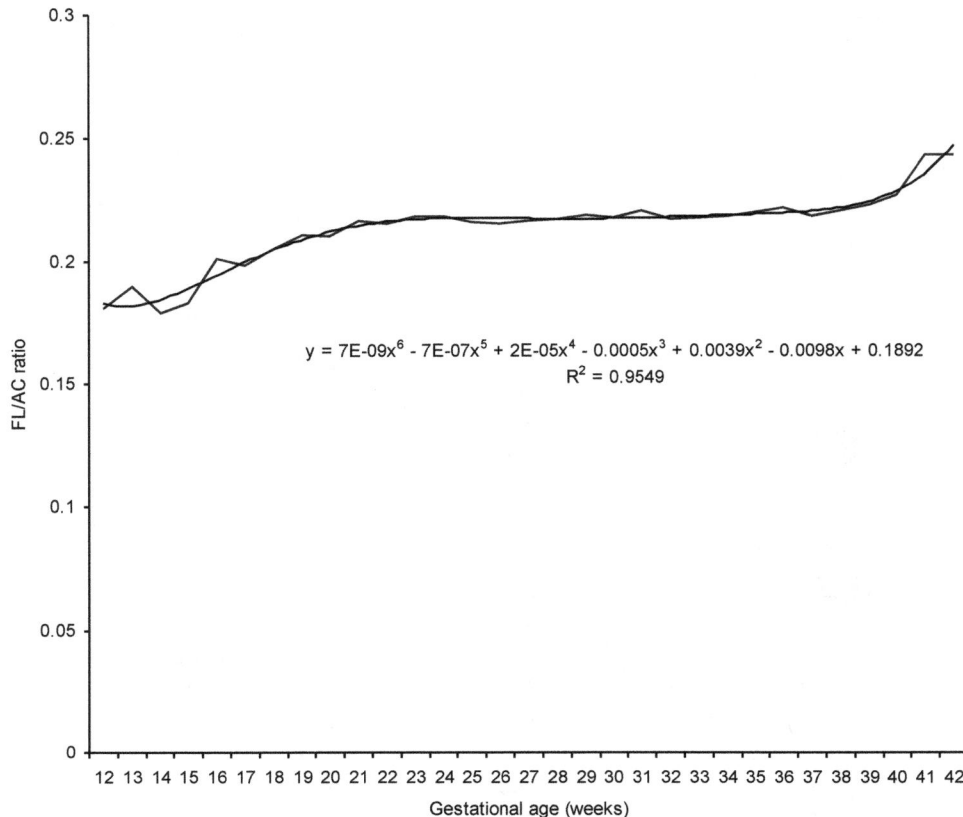

The chart's embedded regression equation:

$$y = 7\text{E-}09x^6 - 7\text{E-}07x^5 + 2\text{E-}05x^4 - 0.0005x^3 + 0.0039x^2 - 0.0098x + 0.1892$$
$$R^2 = 0.9549$$

Figure 6: Graph Showing Correlation and Regression Equation of Mean Femur Length to Abdominal Circumference Ratio Plotted against Gestational Age in Weeks.

95th percentiles of either biparietal diameter, head circumference, occipitofrontal diameter, or abdominal circumference in a certain community in Nigeria is unknown and the attending physician (obstetrician) wants to know if the fetus that he has scanned is macrosomic or not, the parameter in question may be recorded using the ultrasound machine and the 95th percentile of the parameter predicted from the propounded prediction formula of the particular parameter. In a situation where the physicians are attending to a diabetic pregnant woman, they will be monitoring the fetus by regularly checking the weight, head circumference, biparietal diameter and abdominal circumference. When the abdominal circumference increases above the 95th percentile with relatively normal head circumference, then the diagnosis of diabetic macrosomia can be made on that case. The clinician or the clinical anthropologist should have as part of his diagnostic armamentarium charts and nomograms and keep important prediction formulae in his head. With the help of a small pocket calculator he can arrive at highly scientific management of his patients, even in areas far removed from sophisticated clinical gadgetry. Clinical anthropology began as a discipline which recognized the input of medical anthropology in modern medical scientific care (Kleinman, 1975, 1980, 1982). Ogunranti in a series of publications (1986, 1987, 1994) advanced arguments for the use of medical anthropological information in the treatment and diagnosis of diseases in the developing countries. In most cases, this information would be used by the physician working in a particular community for making a diagnosis

9   Conclusion

It is necessary for an attending physician in any community to be conversant with normal values for his community which he/she relies on in order to make diagnosis of ailment and treat his/her patients from that community. The chapter has examined the use of 90th percentile of estimated fetal weight; the use of the 95th percentile of biparietal diameter, head circumference, occipitofrontal diameter, abdominal circumference and FL/AC ratio in the detection of fetal macrosomia in maternal diabetes and has also reported a large cross-sectional study of contemporary growing fetuses in Nigeria from 12 – 42 weeks. A construction of a new percentile chart is made for investigators and clinicians who need them for contemporary growing fetuses. Prediction formulae for obtaining percentile from age are also presented. These values are useful for fetuses all over Africa and obstetricians in Africa (and probably other parts of the developing world) can use the percentile chats as presented in this chapter and the prediction formulae for the diagnosis and treatment of their patients.

References

Alberico S, Businelli C, Wiesenfeld U, Erenbourg A, Maso G, Piccoli M, Ronfani L. Gestational diabetes and fetal growth acceleration: induction of labour versus expectant management (2010). Minerva Ginecol. 62(6):533-9.

Angiolini E, Fowden A, Coan P, Sandovici I, Smith P, Dean W, Burton G, Tycko B, Reik W, Sibley C, et al. (2006). Regulation of placental efficiency for nutrient transport by imprinted genes. Placenta. Suppl A:S98-102.

Ball, R. P. & Marchbanks, S. S. (1935). Roentgen pelvimetry and fetal cephalometry: a new technique. Radiology. 24, 77-84.

Ball, R. P.(1936): Pelvicephalography. American Journal of Obst. & Gynec. 32:249 – 257

Ballard JL, Holroyde J, Tsang RC, Chan G, Sutherland JM, Knowles HC (1984). High malformation rates and decreased mortality in infants of diabetic mothers managed after the first trimester of pregnancy (1956-1978). American Journal of Obstetrics and Gynecology. 148(8):1111 – 1118

Baptiste-Roberts K, Nicholson WK, Wang NY, Brancati FL (2012). Gestational diabetes and subsequent growth patterns of offspring: the National Collaborative Perinatal Project. Matern Child Health J. 16(1):125-32.

Bernstein IM, Catalano PM (1992). Influence of fetal fat on the ultrasound estimation of fetal weight in diabetic mothers. Obstet Gynecol. 79(4):561-3

Boyd ME, Usher RH, McLean FH (1983). Fetal macrosomia: prediction, risks, proposed management. Obstetrics and Gynecology. 61(6):715-22

Butler, N. (1962): Perinatal mortality survey. Brit Med. J. 2: 1463

Campbell, S. & Wilkin, D. (1975). Ultrasonic measurement of fetal abdomen circumference in the estimation of fetal weight. British Journal of Obstetrics and Gynaecology. 82(9): 689 – 697.

Colatrella A, Framarino M, Toscano V, Bongiovanni M, Festa C, Mattei L, Merola G, Bitterman O, Maravalle M, Napoli A (2012). Continuous Glucose Monitoring During Breastfeeding in Women with Recent Gestational Diabetes Mellitus. Diabetes Technol Ther.

Crichton, D. (1952): The Accuracy of X-ray Cephalometry in Utero. Proceeding of the Royal Society of Medicine. 45: 535

Crichton, D. (1962). The intra-uterine growth of the foetal head after the 36th week of pregnancy. An International Journal of Obstetrics & Gynaecology. 60 (2): 233–236

Denman, T. (1795): An Introduction to the Practice of Midwifery. J. Johnson, London

Deter, R. L., Hadlock, F. P., & Harrist., R. B. (1983). Evaluation of fetal growth and the detection of intrauterine growth retardation. In Callen, P. W. (ed): Ultrasonography in Obstetrics and Gynaecology. W. B. Saunders Co., Philadelphia, pp 113 – 140

Deter, R.L. Hadlock. F.P.: Use of ultrasound in the detection of macrosomia: A review. Journal of Clinical Ultrasound 13(1985) 519 – 524.

Divon, M. Y., Chamberlain, P. F., Sipos, L., Manning, F. A. & Platt, L.D. (1986). Identification of the small for gestational age fetus with the use of gestational age-independent indices of fetal growth. American Journal of Obstetrics and Gynaecology. 155: 1197 – 1201

Donakd, I, & Brown, T.G (1961). Demonstration of tissue interfaces within the body by ultrasonic echo sounding. Br J Radiol. 34:539–546

DuBose, T. J., Size/Age analysis. In: DuBose TJ (ed), Fetal Sonography. 1st ED. Philadelphia, WB Saunders. 1996. pp.95 – 156

Dyer JS, Rosenfeld CR. (2011). Metabolic imprinting by prenatal, perinatal, and postnatal overnutrition: a review. Semin Reprod Med. 29(3):266-76.

Fall C (2009). Maternal nutrition: effects on health in the next generation. Indian J Med Res. 130(5):593-9

Farmer RM, Medearis AL, Hirata GI, Platt LD (1992).The use of a neural network for the ultrasonographic estimation of fetal weight in the macrosomic fetus. American Journal Obstetrics of Gynecology. 166(5):1467-72

Fescina, R. H., & Ucieda, F. J. (1980). Reliability of fetal anthropometry by ultrasound. Journal of Perinatal Medicine. 8:93 – 99.

Hadlock FP, Harrist RB, Fearneyhough TC, Deter RL, Park SK, Rossavik IK. Use of femur length/abdominal circumference ratio in detecting the macrosomic fetus. Radiology. 1985 Feb;154(2):503-5

Hadlock FP, Harrist RB, Fearneyhough TC, Deter RL, Park SK, Rossavik IK (1985). Use of femur length/abdominal circumference ratio in detecting the macrosomic fetus. Radiology. 154(2):503-5

Hadlock, F. P., Deter, R. L., Harrist, R. B., Roecker, E., & Park, S. K. (1983). A date-independent predictor of intrau terine growth retardation: Femur length/ abdominal circumference ratio. American Journal of Roentgenology. 141:979 – 984.

Hadlock, F. P., Harrist, R. B., Fearneybough, T. C., Deter, R. L., Park, S. K. & Rossavik, I. K. (1985). Use of femur length/abdominal circumference ratio in detecting the macrosomic fetus. Radiology. 154(2): 503 – 5

Hadlock, F. P., Harrist, R. B., Shah, Y., & Park, S. K. (1984). The femur length/head circumference relation in obstetric sonography. Journal of Ultrasound in Medicine 3:439 – 442.

Hansmann M, Hinckers HJ (1974). Das große Kind. Gynakologe

Jansson T, Powell TL. (2007). Role of the placenta in fetal programming: underlying mechanisms and potential interventional approaches. Clinical Science (Lond). 113(1):1-13.

Kanaka-Gantenbein C (2010). Fetal origins of adult diabetes. Academic Science.1205:99-105

Klebanoff MA, Mills JL, Berendes HW (1985). Mother's birth weight as a predictor of macrosomia. American Journal of Obstetrics and Gynecology. 153(3):253-7

Kleinman, A. (1975). Explanatory in health care relationships . in national council for health: Health of the family. Washinton D.C: National Council for International Health.

Kleinman, A. (1980). Patients and healers in the context of culture: An exploration of the borderland between anthropology, medicine and psychiatry. Berkeley: University of California press

Kleinman, A. (1982)). Clinically applied anthropology on a psychiatric consultation-liaison service. In Clinically applied anthropology, edited by M.J Chrisman and T.

Koukoura O, Sifakis S, Spandidos DA.. (2012). DNA methylation in the human placenta and fetal growth (review). Molecular Medicine Report. 5(4):883-9.

Kwak SH, Kim SH, Cho YM, Go MJ, Cho YS, Choi SH, Moon MK, Jung HS, Shin HD, Kang HM, Cho NH, Lee IK, Kim SY, Han BG, Jang HC, Park KS. (2012). A genome-wide association study of gestational diabetes mellitus in Korean women. Diabetes. 61(2):531-41.

Larkin JC, Speer PD, Simhan HN (2011). A customized standard of large size for gestational age to predict intrapartum morbidity. Am J Obstet Gynecol. 204(6):499.e1-10.

Le Clair C, Abbi T, Sandhu H, Tappia PS (2009). Impact of maternal undernutrition on diabetes and cardiovascular disease risk in adult offspring. Can J Physiol Pharmacol. 87(3):161-79

Lockwood, C., Benacerraf, B., Krinsky, A., Blakemore, K., Belanger, K., Mahoney, M. & Hobbins, J. (1987). A sonographic screening method for Down syndrome. American Journal of Obstetrics Gynecology. 157(1):803 – 808.

Macdonald, I (1952): Growth of Biparietal Diameter of Foetal Head in the Last Weeks of Pregnancy. British Medical Journal. 1(4762): 798–800

Macdonald, I (1954): Hardness and growth of the foetal head. Journal of. Obstetrics and Gynaecology Journal of the British Empire. 61(2):253-8

Mador, E. S., Ekwempu, C. C., Mutihir, J. T., Adoga, G. I. & Ogunranti, J. O. (2011a). Ultrasonographic Biometry: Biparietal Diameter of Nigerian Foetuses. Nigerian Medical Journal. 1(52): 41 – 44

Mador, E. S., Pam, I.C., Mutihir, J. T., Daru, P. H. & Ogunranti, J. O. (2011b). Ultrasound biometry of Nigerian fetuses: Head circumference reference values. African Journal of Natural Sciences. 12: 15 – 23

Mador, E. S., Mutihir, J. T. & Ogunranti, J. O. (2012a). Fetal Head Circumference as an Anthropometric Index. In Preedy, V. R. (ed.): Handbook of Anthropometry: Physical Measures of Human Form in Health and Disease. Springer New York Dordrecht Heidelberg London. pp 477 – 516

Mador, E.S., Ishaya, P., Ekedigwe J.E. & Ogunranti, J. (2012b). Ultrasound Biometry of Nigerian Fetuses, 1: Estimated Fetal Weight. Asian Journal of Medical Sciences 4(2):89 – 93

Mador, E., Ishaya, P., Daru, P. & Ogunranti, J. (2012c). Ultrasound Biometry of Nigerian Fetuses, 3: Abdominal Circumference. Journal of Ultrasound in Medicine. 31(suppl):S35

Mador, E.S., Ishaya, P., Ekedigwe J.E. & Ogunranti, J. (2012d). Ultrasound Biometry of Nigerian Fetuses, 2: Femur Length. Asian Journal of Medical Sciences 4(2):94 – 98

Mador, E. S. (2012). Results. In Fosca, E. (ed): Ultrasonic Fetal Biometry: Anthropometric Reference Values & Predictive Formulae of Fetal Parameters. LAMBERT Academic publishing GmbH & Co.KG, Heinrich-Bocking-str.6-8, 66121 Sacrbruken, Germany. pp 73 – 301

Menger, W.F & Korkmas M. V (1957). Inlet contraction of the pelvis. Amer. J. Obstet. Gynaecol. 74: 151

Modanlou HD, Dorchestet Wl, Thorosian A. Freeman RK. Macrosomia- maternal fetal and neonatal implications. Obstet Gynecol 1980; 55:420. 4

Mulder EJ, Koopman CM, Vermunt JK, de Valk HW, Visser GH (2010). Fetal growth trajectories in Type-1 diabetic pregnancy. Ultrasound Obstet Gynecol. 36(6):735-42.

O'Brien, G. D., Queenan, J. T. & Campbell, S. (1981). Assessment of gestational age in the second trimester by real-time ultrasound measurement of the femur length. American Journal of Obstetrics and Gynaecology. 139(5):540-5.

Ogunranti, J.O (1986). Weight of contemporary Nigerian growing children in clinical anthropology. Journal of Tropical Paediatrics. 32(5): 218 – 224

Ogunranti, J.O (1987). The mid-arm circumference in healthy estern Nierian children. A nutritional – clinical anthropometric paramenter. Child Care, Health and Development. 13: 50 – 67

Ogunranti, J.O (1994). Weight as a Clinical Anthropometric Parameter. Discovery and Innovation. 6(3): 267 – 275

Ott, W. J. (1985). Fetal femur length neonatal crown-heel length and screening for intrauterine growth retardation. Obstetrics and Gynaecology. 65: 460 – 464.

Ozanne SE, Sandovici I, Constância M. (2011). *Maternal diet, aging and diabetes meet at a chromatin loop. Aging (Albany NY). 3(5):548-54.*

Pam I.C, Ekedigwe J.E, Ogunranti J.O, Mador E.S (2012a). *Ultrasound biometry of Nigerian fetuses: 3. Abdominal circumference. Journal of Medical Research and Practice. In press*

Pam, I.C., Ekedigwe, J.E., Ogunranti, J.O., & Mador, E.S (2012b). *Ratio of Femur Length to Abdominal Circumference in Nigerian Fetuses. Highland Medical Research Journal Jos. In press*

Parks DG, Ziel HK (1978). *Macrosomia. A proposed indication for primary cesarean section. Obstetrics and Gynecology. 52(4):407-9*

Pöyhönen-Alho M, Joutsi-Korhonen L, Lassila R, Kaaja R. (2012). *Alterations of sympathetic nervous system, coagulation and platelet function in gestational diabetes. Blood Coagul Fibrinolysis. 2012 May 23.*

Reece, L.N. (1935): *The Estimation of Fœtal Maturity by a New Method of X-ray Cephalometry: Its Bearing on Clinical Midwifery. Proc R Soc Med. 28(5):489-504*

Retnakaran R, Ye C, Hanley AJ, Connelly PW, Sermer M, Zinman B, Hamilton JK. (2012) *Effect of maternal weight, adipokines, glucose intolerance and lipids on infant birth weight among women without gestational diabetes mellitus. CMAJ. 2012 May 22.*

Robinson J, Chidzanja S, Kind K, Lok F, Owens P, Owens J. (1995). *Placental control of fetal growth. Reprod Fertil Dev. 1995; 7(3):333-44.*

Sabrina, Q. R. (2009) *Femur length and Abdominal Circumference Ratio in Bangladesh. Bangladesh Journal of Obstetrics and Gynaecology. 24(2): 52 – 55*

Salbaum JM, Kappen C (2011). *Diabetic embryopathy: a role for the epigenome? Birth Defects Res A Clin Mol Teratol. 91(8):770-80.*

Sandovici I, Hoelle K, Angiolini E, Constância M (2012). *Placental adaptations to the maternal-fetal environment: implications for fetal growth and developmental programming. Reproductive Biomedicine Online. [Epub ahead of print]*

Savage, J. E. (1951): *Clinical and Roentgen Pelvimetry: Correlation. American Journal of Obstetrics & Gynecology. 61:809-823*

Saxena P, Tyagi S, Prakash A, Nigam A, Trivedi SS (2011). *Pregnancy outcome of women with gestational diabetes in a tertiary level hospital of north India. Indian Journal of Community Medicine. 36(2):120-3.*

Scammon, R.E., & Calkins, L.A. (1922). *"Morphometry of the Human Fetus with Special Reference to the Obstetric Measurements of the Head", American Journal of Obstetrics & Gynaecology. 6: 2*

Scammon, R.E., & Calkins, L.A. (1929). *The Development and Growth of the External Dimensions of the Human Body in the Fetal Period. Minneapolis. University of Minnesota Press*

Simonstein F (2006) . *Artificial reproduction technologies (RTs) - all the way to the artificial womb? Med Health Care Philos. 9(3):359-65*

Sjostedt, S., Engleston, G., & Rooth., G (1958). *Dysmaturity. Arch Dis Child. 33(168):123–130*

Smellie, W. (1752): *Treatise on the Theory and Practice of Midwifery. Ed. By A.H. McClintock. The New Syndenham Society, London, 1876. Vol. 1, pp 90, 92*

Stallone LA, Ziel HK (1974). *Management of gestational diabetes. American Journal of Obstetrics and Gynaecology. 119(8):1091-4*

Stevenson DK, Hopper AO, Cohen RS, Bucalo LR, Kerner JA, Sunshine P (1982). *Macrosomia: causes and consequences. Journal of Pediatrics .100(4):515-20*

Tamura RK, Sabbagha RE, Depp R, Dooley SL, Socol ML (1986). *Diabetic macrosomia: accuracy of third trimester ultrasound. Obstet Gynecol. 67(6):828-32*

Tarim E, Cok T (2011). *Macrosomia prediction using different maternal and fetal parameters in women with 50 g glucose challenge test between 130 and 140 mg/dl. Arch Gynecol Obstet. 284(5):1081-5.*

E. S. Mador, J. O. Ogunranti & I. C. Ishaya 229

Timofeev J, Huang CC, Singh J, Driggers RW, Landy HJ (2012). *Spontaneous labor curves in women with pregnancies complicated by diabetes. J Matern Fetal Neonatal Med. 25(1):20-6.*

Udall, J. N., Harrison, G. G., Vaucher, Y., Walson, P. D., &C Morrow, G. (1978). *Interaction of maternal and neonatal obesity. Pediatrics. 62, 17-21*

Welin S (2004). *Reproductive ectogenesis: the third era of human reproduction and some moral consequences. Sci Eng Ethics. 10(4):615-26*

Wheeler MB, Walters EM, Beebe DJ (2007). *Toward culture of single gametes: the development of microfluidic platforms for assisted reproduction. Theriogenology. 1;68 Suppl 1:S178-89.*

Wiedemann, HR, Grosse, KR, & Dibbern, H.: *An Atlas of Characteristic Syndromes. A Visual Aid to Diagnosis. Stuttgart, Wolfe Medical. 1983. 15*

Wilhelm-Benartzi CS, Houseman EA, Maccani MA, Poage GM, Koestler DC, Langevin SM, Gagne LA, Banister CE, Padbury JF, Marsit CJ (2012). *In utero exposures, infant growth, and DNA methylation of repetitive elements and developmentally related genes in human placenta. Environ Health Perspect. 120(2):296-302. Epub 2011 Oct 17.*

Willocks, J (1962a). *The Use of Ultrasonic Cephalometry. Proceedings of Royal Society of Medicine. 55(8): 640*

Yajnik CS, Deshmukh US. *Maternal nutrition, intrauterine programming and consequential risks in the offspring. Endocrine Metabolic Disorder. 9(3):203-11*

Genetic susceptibility to Systemic Lupus Erythematosus is associated with CTLA-4 Gene Polymorphisms in the Chinese Population

Ahmad Taha Khalaf
Dept. of dermatology, Faculty of medicine, Mosul Medical College
University of Mosul, Iraq

Ji-Quan Song, Ting-Ting Gao, and Xiang-Ping Yu
Zhongnan Hospital of Wuhan University
Wuhan University, Wuhan, China

Tie-Chi Lei
Renmin Hospital of Wuhan University
Wuhan University, Wuhan, China

1   Introduction

Systemic lupus erythematosus (SLE) is a chronic multisystem autoimmune disease and is considered to be caused by complex interactions between genetic risk, environmental and hormonal factors that result in an immune dysregulation and autoantibody production ensued (Edberg *et al.*, 2008; Kyttaris *et al.*, 2006; Sawalha *et al.*, 2008). Epidemiological studies reported that SLE is more common in Asians (46.7/100 000) than in Caucasians (20.7/100 000), and ethnicity also influences the age of onset and severity of its manifestations (Lau *et al.*, 2006; Rus *et al.*, 2002).

The precise aetiopathogenesis of SLE is still unclear; however, the search for genes and molecular interactions that influence disease has promoted our understanding of pathogenesis and genetic contributions to autoimmunity in SLE (Sekigawa *et al.*, 2004). Genetic association studies and recent advances in the field of single nucleotide polymorphisms (SNPs) have been highly successful in identifying several loci associated with disease susceptibility (Gregersen & Olsson, 2009; Harley *et al.*, 2006).

The CTLA-4 molecule has a suppressive effect on T-cell activation and might contribute to maintain immune tolerance by blocking CD28-dependent T cell activation through interactions with its ligand CD80/86 on antigen presenting cells (Harley et *al.*, 2006). The CTLA-4/B7 complex can compete with the CD28/B7 complex and convey an inhibitory influence to the T cell affecting T cell development, cytokine production and immune reactions (Gregersen & Olsson, 2009).

CTLA-4 would therefore, be an important negative regulator of T-cell responses, and its dysregulation has the potential to affect the pathogenesis of SLE by altered activation of T cells to self-antigens (Carreno B.M. & Collins M., 2002; Walunas *et al.*, 1996). The CTLA-4 gene is located within the risk region on chromosome 2q33, and several polymorphisms have been reported in this gene. However, only few of them have been studied for association with SLE susceptibility, of which, two are located within the promoter region: a T/C change at position –1722 and an A/G transition at position -1661 (Hudson *et al.*, 2002; Lee *et al.*, 2005; Ueda *et al.*, 2003). The former could alter transcription factor binding sites, whereas the latter may alter the potential response element for myocyte enhancer factor 2 (MEF2)(Ling *et al.*, 1999). Hence, allelic variations of these two sites might lead to a differential susceptibility to SLE resulting from unbalanced or inefficient immune responses.

Although CTLA-4 polymorphism has been shown to be associated with a number of autoimmune diseases, including SLE, Graves' disease, multiple sclerosis and type 1 diabetes, however, the associations have not been always replicated in different populations (Kristiansen *et al.*, 2000; Lee *et al.*, 2005; Ueda *et al.*, 2003). Recent studies showed that the CTLA-4 polymorphism plays an important role in SLE in some populations, which has not been confirmed in Chinese. Using a case-control study design, we have investigated the role of CTLA-4 polymorphism at positions –1661 and –1722 on SLE susceptibility in our Chinese SLE population in central China's Hubei Province.

2   Patients and Methods

2.1   Study Population

A total of 148 patients (17 males and 131 females) meeting the 1997 revised criteria of the American College of Rheumatology (ACR) for SLE (Hochberg, 1997) were recruited from Renmin and Zhongnan Hospitals of Wuhan University, Wuhan, China. Controls were 170 healthy volunteer with no history of autoimmune disease, collected for a case–control study. All patients and controls were Han Chinese residing in the central part of China. The study was approved by the hospitals' Ethics Committee of Wuhan University, and all subjects were consented to participate in the study.

2.2   DNA Extraction and Genotyping

DNA from patients and controls was extracted from peripheral blood with DNA flash kit 2.0 (HaiGene Biotechnolgy Co.Ltd., Gentra Systems Corp.) according to the standard protocol from the manufacturer. The Polymorphisms at positions −1661 and −1722 were analyzed by PCR–RFLP (polymerase chain reaction–restriction fragments length polymorphism), using the specific oligonucleotide primers (Sangon, Shanghai, China), 5' CTAAGAGCATCCGCTTGCACCT 3' and 5'TTGGTGTGATGCACAGAAGCC TTTT 3'. PCR amplification conditions were carried out as follows: initial denaturation at 94 °C for 5 minutes, then thirty cycles at 94°C (15 s), 60°C (30 s), 72°C (45 s), and one final extension at 72°C for 5 min. The products of the PCR were digested with BvbI or MseI at 37°C for 4 h, and then were analyzed by 2% agarose gel electrophoresis stained with ethidium bromide. After resolving, the −1722 T/C polymorphism was determined by detecting a 486 bp digested fragment (T allele) or two fragments of 270 and 216 bp (C allele) (Figure 1). The -1661A/G polymorphism was determined by detecting a 486 bp fragment (G allele) or two fragments of 347 and 139 bp (A allele) (Figure 2).

2.3   Statistical Analyses

We tested for Hardy-Weinberg equilibrium (HWE) among cases and controls. Allelic and genotypic frequencies were calculated by direct counting. The chi-square test with Yates correction and Fisher exact test were used to compare genotypes and alleles frequencies. Statistical significance was defined as $P<0.05$. The odds ratio (OR) was calculated to measure the strength of the association observed.

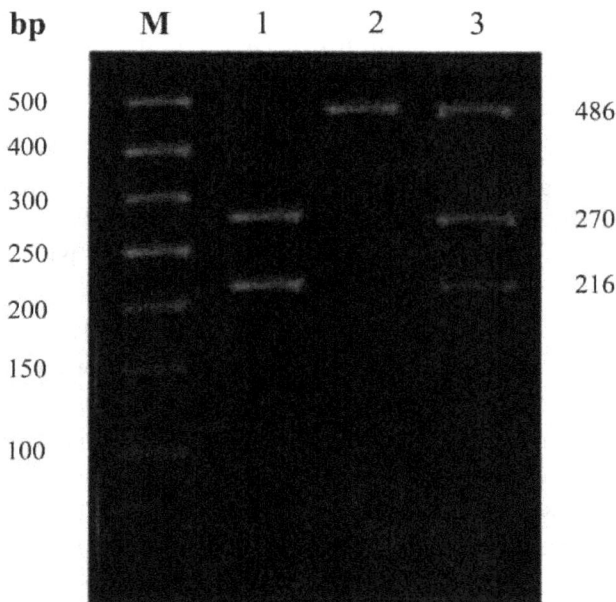

Figure.1: PCR restriction fragment length polymorphism results of −1722 T to C substitution in *CTLA-4* promoter region. 1. CC Genotype; 2. TT Genotype; 3.TC Genotype.

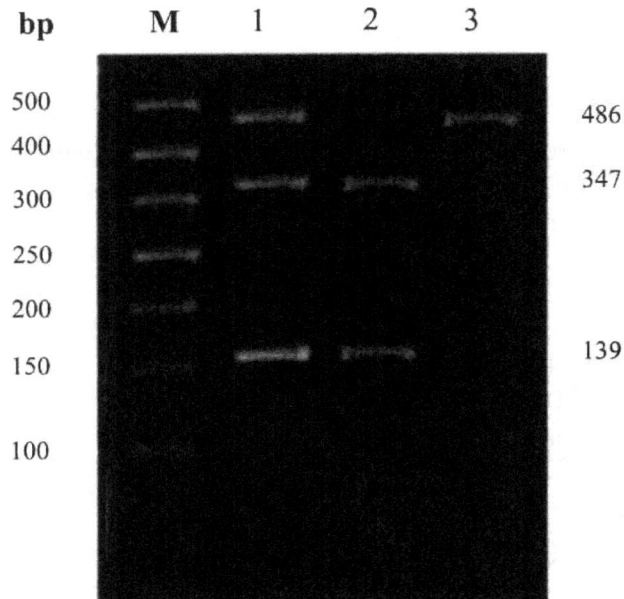

Figure 2: PCR restriction fragment length polymorphism results of -1661 A to G substitution in *CTLA-4* promoter region.1. AG Genotype; 2. AA Genotype; 3. GG Genotype.

3   Results and Discussion

The genotypic frequencies for the two sites tested were not found to be deviated from those predicted from Hardy-Weinberg equilibrium in both SLE patients and controls. Genotype and allele frequencies of the −1722 T/C and 1661 A/G polymorphisms are shown in Table 1 and Table 2. As observed, the genotypes at position −1722 were strongly associated with SLE. The frequency of the T allele on the −1722 SNP was significantly increased in SLE patients: 57.8% versus 40.6% in controls (P < 0.001, OR = 2.002). While the detected C allele frequency in the controls was significantly elevated in comparison with that in the SLE patients (59.4% versus 42.2%).The frequencies of T/T homozygotes and T/C heterozygotes were also significantly higher in patients than in controls (28.4% vs 17.1%, P = 0.016, OR = 1.926; 58.8% vs 47.1%,P=0.037, OR=1.605). Conversely, the frequencies of C/C homozygotes was considerably higher in controls than in patients (35.8% vs 12.8%,P < 0.01, OR = 0.263). We observed no significant difference in the distribution of the alleles and genotypes for the -1661 site between patients and healthy subjects.

Notwithstanding the convincing evidence that CTLA-4 polymorphism plays an important role in susceptibility to SLE, contradictory result has been reported among different populations (Lee *et al.,* 2005). Several studies have observed a significant association of SLE with CTLA-4 gene polymorphisms (Ahmed *et al.,* 2001; Fernandez-Blanco *et al.,* 2004; Hudson *et al.,* 2002; Lee *et al.,* 2005; Ulker *et al.,* 2009). While on the contrary, other studies showed a lack of association with that genetic variation (Aguilar *et al.,* 2003; Liu *et al.,* 2001; Parks *et al.,* 2004). Reasons for the variability in associations are still ambiguous. Thus, investigating the frequencies and distribution of variants CTLA-4 genes across populations are essential for understanding disease association and discovery of population differences,

promoter -1722	SLE n=148	Controls n=170	χ^2	P-value	OR (95%CI)
Genotype frequency					
TT	42(28.4%)	29(17.1%)	5.846	0.016	1.926(1.127-3.293)
TC	87(58.8%)	80(47.1%)	4.362	0.037	1.605(1.028-2.503)
CC	19(12.8%)	61(35.8%)	22.315	< 0.001	0.263(0.148-0.468)
Allele frequency					
T	171(57.8%)	138(40.6%)	18.701	< 0.001	2.002(1.459-2.747)
C	125(42.2%)	202(59.4%)			
Phenotype					
T	129(87.2%)	109(64.1%)	6.182	0.013	1.574(1.100-2.253)
C	106(71.6%)	141(82.9%)			

Abbreviations:
CTLA-4 = cytotoxic T-lymphocyte antigen 4;
SLE =systemic lupus erythematosus;
OR = odds ratios;
95% CI = 95% confidence interval.

Table 1: Genotypic distribution and allelic frequencies of -1722 *CTLA-4* polymorphisms in Chinese SLE patients and healthy controls

promoter -1661	SLE n=148	Controls n=170	χ^2	P-value	OR (95%CI)
Genotype frequency					
AA	59(39.9 %)	63(37.1%)	0.263	0.608	1.126(0.716-1.771)
AG	67(45.2%)	76(44.7%)	0.010	0.920	1.132(0.730-1.755)
GG	22(14.9%)	31(18.2%)	0.647	0.421	0.783(0.431-1.423)
Allele frequency					
A	185(62.5%)	202(59.4%)	0.633	0.426	1.139(0.827-1.568)
G	111(37.5%)	138(40.6%)			
Phenotype					
A	126(85.1%)	139(81.8%)	0.207	0.649	1.090(0.752-1.578)
G	89(60.1%)	107(62.9%)			

Abbreviations:
CTLA-4 = cytotoxic T-lymphocyte antigen 4;
SLE =systemic lupus erythematosus;
OR = odds ratios; 95%
CI = 95% confidence interval

Table 2 Genotypic distribution and allelic frequencies of –1661 *CTLA-4* polymorphisms in Chinese SLE patients and healthy controls.

especially for Chinese as they have a much higher SLE prevalence than the Europeans (Lau *et al.*, 2006; Rus *et al.*, 2002). The interval encompassing the CTLA-4 locus on chromosome 2q33 has been reported to show linkage to SLE in two genome-wide association studies (GWAS) studies (Cantor *et al.*, 2004; Graham *et al.*, 2006). A very recent GWAS has confirmed that variation in the CTLA-4 gene has been associated with a genetic risk of SLE (Budarf *et al.*, 2011). Although, this polymorphism may has not yet reached stringent thresholds of lupus GWAS performed in some Chinese cohorts, however, the association has been observed in multiple independent studies in various ethnic populations including Asian (Ahmed *et al.*, 2001; Barreto *et al.*, 2004; Budarf *et al.*, 2011; Cantor & Collins, 2004; Fernandez-Blanco *et al.*, 2004; Graham *et al.*, 2006; Hudson *et al.*, 2002; Lee *et al.*, 2005; Ulker *et al.*, 2009), and there is strong biological evidence sufficient to conclude that CTLA-4 polymorphism confers susceptibility to SLE through its crucial functions in T cell activation/regulation (Budarf *et al.*, 2011; Graham *et al.*, 2006; Lindqvist *et al.*, 2000; Liu *et al.*, 2003; Ueda *et al.*, 2003; Wong *et al.*, 2005).

Recently, a GWAS study confirmed a SLE susceptibility locus at chromosome 2q32.3 in Chinese population that is near the region 2q33 which encodes the genes for CTLA-4 (Han *et al.*, 2009). As polymorphisms that are near each other have a tendency be inherited together, something worth further pursuit in future studies. In Asian people, positive associations of the CTLA-4 polymorphism with SLE were reported in Korean (Hudson *et al.*, 2002) and Japanese (Ahmed *et al.*, 2001), while no such association was found in Malaysian population (Kek-Heng *et al.*, 2010). Significantly, a meta-analysis by Lee *et al.* found a close association between SLE and exon 1 at +49 of CTLA-4 gene, especially in Asians (Lee *et al.*, 2005). Liu, MF et al did not observe an association of CTLA-4 polymorphism with SLE in Taiwanese, but suggested that it is possible that this polymorphism could affect some specific clinical features (Liu *et al.*, 2001). This discrepancy with the findings of the current study may be partially attributed to the variations among Chinese living in different geographical regions (Xu *et al.*, 2009).

The results of this study confirm the involvement of CTLA-4 polymorphisms at the promoter – 1722 on SLE susceptibility in the Chinese population. Our findings are in agreement with the results of other ethnic groups demonstrating the influence of this polymorphism in the susceptibility to SLE. On the contrary, the genotypic frequencies for the –1661 site were not found to be significantly different between patients and controls. Other studies on –1661 polymorphism in Korean with SLE also could not find a positive correlation (Hudson *et al.*, 2002). In addition, no overall associations were seen between this polymorphism and SLE in African-Americans (Parks *et al.*, 2004). Being inexplicit, despite the short distance between the two locations, only –1722 promoter-region polymorphisms was associated with SLE, while the other –1661 is not. This possibly due to some functional differences between the two sites on regulatory properties of this promoter might affect basal promoter activity and gene expression. Polymorphisms in promoter regions may affect the gene expression quantitatively or qualitatively by altering transcription factor binding sites or other controlling domains (Shastry, 2002).

The significant increase in the C allele observed in the controls is assumed to play a protective role against SLE in Chinese. On the other hand, The T/T and T/C genotypes of –1722 T/C polymorphisms were associated with higher risk to have SLE. Hudson *et al* studied CTLA-4 Polymorphisms at positions T/C –1722 in Korean population and found that T allele was more frequent in SLE patients while C allele was decreased in the controls and suggested that the C allele could contribute protectively to SLE in the Korean population. In contrast, Fernandez-Blanco et al found that the C allele of the –1722 T/C SNP was associated with SLE susceptibility in the Spanish SLE patients. However, another study did not find any significant association between the genetic polymorphisms at the –1722 T/C SNP of the CTLA-4 gene and Spanish SLE patients (Aguilar *et al.*, 2003). Although there were significant associations in two of the three studies described above. However, a published meta-analysis study did not unveil a significantly increased odds ratio for this polymorphism (Lee *et al.*, 2005). Takeuchi *et al.* (2005) also reported a slight increase in the allele frequency of −1722 C in Japanese patients with SLE compared to the controls, but the difference was not statistically significant.

Because there are relatively few studies, it is difficult to explain the contradictories at the promoter −1722 polymorphism in SLE, but they may be due to a different genetic background and a possible role for racial and ethnic influences in the pattern of haplotypes on the CTLA-4 locus between various populations in SLE predisposition (Lau *et al.*, 2006; Rus *et al.*, 2002). Variations in associations among populations maybe also related to difference in patient characteristics or the distribution of other risk factors that interact with CTLA-4 concerning SLE. Moreover, genetic evidence suggests that genetic heterogeneity, a common phenomenon in complex diseases, are responsible for a considerable portion of this variability. We believe that there is not sufficient research on CTLA-4 polymorphisms to identify and demonstrate the role of these important genetic variants that confer susceptibility to SLE susceptibility among different populations.

Whereas some polymorphisms on the CTLA-4 gene have been analyzed in various populations for investigating an association with SLE, only one of these, the CTLA-4 A/G polymorphism at position +49 in exon 1 has been widely studied, mainly in European populations (Lee *et al.*, 2005). Accordingly, we expect that the results of our study to reinforce the interest of focusing on analyzing the role of CTLA-4 polymorphism in increased susceptibility to SLE. Furthermore, an elevated level of soluble CTLA-4 in sera has been described in SLE, with a positive and significant correlation between plasma sCTLA-4 concentration and SLE activity (Liu *et al.*, 2003; Wong *et al.*, 2005). Besides, the therapeutic use of CTLA4Ig which is a soluble fusion protein that interferes with T cell activation by inhibiting the B7/CD28 costimulatory interaction, appears to delay or extenuate disease development in experimental models of lupus (Dall'Era & Davis, 2004). In this way, the results observed should provide new postulates for the immunological role of this co-stimulatory molecule in the pathogenesis of SLE and should facilitate recent advances in the exploration of therapeutic agents targeting T-cell activation in this disease (Liu *al.*, 2003).

Other polymorphisms have also been described in the promoter region (-658 and-318), the CT60 (A/G) and at the 3-end of the gene as well as the microsatellite (AT)(n) in the 3'-untranslated region (3'-UTR) of the CTLA-4 gene. Nevertheless, the reported results have been inconsistent across different ethnic populations [27,39]; (Johnson *et al.*, 2001; Torres *et al.*, 2004). Hence, further explorations of these polymorphisms are needed in order to more fully examine SLE associations with CTLA-4 locus in Chinese population. Allelic and genotypic frequencies may vary between the populations; therefore, disease association studies and interpreting their results offer a possible route to understanding the influence of these genetic variants on disease aetiology and potentially to the development of new treatments.

4   Conclusions

CTLA-4 polymorphism at positions −1722 was significantly associated with SLE and may be a risk factor for SLE susceptibility in Chinese. Our results concur with the majority of those published supporting the important influence of CTLA-4 polymorphisms in the susceptibility to SLE. Nevertheless, further study in terms of the functional analysis of polymorphisms on the CTLA-4 gene needs to be done, and larger population studies in different ethnic groups should be performed in the future.

Acknowledgements

This study was supported by Department of Dermatology, Renmin and Zhongnan hospitals of Wuhan University. The authors like to thank Dr Ahmed N. Abdalla for his kind help. Special thanks and appreciation are extended to our laboratory colleagues for preparing samples.

References

Aguilar F., Torres B., Sanchez-Roman J., Nunez-Roldan A., Gonzalez-Escribano M.F.(2003). CTLA4 polymorphism in *Spanish patients with systemic lupus erythematosus. Hum Immunol. 64:936-40.*

Ahmed S, Ihara K, Kanemitsu S, Nakashima H, Otsuka T, Tsuzaka K, Takeuchi T, Hara T.(2001). Association of CTLA-4 but not CD28 gene polymorphisms with systemic lupus erythematosus in the Japanese population. Rheumatology. 40:662–667

Barreto M., Santos E., Ferreira R., et al.(2004). Evidence for CTLA4 as a susceptibility gene for systemic lupus erythematosus," Eur. J. Hum. Genet. 12, 620-626.

Barreto M., Santos E., Ferreira R., et al.(2004). Evidence for CTLA4 as a susceptibility gene for systemic lupus erythematosus. Eur J Hum Genet. 12: 620–626.

Budarf M.L., Goyette P., Boucher G., et al.(2011). A targeted association study in systemic lupus erythematosus identifies multiple susceptibility alleles. Genes Immun. 12(1):51-8

Cantor R.M., Yuan J., Napier S., et al.(2004). Systemic lupus erythematosus genome scan: support for linkage at 1q23, 2q33, 16q12-13, and 17q21-23 and novel evidence at 3p24, 10q23-24, 13q32, and 18q22-23. Arthritis Rheum. 50:3203–10.

Carreno B.M., Collins M.(2002). The B7 family of ligands and its receptors: new pathways for costimulation and inhibition of immune responses. Annu Rev Immunol. 20:29–53.

Dall'Era M., Davis J.(2004). CTLA4Ig: a novel inhibitor of costimulation. Lupus. 13: 372-376

Edberg J.C., Wu J., Langefeld C.D., et al.(2008). Genetic variation in the CRP promoter:association with systemic lupus erythematosus. Hum Mol Genet.17:1147–55.

Fernandez-Blanco L., Perez-Pampin E., Gomez-Reino J.J., and Gonzalez A.(2004). A CTLA-4 polymorphism associated with susceptibility to systemic lupus erythematosus. Arthritis & Rheumatism. 50: 328–329.

Graham D.S., Wong A.K., McHugh N.J., Whittaker J.C., Vyse T.J.(2006). Evidence for unique association signals in SLE at the CD28-CTLA4-ICOS locus in a family-based study. Hum Mol Genet. 1;15(21):3195-205.

Gregersen P.K., Olsson L.M.(2009). Recent advances in the genetics of autoimmune disease," Annu Rev Immunol. 27:363–91.

Han J.W., Zheng H.F., Cui Y. et al.(2009). Genome-wide association study in a Chinese Han population identifies nine new susceptibility loci for systemic lupus erythematosus. Nat Genet. 41:1234_7.

Harley J.B., Kelly J.A., Kaufman K.M.(2006). Unraveling the genetics of systemic lupus erythematosus. Semin Immunopathol. 28:119–130.

Hochberg M.C.(1997). Updating the American College of Rheumatology revised criteria for the classification of systemic lupus erythematosus. Arthritis Rheum. 40: 1725-1728.

Hudson LL, Rocca K., Song Y.W., Pandey J.P.(2002). CTLA-4 gene polymorphisms in systemic lupus erythematosus: a highly significant association with a determinant in the promoter region. Hum Genet. 111:452-5.

Johnson GC, Esposito L, Barratt BJ et al.(2001). Haplotype tagging for the identification of common disease genes. Nat Genet. 29: 233–237.

Kek-Heng C., Suat-Moi P., Ching-Hoong C., et al.(2010). Study of the CTLA-4 gene polymorphisms in systemic lupus erythematosus(SLE) samples from Malaysia,"Annals of Human Biology. 37: 275-281

Kristiansen O.P., Larsen Z.M., Pociot F.(2000). CTLA-4 in autoimmune diseases—A general susceptibility gene to autoimmunity?. Genes Immun. 170– 184.

Kyttaris V.C., Krishnan S., Tsokos G.C.(2006). Systems biology in systemic lupus erythematosus: integrating genes, biology and immune function. Autoimmunity. 39:705–9.

Lau C.S., Yin G., Mok M.Y.(2006). Ethnic and geographical differences in systemic lupus erythematosus, an overview. Lupus. 15:715–719.

Lee Y.H., Harley J.B., Nath S.K.(2005). CTLA-4 polymorphisms and systemic lupus erythematosus (SLE): a meta-analysis. Hum Genet. 116: 361–7.

Lindqvist A.K., Steinsson K., Johanneson B., et al.(2000). A susceptibility locus for human systemic lupus erythematosus (hSLE1) on chromosome 2q. J. Autoimmun.14, 169-178.

Ling V., Wu P.W., Finnerty H.F., Sharpe A.H., Gray G.S., Collins M.(1999). Complete sequence determination of the mouse and human CTLA4 gene loci: cross-species DNA sequence similarity beyond exon borders. Genomics. 60: 341– 355.

Liu M.F., Wang C.R., Chen P..C, Fung L.L.(2003). Increased expression of soluble cytotoxic T-lymphocyte-associated antigen-4 molecule in patients with systemic lupus erythematosus. Scand J Immunol. 57:568-72.

Liu M.F., Wang C.R., Lin L.C., Wu C.R.(2001). CTLA-4 gene polymorphism in promoter and exon-1 regions in Chinese patients with systemic lupus erythematosus. Lupus. 10:647–9.

Parks C G, Hudson L L, Cooper G S, Dooley M A, Treadwell E L, Clair E W St, Gilkeson G S, and Pandey J P.(2004). CTLA-4 gene polymorphisms and systemic lupus erythematosus in a population-based study of whites and African-Americans in the southeastern United States. Lupus. 13: 784-791.

Rus V., Hochberg M.C., "In Wallace,D.J., Hahn,B.H. (eds.).(2002). Dubois' Lupus Erythematosus. Lippincott,"Williams and Wilkins, Baltimore. 65-83.

Sawalha A.H., Kaufman K.M., Kelly J.A., et al.(2008). Genetic association of interleukin-21 polymorphisms with systemic lupus erythematosus. Ann Rheum Dis. 67:458–61.

Sekigawa I., Naito T., Hira K. et al.(2004). Possible mechanisms of gender bias in SLE: a new hypothesis involving a comparison of SLE with atopy. Lupus. 13: 217–22.

Shastry B.S.(2002). SNP alleles in human disease and evolution. J Hum Genet. 47:561–566.

Takeuchi F. , Kuwata S. , Mori M.(2005). CTLA-4 -1661A/G and -1772T/C dimorphisms in Japanese patients with systemic lupus erythematosus. J Rheumatol. 32(10):2062.

Torres B., Aguilar F., Franco E., Sánchez E., Sánchez-Román J., Jiménez J. Alonso, Núñez-Roldán A., Martín J., González-Escribano M.F.(2004). Association of the CT60 marker of the CTLA4 gene with systemic lupus erythematosus. Arthritis Rheum. 50(7):2211-5.

Ueda H., Howson J.M., Esposito L. et al.(2003). Association of the T-cell regulatory gene CTLA4 with susceptibility to autoimmune disease. Nature. 423: 506–511.

Ulker M., Yazisiz V., Sallakci N., Avci A.B, Sanlioglu S., Yegin O., Terzioglu E.(2009). CTLA-4 gene polymorphism of exon 1(+49 A/G) in Turkish systemic lupus erythematosus patients. Int J Immunogenet. 36(4):245-50.

Walunas T.L., Bakker C.Y., Bluestone J.A. (1996). CTLA-4 ligation blocks CD28-dependent T cell activation. J Exp Med. 183:2541–2550.

Wandstrat A.E., Nguyen C., Limaye N., et al.(2004). Association of extensive polymorphisms in the SLAM/CD2 gene cluster with murine lupus. Immunity. 21:769-780.

Wong C.K., Lit L.C., Tam L.S., et al.(2005). Aberrant production of soluble costimulatory molecules CTLA-4, CD28, CD80 and CD86 in patients with systemic lupus erythematosus. Rheumatology (Oxford). 44: 989.

Xu S., Yin X, Li S., et al.(2009). Genomic Dissection of Population Substructure of Han Chinese and Its Implication in Association Studies. Am J Hum Genet. 85:762-74

The Role of Viruses, Bacteria, and *Mycobacterium Avium* Subspecies *Paratuberculosis* Infection in the Etiology of Diabetes Mellitus

Anna Rita Attili
School of Biosciences and Veterinary Medicine
University of Camerino, Italy

Victor Ngu Ngwa
School of Veterinary Medicine and Sciences
University of Ngaoundere, Cameroon

Vincenzo Cuteri
School of Biosciences and Veterinary Medicine
University of Camerino, Italy

1   Pathogens and Diabetes

Convincing evidence to date indicates that microorganisms are associated with Type 1 diabetes (T1D) development and progression. Insulin-dependent T1D is a prototypic organ-specific autoimmune disease resulting from the selective destruction of insulin-secreting β cells within pancreatic islets of Langerhans by an immune-mediated inflammation involving autoreactive CD4$^+$ and CD8$^+$ T lymphocytes which infiltrate pancreatic islets.

T1D is a paradigmatic example of chronic multi-factorial disease determined by the interaction of genetic, environmental and immunologic factors with consequent destruction or damaging of the β-cells in the islets of Langerhans, insulin deficiency and hyperglycemia (Coppieters *et al.*, 2012). T1D is a polygenic disease, in which the genetic background is essential but not sufficient in causing the disease (Patterson *et al.*, 2009). Indeed, approximately 85-90% of new onset T1D patients do not have a first degree relative with the disease, this implies a strong environmental component to contribute to the development of T1D (Coppieters *et al.*, 2012). While several genetic susceptibility loci have been pinpointed by genome-wide association studies (Concannon *et al.*, 2009), the environmental factors at play remain boldly elusive. Yet, environmental factors play a prominent role in T1D pathogenesis, as suggested by the incomplete (~65%) T1D concordance between monozygotic twins (Redondo *et al.*, 2009), by migrant studies (Bodansky *et al.*, 1992; Kondrashova *et al.*, 2007) or by the decreasing weight of susceptible and protective HLA Class II haplotypes over the last decades (Hermann *et al.*, 2003; Gillespie *et al.*, 2004).

One of the environmental risk factors identified by a series of independent studies is represented by pathogens, with strong evidence showing that viruses and bacteria can infect pancreatic beta cells with consequent effects ranging from functional damage to cell death. Many experimental studies support the potential participation of viral infections to T1D pathogenesis, with a particular emphasis on virus-triggered islet inflammation, beta cell dysfunction and autoimmunity. Evidence from animal models suggests that viruses can trigger T1D in some cases. Viruses have also been implicated as possible triggers of other autoimmune disorders, including multiple sclerosis, autoimmune chronic active hepatitis, Sjögren's syndrome, juvenile rheumatoid arthritis and systemic lupus erythematosus (Schattner & Rager-Zisman, 1990; Talal *et al.,* 1992). Several mechanisms have been proposed for virus-mediated autoimmunity.

First, a virus could alter the target tissue of the host such that the tissue becomes recognized as foreign by the host's immune system, thus triggering an autoimmune response. These alterations could include modification of surface antigens into immunogenic forms, induction of new antigens, release of sequestered antigens during host cell lysis, incorporation of cellular antigens with viral envelope, or upregulation of MHC class I and/or class II molecules on the target tissue of the host. Second, the virus could alter the immune system of the host, resulting in autoimmune attack of beta cells. These alterations could include: - polyclonal B cell activation leading to production of autoantibodies, - release of lymphokines such as interferon (IFN)-α and tumor necrosis factor (TNF), which in turn recruit immunocytes to the host's tissues, - activation of immune cells that results in a breakdown of immune tolerance, or - disruption of the Th1/Th2 immune balance. Third, antigenic epitopes on the virus could be similar to molecules on the host tissue (molecular mimicry), thus causing the generation of antigen-specific T effector cells and/or antibodies that recognize the host target cell, leading to the development of autoimmunity. Fourth, it has been proposed that antiviral antibodies arising as a result of viral infection could lead to the formation of anti-idiotypic antibodies. These secondary antibodies could be autoreactive if the first antibody was produced against the part of the virus that reacts with the host (Jun & Yoon, 2003).

1.1   Viral Infections

Might persistent viral populations play a role in human T1D?

Viruses have long been suspected to contribute to the onset of T1D, based on detection frequencies around clinical onset in patients and their ability to rapidly trigger hyperglycaemia in the non-obese diabetic (NOD) mouse. Figure 1 shows a point–counterpoint type of approach about deciphering the etiology of human T1D (Coppieters *et al.*, 2012).

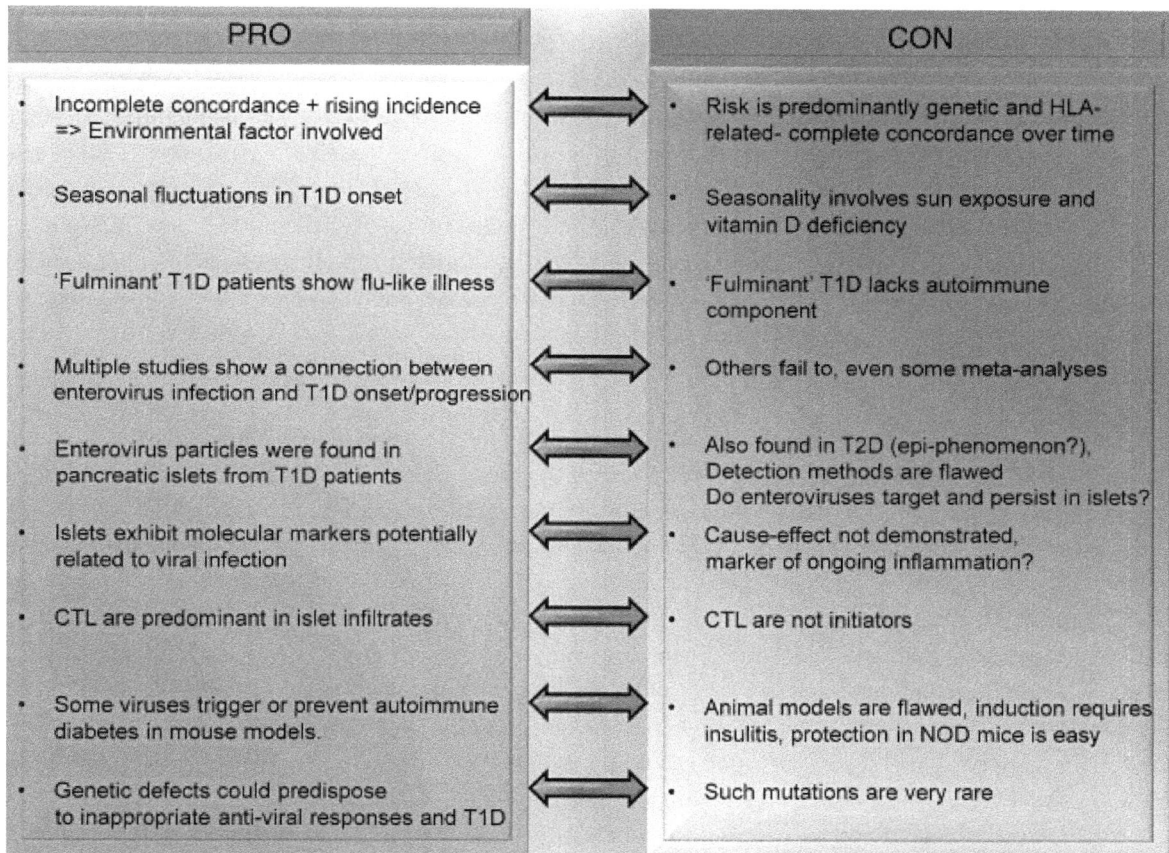

PRO		CON
• Incomplete concordance + rising incidence => Environmental factor involved	⟷	• Risk is predominantly genetic and HLA-related- complete concordance over time
• Seasonal fluctuations in T1D onset	⟷	• Seasonality involves sun exposure and vitamin D deficiency
• 'Fulminant' T1D patients show flu-like illness	⟷	• 'Fulminant' T1D lacks autoimmune component
• Multiple studies show a connection between enterovirus infection and T1D onset/progression	⟷	• Others fail to, even some meta-analyses
• Enterovirus particles were found in pancreatic islets from T1D patients	⟷	• Also found in T2D (epi-phenomenon?), Detection methods are flawed Do enteroviruses target and persist in islets?
• Islets exhibit molecular markers potentially related to viral infection	⟷	• Cause-effect not demonstrated, marker of ongoing inflammation?
• CTL are predominant in islet infiltrates	⟷	• CTL are not initiators
• Some viruses trigger or prevent autoimmune diabetes in mouse models.	⟷	• Animal models are flawed, induction requires insulitis, protection in NOD mice is easy
• Genetic defects could predispose to inappropriate anti-viral responses and T1D	⟷	• Such mutations are very rare

Figure 1: Point–counterpoint argument for a viral etiology in T1D.

The earliest observations were that the onset of T1D sometimes followed acute infections (Harris, 1898) and occurred with greater frequency at certain times of the year (Adams, 1926; Gamble & Taylor, 1969) which often indicates a viral cause. Then, epidemiological studies have shown the presence of virus-specific IgM antibodies in recent-onset T1D patients (Banatvala *et al.*, 1985; Friman *et al.*, 1985; Szopa *et al.*, 1993). The most convincing evidence comes from studies in which viruses isolated from the pancreas of patients that died from acute T1D caused diabetes in animals by the destruction of beta cells (Yoon *et al.*, 1979; Champsaur *et al.*, 1982).

The most well studied environmental factor and the most robust association with viruses and T1D involves *Enterovirus* species, of which some strains have the ability to induce or accelerate disease in animal models (Tracy *et al.*, 2010; Getts & Miller, 2010; Stene &Rewers, 2012). A possible link was first reported by Gamble *et al.* (1969) with many subsequent studies, in humans and animal models of diabetes, showing an association, particularly with *Coxsackie virus* B-4. Higher rates of *Enterovirus* infection, defined by detection of enterovirus IgM or IgG, or both, viral RNA with reverse transcription polymerase chain reaction (RT PCR), and viral capsid protein, have been found in patients with diabetes at diagnosis compared with controls (Andreoletti *et al.*, 1997; Lönnrot *et al.*, 2000; Craig *et al.*, 2003; Sarmiento *et al.*, 2007; Richardson *et al.*, 2009). Prospective studies have also shown more enterovirus infections in children who developed islet autoantibodies or subsequent diabetes, or both; as well as a temporal relation between infection and autoimmunity (Hyöty *et al.*, 1995; Hiltunen *et al.*, 1997; Lönnrot *et al.*, 2000; Salminen *et al.*, 2003). The extreme difficulty in biopsying pancreas has made it almost impossible to assay for viruses (or any other pathogen) in the pancreas at the time of T1D onset, a scientifically sound type of observation for associating specific pathogens with a disease. Associations of viruses other than *Enterovirus* with a T1D etiology (e.g. *Rubella virus*) (Menser *et al.*, 1978) or in mouse models (Oldstone, 1988; Wilberz *et al.*, 1991), as well as diverse reports of involvement of different Human Enteroviruses (HEV) in T1D onset (Tracy *et al.*, 2010; Okada *et al.*, 2010), continues to fuel debate as to either a specific role for diverse viruses in T1D onset or a role for specific viruses themselves. Further confounding the issue are data from the non-obese diabetic (NOD) mouse model showing that Human Enteroviruses can induce long-term protection from the onset of host-driven autoimmune T1D onset (Tracy *et al.*, 2002; Tracy *et al.*, 2010; Chatenoud *et al.*, 2010).

Over a half-dozen human viruses have been reported to be associated with human T1D. These include *Coxsackie B virus* (Jensen *et al.*, 1980; Yoon & Kominek, 1996), *Rubella virus* (Ginsberg-Fellner *et al.*, 1984; Ginsberg-Fellner *et al.*, 1986), *Mumps virus* (Gamble, 1980; Helmke *et al.*, 1980), *Cytomegalovirus* (Ward *et al.*, 1979; Pak *et al.*, 1988; Yasumoto *et al.*, 1992), *Epstein-Barr virus* (*EBV*) (Chikazawa *et al.*, 1985; Surcel *et al.*, 1988), *Varicella zoster virus* (Jali *et al.*, 1990), *Retrovirus* (Conrad *et al.*, 1997; Stauffer *et al.*, 2001) and *Rotavirus* (Honeyman *et al.*, 2000). The finding that *Saffold viruses*, a relatively recently characterized group of human cardioviruses (Chiu *et al.*, 2008), are apparently widespread in the human population (Zoll *et al.*, 2009) alters this dynamic and raises the question: could there be other viruses associated more commonly and more specifically with human T1D than HEV? It will be worthwhile to explore this topic, perhaps initially by utilizing microarray tools (Wang *et al.*, 2002) which can assay for diverse species of viruses within a single sample.

About ten viruses have been reported to be associated with the development of T1D in animals. These include *Encephalomyocarditis virus* (*EMCV*) (Craighead *et al.*, 1968; Yoon J *et al.*, 1980), *Mengo virus* (Yoon *et al.*, 1984), *Reovirus* (Onodera *et al.*, 1978) and *Retrovirus* (Suenaga & Yoon, 1988; Gaskins *et al.*, 1992; Nakagawa *et al.*, 1992) in mice; *Coxsackie B virus*, particularly B4, in mice (Yoon *et al.*, 1978; Hou *et al.*, 1993) and nonhuman primates (Yoon *et al.*, 1986); *Foot-and-Mouth Disease virus* in pigs and cattle (Barboni *et al.*, 1966); *Rubella virus* in hamsters and rabbits (Menser *et al.*, 1978; Rayfield *et al.*, 1986); *Bovine viral diarrhea virus* in cattle (Tajima *et al.*, 1992) and *Kilham's rat virus* in rats (Guberski *et al.*, 1991). As well as triggering beta cell-specific autoimmunity, three picornaviruses are may cause T1D by directly infecting and destroying beta cells: *EMC virus*, *Mengovirus*, and the *Coxsackie viruses*. When susceptible cells are infected with picornaviruses, the cells are destroyed because of the inhibition of RNA and protein synthesis of the infected cells.

On the contrary, there is also some evidence that viruses such as *Lymphocytic choriomeningitis virus* (*LCMV*) (Oldstone, 1988; Dyrberg *et al.*, 1988) and *Mouse hepatitis virus* (*MHV*) (Wilberz *et al.*, 1991) can protect against the development of autoimmune T1D in two spontaneously diabetic animals, the BioBreeding (BB) rat and the NOD mouse. Furthermore, in view of the disease's globally rising incidence, it is hypothesized that improved hygiene standards may reduce the immune system's ability to appropriately respond to viral infections. The hygiene hypothesis proposes that increased hygiene may cause changes in the composition of gut bacterial flora (Wen *et al.*, 2008), influencing the maturation of the immune system, facilitating imbalance and thereby autoimmune reactions in genetically predisposed individuals (Ludvigsson *et al.*, 2006). In some studies, the frequency of childhood infections correlated inversely with the incidence of T1D (Gibbon *et al.*, 1997; Pundziute *et al.*, 2000).

Arguments in favour of and against viral infections as major aetiological factors in T1D will now be discussed in conjunction with potential pathological scenarios.

1.1.1   Arguments in Favour of Viral Involvement in the Pathogenesis of T1D

What could be the pathological mechanisms that link viral infection to the onset of islet autoimmunity and eventually development of T1D?

One possibility that was put forward by the work of Foulis and co-workers (1987) is that a beta cell-specific viral infection could have the ability to persist and initiate islet inflammation. It was demonstrated that recently diagnosed T1D patients harboured pancreatic islets that expressed aberrantly major histocompatibility complex (MHC) class I and interferon (IFN)-α. Both molecules are up-regulated typically in response to viral infection and could be envisioned to cause recognition and killing of beta cells by infiltrating CD8 T cells. Some reports have indeed documented enterovirus infection specifically within pancreatic islets, and there seems to be a connection with an atypical "fulminant" subtype of T1D (Dotta *et al.*, 2007; Richardson *et al.*, 2009; Tanaka *et al.*, 2009). Nevertheless, these results are in need of further confirmation using complementary detection techniques in order to gauge the precise frequency of beta cell-specific viral infection in T1D *versus* controls.

The concept of "molecular mimicry" suggests that viruses expressing epitopes resembling certain beta cell structures have the potential to induce cross-reactive immune responses (Coppieters & von Herrath, 2010). Proof of concept was offered with the design of rat insulin promoter-lymphocytic choriomeningitis virus glycoprotein (RIP-*LCMV*.GP) transgenic mice, which develop diabetes after infection with *LCMV* (Ohashi *et al.*, 1991; Oldstone *et al.*, 1991). Some potential cross-reactivity has been documented in the past between *Coxsackie virus* constituents and glutamic acid decarboxylase (GAD) (Kaufman *et al.*, 1992; Atkinson *et al.*, 1994), a major autoantigen in T1D, but this correlation has since been challenged by others (Richter *et al.*, 1994; Horwitz *et al.*, 1998; Schloot *et al.*, 2001). An alternative scenario was proposed based on results in the RIP-*LCMV* model showing that sequential viral mimicry events can accelerate disease onset (Christen *et al.*, 2004), but such hypotheses are difficult to test in a patient setting.

In contrast, "bystander activation" explains the recruitment and activation of auto aggressive cells to the islet milieu as a consequence of localized viral infection. Virus could lead to activation and maturation of antigen-presenting cells (APCs), which would then shuttle antigen to the pancreatic draining lymph nodes resulting in priming of autoaggressive T cells (von Herrath *et al.*, 2003). The theory was strengthened by the finding that *Coxsackie virus* infection acts primarily by enhancing the release of islet antigens which, in turn, stimulate resting autoreactive T cells (Horwitz *et al.*, 1998). Bystander activation, caused merely by cytokine released from inflammatory cells and infected cells, is unlikely to be enough to break tolerance (von Herrath *et al.*, 1995; Holz *et al.*, 2001) and by itself give rise to diabetes induction, as studies show that activation of APCs in the pancreas is required for T1D initiation in RIP-*LCMV* mice (von Herrath *et al.*, 1997; Garza *et al.*, 2000). The observation that enteroviruses are found predominantly around clinical diagnosis may support indirectly the idea that viral infection serves only as a non-specific, one-time trigger to allow pre-existing autoreactive T cells to reach their targets. Studies in the NOD mouse also revealed that a critical mass of autoimmunity is required for *Coxsackie virus* infections to be diabetogenic (Serreze *et al.*, 2000; Drescher *et al.*, 2004). One attractive mechanism would be that pancreotropic viruses can precondition the local vasculature to allow entry of effector T cells.

The "fertile-field hypothesis" was conceived to explain how multiple microbial agents could culminate in potentially a single autoimmune disorder. Applied to T1D, the idea is that a viral infection with the right timing may give rise to a transient period, during which the pancreas becomes a fertile field for the development of autoimmune cells. Through induction of beta cell stress and activation of antigen drainage, self-epitopes are then released and presented to self-reactive T cells. In this context, it was found that the contribution of apoptosis-related epitopes during spontaneous development in the NOD mouse, appears to be limited, but this pathway could become enhanced after viral infection (Coppieters *et al.*, 2011). The observation that diabetes acceleration in NOD mice by *Coxsackie virus* requires a critical level of inflammation contradicts this hypothesis, and indicates that insulitis may, in fact, serve as the "fertilizer" for viruses to inflict any meaningful damage (Serreze *et al.*, 2000; Drescher *et al.*, 2004).

"Genetic predisposition" is obviously a major factor in T1D development. Could it be that individuals with susceptibility genes for T1D possess a greater risk of productive infection or an inability to accurately respond to, e.g. enteroviral infections? Genetic studies indeed suggest that mutations in IFN-response genes might lay at the basis of an exaggerated response to viral infection in type 1 diabetes patients. It should therefore be considered that the observed co-occurrence of enteroviruses and T1D reflects the host's inability to deal appropriately with a common, normally harmless infection (Jaïdane *et al.*, 2012; Hober *et al.*, 2012).

Finally, it is relevant to mention the aggressive T1D subtype known as "*fulminant*" T1D. Viral infection is associated primarily with non-autoimmune subtypes of T1D. It is reported predominantly in the Japanese population and is characterized by the absence of autoantibodies, acute onset - often with ketoacidosis - and the almost complete destruction of beta cells at diagnosis. Patients with *fulminant* T1D often show symptoms of *Enterovirus* infection prior to onset (Hanafusa *et al.*, 2007), and histological data demonstrate that a significant fraction of pancreas contain enteroviral particles (Tanaka *et al.*, 2009). The apparently strong correlation between enteroviruses and this unconventional, non-autoimmune disease phenotype could mean that at least some less-characterized donors may have been affected by this disease subtype (Richardson *et al.*, 2009).

1.1.2   Arguments Opposed to a Viral Involvement in the Pathogenesis of T1D

"Viral" or "inflammatory" signature? Up-regulation of MHC class I as well as type 1 IFN and IFN-inducible chemokines such as CXCL10 has been observed in pancreas from T1D patients. All these markers are expressed typically in response to viral infection, but also as a consequence of generalized local inflammation. In mouse models, Seewald *et al.* (2000) demonstrated persistent up-regulation of MHC class I long after viral clearance in diabetic RAT-LCMV.GP transgenic mice. This raises the question of whether MHC class I hyperexpression may be a mere consequence of ongoing inflammation rather than a result of ongoing infection. Can virus persist at all in the pancreas? Although shown only in cardiac tissue to date, it is not known whether a similar persistence can occur in other tissues, although there is no reason at this point to doubt that it could. The question devolves to how long might an HEV persist in any given tissue. It was found MHC class I hyperexpression but no evidence of viral infection in any of the long-standing T1D donor pancreas, thus suggesting that up-regulation is not caused by any known virus (Kim *et al.*, 2005; Chapman *et al.*, 2008).

Another opinion is that viral agents may represent a minor environmental component in T1D. Throughout history, many inconsistencies have accumulated in the literature with regard to studies linking detection of viral RNA or protein in blood, stool or pancreatic tissue to T1D onset. A recent meta-study by Yeung *et al.* (2011) that included measurements of *Enterovirus* RNA or viral capsid protein in blood, stool or tissue of patients with pre-diabetes and diabetes found a significant correlation. An earlier meta-study, in contrast, claimed that no convincing evidence existed for an association between *Coxsackie B virus* serology and T1D from the 26 examined studies that were included (Green *et al.*, 2004). These discrepancies could be explained by the involvement of several viral strains, many of which are still undiscovered, all of which may affect certain populations differently. Further, it is possible that not a single event, but rather a series of infections is required and that transient infection stages escape detection in cross-sectional studies. Importantly, detection methods are far from standardized, and sensitivity thresholds can be expected to vary wildly. The option should be considered that viral agents represent only a small percentage of the environmental component in T1D and that significance is achieved only within certain susceptible populations. Finland, with its staggering T1D incidence, might be such a region where enteroviral strains contribute more aggressively compared to other countries. Moreover, viral infections could be an epiphenomenon. In a study by Richardson *et al.* (2009) the observation that 40% of type 2 diabetics showed that the presence of virus in their pancreatic islets may indicate that viral infection is an epiphenomenon to conditions of general beta cell stress. The true infection frequency in T1D should therefore be considered *vis-à-vis* with other forms of diabetes in order to exclude any secondary effects.

1.1.3 *Retrovirus* and Diabetes

As most mammalian species contain endogenous retroviruses as part of their DNA, the expression of endogenous retroviruses by beta cells could be associated with insulitis and T1D in NOD mice (Suenaga & Yoon, 1988; Gaskins *et al.*, 1992; Nakagawa *et al.*, 1992). In NOD mice, the islet cells express various retroviral messenger RNAs (mRNAs) encoded by the *gag*, *pol* and *env* genes, and the beta cells in particular express the group-specific antigen p73 of the A-type *retrovirus* (Pak *et al.*, 1995). In addition, the presence of both A-type and C-type retroviral particles was found in the pancreatic beta cells of NOD mice and was considered to be associated with the development of autoimmune T1D in these animals (Fukino-Kurihara *et al.*, 1985). It is not certain how retroviruses may be involved in the pathogenesis of autoimmune T1D in NOD mice. The presentation of a retroviral antigen on the beta cells by antigen-presenting cells, such as macrophages and dendritic cells may be the initial step in the autoimmune destruction of beta cells. An immune response to a specific antigen on a target cell involves the activation of CD4[+] T cells by antigens presented on the surface of a macrophage or other antigen-presenting cells. Studies support this possibility, as elimination of macrophages resulted in the prevention of beta cell-specific autoimmune processes in NOD mice (Lee *et al.*, 1988; Charlton *et al.*, 1988; Jun *et al.*, 1999; Jun & Yoon, 2003). Another possible mechanism whereby retroviruses could be involved in the initiation of autoimmune T1D in NOD mice is the alteration of the expression of cellular genes by the retroviral genomes in the beta cells, possibly resulting in a beta cell-specific altered antigen(s). An altered antigen might be recognized as foreign by immunocytes, leading to beta cell-specific autoimmunity. Besides, it is possible that cellular proteins taken up in the retroviral envelope may elicit an autoimmune response or that IFN-γ-induced expression of HLA-II may trigger autoimmunity through CD4[+] lymphocytes.

In addition to animal models such as the NOD mouse, endogenous retroviruses have also been implicated in human T1D. Anti-insulin autoantibodies from T1D patients and their non diabetic, first-degree relatives have been found to cross-react with the retroviral p73 antigen in up to 75% of cases, whereas only 3% of non diabetic unrelated controls had p73-binding antibodies, confirming that anti-insulin auto-antibody-positive sera contain antibodies that recognize both insulin and p73 (Hao *et al.*, 1993). In other autoimmune diseases, nucleotide sequence homologies are being discovered between human retroviruses and self-antigens, in particular between ribonucleoproteins and the p30 C-type retroviral gag-gene product (Query & Keene, 1987; Nyman *et al.*, 1990; Brookes *et al.*, 1992). Moreover, electron microscope studies demonstrated *Retrovirus*-like particles in the cytoplasm of beta cells of T1D patients who died shortly after the onset of diabetes, and in none of the non diabetic controls. All diabetic pancreases showed islet destruction with insulitis. Retroviral antigens released from beta cells during beta cell turnover might be processed by antigen-presenting cells such as macrophages, dendritic cells or B cells and presented to T-helper cells (CD4$^+$) in association with HLA class II antigens. The activated CD4$^+$ T cells secrete interleukin (IL)-2, which amplifies retroviral antigen-specific CD8$^+$ cytotoxic T cells. These cells could recognize retroviral antigens expressed on beta cells in conjunction with MHC class I antigen, resulting in CD8$^+$ cytotoxic T cell-mediated beta cell destruction. A novel human endogenous retroviral gene, designated IDDMK$_{1,2}$22, thought to belong to the mouse mammary tumor virus-related family of human endogenous retroviruses (HERV)-K, was reported to be expressed in the plasma of recent-onset T1D patients but not in nondiabetic control subjects (Conrad *et al.*, 1997). However, careful studies have shown that a sequence identical to that of IDDMK$_{1,2}$22 was not present in either the plasma or peripheral lymphocytes from either diabetic or control subjects (Kim *et al.*, 1999). Instead, a related human endogenous retrovirus with 90% to 93% sequence homology with IDDMK$_{1,2}$22 was present equally in both diabetic and non diabetic subjects, indicating that this identified human endogenous *Retrovirus* is unlikely to be associated with the development of autoimmune T1D in humans (Lower *et al.*, 1998). Even though it appears that the endogenous retroviral gene homologous with IDDMK$_{1,2}$22 is not associated with T1D, it does not necessarily exclude the involvement of other human retroviruses or endogenous *Retrovirus* genes in the pathogenesis of autoimmune diabetes. An interesting report showed that the expression of the defective retroviral gene, the HERV-K18 provirus encoding super antigen, is induced by IFN-α and subsequently stimulates Vβ7 T cells, which was correlated with the onset of T1D. Whether the HERV-K18 provirus is truly involved in the development of autoimmune diabetes remains to be determined (Stauffer *et al.*, 2001).

1.1.4 *Reovirus* and Diabetes

Reovirus is a double-stranded RNA virus that is believed to cause mild infections of the upper respiratory and gastrointestinal tract of humans.

It has also been associated with T1D in animals; however its mode of action is not known. Mice infected with beta cell-passaged *Reovirus type 3* showed abnormal glucose tolerance tests within 10 days after infection, but glucose tolerance returned to normal after three weeks (Onodera *et al.*, 1978). Specific viral antigens were present in some beta cells as well as in acinar cells of these animals, and viral particles were detected by electron microscopy in the cytoplasm of some beta cells, suggesting that the diabetic symptoms were caused by direct infection of the beta cells. Other evidence suggests that *Reovirus* might cause transient diabetes through an immune reaction. Mice infected with beta cell-passaged *Reovirus type 1* developed transient diabetes, and their sera contained auto-antibodies that reacted with cytoplasmic antigens from the islets of Langerhans, the anterior pituitary, and the gastric mucosa of uninfected mice (Onodera *et al.*, 1981). An autoimmune mechanism might be involved in the disease because of the administration of immunosuppressive drugs to *Reovirus*-infected SJL and NFS mice reduced or prevented the development of *Reovirus*-induced diabetes and mortality. Moreover, other studies suggest that a Th1 response induced by the increased expression of IL-12 may be responsible for the development of diabetes in newborn DBA/1 mice infected with *Reovirus* (Hayashi *et al.*, 2001). Human beta cells are also susceptible to *Reovirus type 3* infection *in vitro* (Yoon *et al.*, 1981); however there is little evidence for the involvement of *Reovirus* in the pathogenesis of human T1D.

1.1.5 *Kilham Rat Virus* and Diabetes

Kilham rat virus (*KRV*) belongs to the *Parvoviridae* family and it was originally isolated from a rat sarcoma, it has been found to cause a fatal neonatal disease, physical deformities and mental retardation in newborn rats.

KRV has been shown to induce diabetes by provoking autoimmune responses against the beta cells, rather than by direct beta cell infection in diabetes-resistant BB (DR-BB) rats (Guberski *et al.*, 1991; Brown *et al.*, 1993). Diabetes-prone (DP)-BB rats, like NOD mice, spontaneously develop a diabetic syndrome that resembles human T1D in many respects (Marliss, 1983). DP-BB rats are lymphopenic and 80% to 100% of the animals become diabetic at about 120 days of age. DR-BB rats are derived from DP-BB rats, but do not normally develop diabetes. When DR-BB rats were infected with *KRV* at three weeks of age, about 30% of these animals developed autoimmune diabetes within two to four weeks after infection and a further 30% showed insulitis without diabetes (Guberski *et al.*, 1991). Because of the inactivation of macrophages with liposomal dichloromethylene diphosphonate (lip-Cl$_2$MDP), which selectively destroys macrophages by apoptosis, results in the near complete prevention of insulitis and diabetes in *KRV*-infected DR-BB rats, macrophages and macrophage-derived cytokines play a critical role in the cascade of events leading to the destruction of pancreatic beta cells, culminating in the development of autoimmune diabetes in *KRV*-infected DR-BB rats (Chung *et al.*, 1997). Experimental data suggests that *KRV* infection leads to the activation of silent autoreactive T cells that are specific for beta cells in DR-BB rats (Ellerman *et al.*, 1996). However, the precise mechanism by which *KRV* induces autoimmune T1D without the infection of beta cells is poorly understood. In addition, it was unclear how *KRV*-specific autoreactive T cells destroy pancreatic beta cells without direct infection of the cells by *KRV*. It was hypothesized that *KRV* antigen-specific T cells generated by *KRV* peptides might cross-react with pancreatic beta cells and attack them, resulting in the development of insulitis and, subsequently, diabetes. Chung and colleagues (2000) indicated that molecular mimicry between *KRV* peptides and beta cell-specific autoantigens in DR-BB rats is unlikely to be a mechanism by which *KRV* induces beta cell-specific autoimmune diabetes.

Another possibility is that *KRV* infection of DR-BB rats might disturb the finely tuned immune balance and activate autoreactive T cells that are cytotoxic to beta cells, resulting in T cell-mediated autoimmune diabetes similar to that seen in DP-BB rats. To test this hypothesis, the CD4$^+$ and CD8$^+$ T-cell populations were examined in the splenocytes of DR-BB rats after KRV infection. The percentage of CD8$^+$ T cells increased considerably, whereas the percentage of CD4$^+$ T cells decreased, although the absolute number of both CD4$^+$ and CD8$^+$ T cells was increased during *KRV* infection. In addition, CD8$^+$ T cells preferentially proliferated as compared with CD4$^+$ T cells in *KRV*-infected DR-BB rats (Chung *et al.*, 2000). Moreover treatment of *KRV*-infected DR-BB rats with OX-8 monoclonal antibody significantly decreased the incidence of diabetes, indicating that CD8$^+$ T cells are clearly involved in the destruction of beta cells. It has been reported that the treatment of DP-BB rats with anti-NK cell antibody failed to prevent diabetes, while OX-8 monoclonal antibody treatment successfully prevented diabetes (Ellerman *et al.*, 1993). Therefore, it is more likely that CD8[+] T cells may play a major role in *KRV*-induced diabetes, although the possibility of the involvement of NK cells cannot be absolutely excluded, because OX-8 monoclonal antibody also depletes NK cells.

It has been suggested that the dominance of Th1 cells over Th2 cells is associated with the development of autoimmune T1D, whereas the dominance of Th2 cells over Th1 cells is associated with the prevention of T1D (Rabinovitch, 1994; Liblau *et al.*, 1995; Delovitch & Singh, 1997). *KRV* infection in DR-BB rats increased the expression of Th1-type cytokines in the splenocytes and pancreatic infiltrates (Chung *et al.*, 1997); therefore, it is possible that the proportions of Th1 and Th2 cells are altered during *KRV* infection in DR-BB rats. Subsequent experiments showed that the number of Th2-like CD45RC⁻ CD4[+] T cells was significantly decreased and the number of Th1-like CD45RC[+] CD4[+] T cells significantly increased in the splenocytes of *KRV*-infected DR-BB rats as compared with PBS-treated controls. In addition, Th1-like CD45RC[+] CD4[+] and CD8[+] T cells isolated from DR-BB rats after infection with *KRV* could induce diabetes in 88% of recipient DP-BB rats when both CD45RC[+] CD4[+]and CD8[+] T cells were transferred (Chung *et al.*, 2000). This result indicates that CD45RC[+] CD4[+] and CD8[+] T cells are major effector T cells that can induce autoimmune diabetes. The incidence of diabetes in DP-BB rats that received either CD45RC[+] CD4[+] or CD8[+] T cells alone was, however, significantly lower as compared with that in rats that received a combination of CD45RC[+] CD4[+] and CD8[+] T cells. These results indicate that Th1-like CD4[+] and CD8[+] T cells from *KRV*-infected rats work synergistically to destroy pancreatic beta cells, as proposed previously (Chung et al., 1997). In contrast, none of the recipients of both CD45RC⁻ CD4[+] and CD8[+] T cells developed diabetes, indicating that CD45RC⁻ CD4[+] T cells play a role as regulatory T cells. Therefore, infectious *KRV*, rather than *KRV* proteins expressed in rVVs, is absolutely required to disturb or breakdown the finely tuned immune balance, resulting in the upregulation of preexisting beta cell-specific autoreactive T cells that can destroy beta cells.

1.1.6   *Bovine Viral Diarrhea Virus* and Diabetes

Bovine viral diarrhea virus (*BVDV*) belongs to *Pestivirus* genus of the *Flaviviridae* family and is widespread in livestock such as cattle. *BVDV* has been reported to be associated with T1D in cattle, however not all animals with *BVDV* infection develop diabetes (Tajima *et al.*, 1992). This may be attributable to the existence of different variants of the virus or to genetic differences among the hosts. In a more recent study, *BVDV* infected cattle with T1D showed the presence of *BVDV* genes in the pancreas, however, not in the islet cells. Many of these cattle also had islet cell autoantibodies, suggesting that T1D associated with *BVDV* is not a direct effect of *BVDV* on islet cells (Tajima *et al.*, 1999).

1.1.7   *Mumps Virus* and Diabetes

The *Mumps virus* is an enveloped single-stranded virus belonging to the *Paramyxoviridae* family. *Mumps virus* was one of the first viruses implicated in the development of human T1D; several cases were reported in which mumps infection appeared to precede the onset of T1D (Gamble, 1980).

It has been hypothesized that infection with *Mumps virus* may induce autoimmunity, as some children appear to develop islet cell autoantibodies during parotiditis (Helmke *et al.*, 1980), however the mechanisms by which this might occur are unknown. *In vitro* studies have shown that human beta cells could be infected with *Mumps virus* (Prince *et al.*, 1978), that mumps infection of a human insulinoma cell line induced the release of IL-1 and IL-6 and upregulated the expression of HLA class I and II antigens (Cavallo *et al.*, 1992), and that pancreatic beta cells infected had increased expression of only HLA class I molecules (Parkkonen *et al.*, 1992). In addition, *Mumps virus* has been shown to be capable of replicating in the exocrine pancreas (Vuorinen *et al.*, 1992). On the basis of these studies, it may be suggested that cytokines released by *Mumps virus*-infected cells and increased expression of HLA molecules by infected beta cells may lead to an immune response against the beta cells or may increase preexisting autoimmune processes directed against beta cells. Several studies have explored the impact of mumps vaccinations on either increasing or decreasing the incidence of T1D. One investigation concluded that the elimination of natural mumps infections by vaccination may have been responsible for the decreased risk of developing T1D (Hyöty *et al.*, 1993). Other studies concluded that there is no association with childhood mumps vaccinations and the development of islet autoimmunity (Hummel *et al.*, 2000) or T1D (De Stefano *et al.*, 2001).

1.1.8 *Rubella Virus* and Diabetes

Rubella virus is a non-segmented, single-stranded RNA enveloped virus that belongs to the *Togaviridae* family. It has been implicated in T1D. Patients with congenital rubella syndrome (CRS) had a higher incidence of T1D than the general population, with approximately 10% to 20% developing diabetes between the ages of 5 to 20 years (McEvoy *et al.*, 1986). Islet cell and anti-insulin antibodies were found in 50% to 80% of diabetic patients with CRS, whereas these antibodies were present in about 20% of non diabetic patients with CRS (Ginsberg-Fellner *et al.*, 1984), suggesting an underlying autoimmune disorder. Genetic susceptibility may also be involved (Ginsberg-Fellner *et al.*, 1986).

Rubella virus appears to be able to directly infect beta cells, as shown by *in vivo* and *in vitro* studies. Neonatal golden Syrian hamsters infected with beta cell-passaged *Rubella virus* developed hyperglycemia and hypoinsulinemia between 7 and 10 days of age, and their beta cells were positive for *Rubella virus* antigen. An autoimmune process may be involved, as 40% of infected animals had cytoplasmic islet cell antibodies and 34.5% had insulitis (Rayfield *et al.*, 1986). Human islets are also susceptible to direct *Rubella virus* infection under culture conditions. Human fetal islets exposed to *Rubella virus* contained rubella viral antigens in both beta and non beta cells and had lowered levels of insulin production (Numazaki *et al.*, 1989), although without any demonstrable cytopathology (Numazaki *et al.*, 1990). It is possible that the virus may insert, expose, or alter antigens in the plasma membrane of the infected host as it buds through the cell membrane. Rubella viral antigens on beta cells or *Rubella virus*-altered antigens on the surface of beta cells may be perceived as foreign by the host's immune system, leading to beta cell-specific autoimmunity.

Alternatively, *in vitro* studies suggest that *Rubella virus* may induce autoimmune T1D by molecular mimicry. When a panel of monoclonal antibodies that recognize rubella virus capsid and envelope glycoproteins were tested for reactivity with islet cell antigens, one monoclonal antibody that recognized a domain within the *Rubella virus* capsid protein was found to react with extracts from rat and human islets, as well as with extracts from a rat insulinoma line (Karounos *et al.*, 1993). Further testing showed that the shared epitope was on a 52-kD protein. In addition, it was reported that T cells of diabetic patients recognize cross-reactive protein determinants from *Rubella virus* and glutamic acid decarboxylase (GAD) 65 and 67 (Ou *et al.*, 2000), which is considered to be an important β-cell autoantigen in the pathogenesis of T1D. This suggests that *Rubella virus* exposure may lead to the generation of viral antigen-specific cytotoxic T cells that also recognize beta cell-specific antigen(s) in susceptible individuals.

1.1.9   *Cytomegalovirus* and Diabetes

Cytomegalovirus (*CMV*) belongs to the *Herpesviridae* family and is a double-stranded DNA enveloped virus. Like *Rubella virus*, human *CMV* can be congenital, although the disease may not appear until later in life. *CMV* infections can also be transmitted perinatally or postnatally through close contact or breast milk, as the immaturity of infant immune systems favors the establishment of persistent viral infections.

   CMV has been implicated in T1D by a number of clinical studies. Case reports describe a child with congenital *CMV* infection (Ward *et al.*, 1979) and a woman with *CMV* infection (Yasumoto *et al.*, 1992) who both developed T1D, the latter after extensive pancreatitis. In a study of children with fatal viral infections, viral cytopathology of the pancreas and characteristic inclusion bodies in the beta cells were found in 20/45 cases of *CMV* infection (Jensen *et al.*, 1980), indicating that *CMV* can infect pancreatic beta cells. In another study following 73 infants with congenital *CMV* infection, one developed T1D, compared to 38/19,483 non infected control subjects, which the investigators believed indicated no statistical correlation between *CMV* infection and the development of T1D (Ivarsson *et al.*, 1993). Correlations between *CMV* infection and T1D also have been found by studies using molecular biological methods. A research using both dot and *in situ* hybridization techniques showed that 20% of T1D patients had cytomegalovirus genomic DNA in their lymphocytes, compared to only 2% of normal controls. Furthermore, 80% of patients who had both anti-*CMV* antibodies and the *CMV* genome also had islet cell autoantibodies (Pak *et al.*, 1988). Nicoletti *et al.* (1990) found that non diabetic siblings of T1D patients had a significant association between high titers of anti-*CMV* antibodies and islet cell auto-antibodies, but no correlation between anti-*CMV* antibodies with HLA-DR antigens. These findings suggest that chronic *CMV* infection may be associated with islet cell autoantibody production, but that other factors may be needed for the development of clinical T1D. It is possible that molecular mimicry may be involved in some cases of *CMV*-induced diabetes. In this situation, immune responses against similar epitopes shared by antigenic determinants of *CMV* and islet cell-specific proteins may lead to islet cell-specific autoimmunity. Evidence for this is the finding that human *CMV* can induce an islet cell antibody that reacts with a 38-kD auto-antigen expressed in human pancreatic islets (Pak *et al.*, 1990). Also, a work showed that a CD4$^+$ T-cell clone reactive to GAD65 isolated from a prediabetic Stiffman syndrome patient cross-reacted with a peptide of human *CMV* major DNA binding protein, suggesting that human *CMV* may be involved in the induction of autoimmunity by molecular mimicry of the beta cell autoantigen, GAD65 (Hiemstra *et al.*, 2001). Further studies are needed to determine whether *CMV* is actually involved in the development of T1D in man and/or animals because the evidence of the association of *CMV* with T1D remains circumstantial.

1.1.10   *Epstein-Barr Virus* and Diabetes

Epstein-Barr virus (*EBV*) is a double-stranded DNA enveloped virus that belongs to the *Herpesviridae* family. *EBV* has been implicated in the etiology of autoimmune diseases (Hyöty *et al.*, 1991; Parkkonen *et al.*, 1994). A temporal link between *EBV* infection and the onset of T1D has been reported in a rare number of cases, including one in which the child also had concurrent *Adenovirus* and *Coxsackie B* viral infections (Surcel *et al.*, 1988).

   There is some evidence that *EBV* may be potentially capable of triggering autoimmune T1D by molecular mimicry. An 11 amino acid sequence of the *EBV* protein, BOLF1, was found to be homologous to residues in the Asp-57 region of the HLA-DQw8 beta chain peptide, although sera from the diabetic patients tested by Sairenji *et al.* (1991) did not bind to DQw8 beta. It was also found that a pentapeptide sequence in the Asp-57 region of the HLA-DQβ chain is successively repeated six times in the EBV-BERF4-encoded epitope (Horn *et al.*, 1988). Two patients who produced antibodies against this epitope during acute *EBV* infection soon developed T1D, while five individuals also acutely infected but not producing antibodies against this epitope did not develop T1D (Parkkonen *et al.*, 1994).

1.1.11 *Encephalomyocarditis Virus* and Diabetes

There is unequivocal evidence that diabetogenic variants of *Encephalomyocarditis virus* (*EMCV*), a member of *Picornaviridae* family, can induce diabetes in animals (Yoon J *et al.*, 1980), although there is little evidence that this occurs in humans. Infection of genetically susceptible mice with the M variant of *EMCV* virus resulted in the selective destruction of pancreatic beta cells (Stefan *et al.*, 1978). Further searches found that beta cell destruction in *EMCV*-infected mice is dependent on the genetic makeup of the virus and the genetic background of the host (Kang *et al.*, 1993; Jun & Yoon, 2001). Two different animal models for *EMCV*-induced diabetes are supposed. The first model involves animals infected with a high dose (10^5 PFU/mouse) of *EMCV*-induced diabetes, in which replication of *EMCV* within the beta cells plays a major role, whereas recruitment of macrophages plays a minor role in beta cell destruction. In contrast, the second model involves animals infected with a low dose ($<10^2$ PFU/mouse) of *EMCV*-induced diabetes, in which activated macrophages that are recruited to the beta cells play a major role, whereas replication of the virus within the beta cells plays a minor role in beta cell destruction. The development of diabetes in these infected mice is mainly due to the replication of the *EMCV* within the beta cells, rather than to the involvement of humoral and/or cell-mediated immune responses. Although T cells do not appear to be involved, it is possible that macrophages might contribute to the destruction of pancreatic beta cells in mice infected with a high dose of *EMCV*. Macrophages predominate in the pancreatic islets during the early stages of *EMC* viral infection (Baek & Yoon, 1990), and it is possible that activated macrophages might migrate to *EMCV*-infected beta cells as scavengers and secrete cytotoxic cytokines such as IL-1, TNF-α and IFN-γ and nitric oxide. In this way, the active replication of *EMCV*-induced diabetes within the beta cells and the production of cytokines and oxygen free radicals from activated macrophages could act synergistically to destroy beta cells, leading to the development of diabetes.

As natural viral infections in animals and man generally involve exposure to relatively low numbers of virus, and exposure to the high viral titers would be unlikely in nature, another animal model was established to study the immune mechanisms involved in the destruction of beta cells, in which mice were infected with a low dose (100 PFU/mouse) of *EMCV*-induced diabetes. In mice infected with a low dose of *EMCV*-induced diabetes, macrophages play a central role in the destruction of pancreatic beta cells, as activation of macrophages prior to viral infection results in a statistically significant increase in the incidence of diabetes, and inactivation of macrophages prior to viral infection almost completely prevents *EMCV*-induced diabetes (Baek & Yoon, 1991). Additional studies showed that the selective *EMCV*-induced diabetes viral infection of pancreatic beta cells results in an initial recruitment of macrophages into the islets, followed by infiltration by other immunocytes including T cells, NK cells and B cells (Baek & Yoon, 1990). Further study revealed that *EMCV*-induced diabetes infects macrophages and activates them, but does not replicate within the macrophages (Hirasawa *et al.*, 1999). The expression of IL-1β, TNF-α and inducible nitric oxide synthase (iNOS) was selectively detected in the pancreatic islets of mice infected with a low dose of *EMCV*-induced diabetes. In addition, treatment of *EMCV* infected mice with antibody against IL-1β or TNF-α or with the iNOS inhibitor, aminoguanidine, exhibited a significant decrease in the incidence of diabetes (Hirasawa *et al.*, 1997). These results suggest that macrophage-derived soluble mediators play a critical role in the destruction of pancreatic beta cells resulting in the development of diabetes in mice infected with a low dose of *EMCV*-induced diabetes. Further investigations regarding the mechanisms that activate macrophages found that tyrosine kinase signaling pathways are involved in the *EMCV*-induced activation of macrophages. It was recently found that an Src family kinase, hematopoetic cell kinase (*hck*), showed a dramatic increase in autophosphorylation and phosphorylation of Sam 68 (a substrate for Src kinase) in EMC-D virus-infected mice. The protein level of *hck* had a peak at 48h after the infection of *EMCV*, suggesting that *hck* is involved in the activation of macrophages in mice infected with EMC-D virus. Treatment of EMC-D virus-infected mice with an *Src* kinase inhibitor, PP2, resulted in the inhibition of *hck* activity, a decrease in the production of TNF-α and iNOS in the macrophages and the subsequent prevention of diabetes (Choi *et al.*, 2001).

1.1.12 *Mengovirus* and Diabetes

Mengovirus is a member of the *Cardiovirus* genus of *Picornaviridae* family, like *EMCV*, and produces fatal encephalitis in mice. While *Mengovirus* is antigenically similar to *EMCV*, it is more neuropathic and lethal and has different tissue tropisms (Morishima *et al.*, 1982). Plaque purification of *Mengovirus* resulted in the isolation of a clone, *Mengovirus*-2T, which caused diabetes in strains of mice resistant to *EMCV*-induced diabetes infection. Pancreas from *Mengovirus* 2T-infected mice revealed marked beta cell necrosis, severe inflammatory infiltration of the islets, and decreased insulin content, without evidence of autoimmune responses (Yoon *et al.*, 1984). It appears that *Mengovirus*-2T acts by directly infecting beta cells, and it may bind to a different beta cell receptor than *EMCV*, thus accounting for the difference in strain susceptibility between the two viruses.

1.1.13 *Coxsackie Virus* and Diabetes

There is considerable information that T1D may be associated with *Enterovirus* infection, including infection with *Coxsackie viruses* and *Echoviruses*.

There have been many epidemiological studies linking recent-onset T1D with *Coxsackie A* and *B* viral infections in humans (Fohlman & Friman, 1993; Yoon *et al.*, 1996). Several studies have reported that patients with recent-onset T1D had significantly higher titers of antibody to *Coxsackie virus*, especially the B4 serotype, than did non diabetic controls (Friman *et al.*, 1985; Frisk *et al.*, 1992). In addition, it was reported that T-cell responses to *Coxsackie* B4 nonstructural protein of the virus increased in new-onset T1D patients (Juhela *et al.*, 2000). While these studies support *Coxsackie B* viral involvement in the development of human T1D, results from epidemiological studies have been inconsistent. Some works have found no evidence of a correlation between the onset of T1D and *Coxsackie B* viral infections (Pato *et al.*, 1992; Marttila *et al.*, 2001), while other studies have found higher levels of anti-*Coxsackie B* virus-specific antibodies in non diabetic control subjects than in recent-onset T1D patients (Tuvemo *et al.*, 1989). The interpretation is complicated by the fact that there are many variants of *Coxsackie B4* virus (Prabhakar *et al.*, 1982), and only a minority is likely to cause diabetes: four *Coxsackie B4* variants were tested and only one proved to cause diabetes in mice, while the remaining three variants did not (Yoon *et al.*, 1986). Moreover, the lack of correlation may depend on the genetic makeup of the virus and differences in immune responses among individuals. Many anecdotal reports described the development of T1D in patients with recent or concurrent *Coxsackie B* viral infections (Nigro *et al.*, 1986; Andreoletti *et al.*, 1997). There are several direct supporting evidences on the association of Coxsackie B viral infection with the onset of T1D (Dotta *et al.*, 2007). *In vitro* studies have shown that *Coxsackie B3 virus* and *Coxsackie B4 virus* can infect and impair human islet beta cells metabolism (Szopa *et al.*, 1986). These works have shown that the insulin content of infected beta cells decreased rapidly, beginning at 24h after infection, and that the decrease in insulin roughly paralleled the increase in viral titer.

Not all variants of *Coxsackie B4 virus* cause overt diabetes in susceptible animals explaining why T1D appears to be associated with *Coxsackie B* viral infection in infrequent isolated cases. In early studies, mice inoculated with *Coxsackie B4 virus* did not develop diabetes; however repeated passaging of *Coxsackie B4* in murine-enriched pancreatic beta cell cultures resulted in the virus acquiring more diabetogenic capacity (Yoon *et al.*, 1978). Mice infected with this virus showed lymphocytic infiltration of the islets and beta cell destruction, which lead to hypoinsulinemia and hyperglycemia. An inverse correlation was observed between the reduction in immunoreactive insulin and the elevation in blood glucose levels (Yoon *et al.*, 1978; Toniolo *et al.*, 1982). In the majority of animals, hyperglycemia is transient. It is possible that sufficient beta cells remain intact after some *Coxsackie B4* viral infections so that proliferation and/or hypertrophy of these cells results in metabolic compensation. During the acute phase of *Coxsackie B4* viral infection, viral antigens have been found in the islets of Langerhans. Genetic susceptibility of the host plays an important role in *Coxsackie B*-induced diabetes in animals, as is the case with *EMCV*. Genetic studies showed that the 'db' diabetic mutation on chromosome 4 exerted the most effect on susceptibility and host response to *Coxsackie B4 virus* and was associated with an impaired humoral response to *Coxsackie B4* viral infection as infected mice did not develop an adequate level of anti-*Coxsackie B4* IgM and IgG antibodies. The animals were also found to be deficient in absolute and relative numbers of splenic lymphocyte subsets. It has also been reported that *Coxsackie B4* viral infection alters thymic, splenic, and peripheral lymphocyte repertoire before the onset of hyperglycemia in mice (Chatterjee *et al.*, 1992).

Coxsackie B viruses may induce diabetes through several mechanisms. Coxsackie B viruses affect glucose homeostasis. The virus has cytolytic activity, and in animals, may directly destroy enough of the beta cell mass to cause T1D (Toniolo *et al.*, 1982). Autoimmune mechanisms may also be involved, perhaps because the immune response rose against the virus cross-reacts with specific beta cell antigens. P2-C, a non-capsid protein of *Coxsackie B4*, has sequence homology with GAD, which is expressed by beta cells and is a putative autoantigen (Kaufman *et al.*, 1992). Moreover, infection with the virus increases expression of GAD by beta cells (Hou *et al.*, 1993). Antibodies have been detected in T1D patients that react with both P2-C and GAD (Hou *et al.*, 1994), suggesting that this 'molecular mimicry' could underlie the autoimmune damage to the beta cells. However, this hypothesis is not supported by studies that characterized antibodies produced by lymphocytes isolated from a newly diagnosed T1D patient. Four of six antibodies studied recognized and bound to the region of GAD65 that is homologous to P2-C, but none cross-reacted with P2-C itself or with any other *Coxsackie* B4 viral proteins. The lack of cross-reactivity between these two proteins may be due to differences in secondary or tertiary structure (Richter *et al.*, 1994). On the other hand, the capacity of murine T lymphocytes to cross-react with P2-C and GAD is associated with a diabetes susceptibility allele; cross-reactive T-cell recognition of GAD65 may therefore contribute to the initiation or amplification of autoimmune responses against the beta cell, and perhaps to the association of T1D with certain HLA alleles (Tian *et al.*, 1994). *Coxsackie B virus* may also induce diabetes by bystander activation of autoreactive T cells against islet antigens. Mice with susceptible MHC alleles had no viral acceleration of diabetes, but mice with a T-cell receptor transgene specific for a different islet autoantigen rapidly developed diabetes. This suggests that Coxsackie B virus-induced diabetes by a direct local infection leading to inflammation, tissue damage and the release of sequestered islet antigens resulting in the restimulation of resting autoreactive T cells (Horwitz *et al.*, 1998). A further possibility is that a defective *Coxsackie B virus*, lacking the usual high lytic activity, could cause persistent infection of beta cells, resulting in autoimmune beta cell destruction (Foulis *et al.*,   1990). In addition, it was reported that the level of IFN-α was elevated in the plasma of T1D patients, and this was associated with *Coxsackie B virus* infection (Chehadeh *et al.*, 2000). The persistent infection of beta cells with *Coxsackie B viruses* may result in expression of IFN-α, which in turn could induce HLA class I antigen hyperexpression and expression of chemokines that recruit and activate macrophages and T cells. These activated immunocytes could kill beta cells, resulting in T1D. Finally, *Coxsackie* viral infections may be involved in the pathogenesis of T1D by acting as the terminal insult in individuals who have already lost substantial beta cell mass through ongoing autoimmune damage. Destruction of a critical number of residual cells would result in the clinical onset of T1D.

1.1.14   *Hepatitis C virus* and Diabetes

While patients with liver disease are known to have a higher prevalence of glucose intolerance, studies suggest that infection with *Hepatitis C virus* (*HCV*), a member of *Flaviviridae* family, may be an additional risk factor for the development of diabetes mellitus (Mason *et al.*, 1999).

Humans with various forms of liver disease can be predisposed to impaired glucose tolerance because of corticosteroid and hydrochlorthiazide therapy or hemochromatosis (Muting *et al.*, 1969; Petrides, 1994; Niedereau *et al.*, 1985). In addition, glucose intolerance is observed more often in patients with *HCV* infection compared with controls with liver disease (Allison *et al.*, 1994; Ozyilkan & Arslan, 1996), and the frequency of *HCV* infection in European populations with type II diabetes has been reported to be higher than expected compared with the general population (Ozylikan *et al.*, 1994; Gray *et al.*, 1995; Simo *et al.*, 1996). *HCV* infection cannot be considered to be a cause of diabetes without establishing a temporal relationship for the development of disorder.

1.2   Bacterial Infections

The bacterial composition of the intestine has long been acknowledged as an important variable affecting T1D development. Direct evidence exists in rodents, for example, feeding probiotic bacterial strains, usually lactic acid bacteria, to non-obese diabetic (NOD) mice or bio breeding diabetes-prone (BB-DP) rats can delay or prevent diabetes (Matsuzaky *et al.*, 1997; Calcinaro *et al.*, 2005; Yadav *et al.*, 2007). Feeding antibiotics to NOD mice or BB-DP rats can also increase survival in these models (Brugman *et al.*, 2006; Schwartz *et al.*, 2007). In addition, pathogen-free NOD mice lacking an adaptor protein for multiple toll-like receptors known to bind to bacterial ligands fail to develop diabetes (Wen *et al.*, 2008). Perhaps autoimmunity ensues whenever the intricate microbial balance in the intestine is disturbed. Additionally, the intestinal wall does not seem to have the same capacity to form a coherent barrier separating luminal bacteria and the immune system in T1D models and patients versus controls. This so-called-leaky gut phenotype is thought to enhance the exposure of bacterial antigens to the immune system. In the intestine of T1D patients, subclinical immune activation (Westerholm *et al.*, 2003) and evidence for an impaired regulatory T cells (T *reg*) subset (Tiittanen *et al.*, 2008) were found. T *reg* are a specialized subpopulation of T cells which suppresses activation of the immune system and thereby maintains tolerance to self antigen. Thus, both antibiotics and probiotics may influence T1D development by altering the balance of gut microbiota toward either a tolerogenic or nontolerogenic state, depending on constitution of the intestinal microflora at the time of administration (Vaarala *et al.*, 2008).

Chronic bacterial infections could be contributing to the socioeconomic gradient in chronic diseases. Although chronic infections have been associated with increased levels of inflammatory cytokines and cardiovascular disease, there is limited evidence on how infections affect risk of diabetes. Studies suggest that *Chlamydia pneumoniae*, and *Helicobacter pylori*, may have an impact on cardiovascular conditions and metabolic syndrome (Georges *et al.*, 2003; Nabipour *et al.*, 2006) potentially mediated by elevations in inflammatory markers such as C-reactive protein (CRP) and interleukin (IL)-6 (Georges *et al.*, 2003). Inflammation and activated innate immunity have also been implicated in the pathogenesis of diabetes through insulin resistance. Elevated levels of inflammatory cytokines may lead to phosphorylation of serine residues on the insulin receptor substrate, which prevents its interaction with insulin receptors, inhibiting insulin action (Wellen & Hotamisligil, 2005).

1.2.1   *Helicobacter Pylori* and Diabetes

There are little, equivocal available contradictory data on *Helicobacter pylori* prevalence and its relationship to Type 2 diabetes mellitus (T2D) in the literature (Gasbarrini *et al.*, 1998; Oldensbury *et al.*, 1996; Ko *et al.*, 2001; Gulcelik *et al.*, 2005).

Many authors reported high prevalence of *H. pylori* infection among patients with T2D, suggesting that delayed gastric clearance could be attributed to bacterial colonization or overgrowth in the gastrointestinal tract as a result of autonomic neuropathy (Albaker, 2011). Some works, based on serologic antibody detection, have found a high prevalence of *H. pylori* infection among diabetics as compared to the general population (Gasbarrini *et al.*, 1998; Gulcelik *et al.*, 2005). On the other hand, another study with histopathological demonstration of microorganism, described a minor role of *H. pylori* infection among upper gastrointestinal pathologies (Malecki *et al.*, 1996), while other reports did not detect a relationship between *H. pylori* infection and diabetes mellitus (Woodward *et al.*, 2000; Hia *et al.*, 2001; Ko *et al.*, 2001; Demir *et al.*, 2008; Lutsey *et al.*, 2009). Jeon and colleagues (2012) found a positive association between *H. pylori* infection and the prevalence of T2D in cross-sectional studies, in accord with the results from previous studies carried out by Gasbarrini *et al.* (1998) and So *et al.* (2009). They were able to establish the relative timing of seropositivity and development of diabetes, giving more credence to a potential causal relationship. The mechanism by which *H. pylori* infection increases the risk of diabetes remains to be elucidated but may involve inflammation or dyspepsia. Infection with *H. pylori* was found in previous studies to be correlated with elevated levels of CRP (Diomedi *et al.*, 2008), IL-6, and TNF-α (Hamed *et al.*, 2008), which are markers of inflammation implicated in insulin resistance and development of diabetes. Furthermore, the presence of Gram-negative bacteria, such as *H. pylori*, in the gut microbiota leads to increased production of lipopolysaccharide, which also activates innate inflammatory processes (Manco *et al.*, 2010). An alternative hypothesis is that gastroduodenal conditions resulting from *H. pylori* infection could delay gastric emptying (Ojetti *et al.*, 2010), which has been postulated to cause poor glucose control in insulin-dependent children with diabetes. The biological impact of *H. pylori*-associated disorders on glucose metabolism and insulin sensitivity should be further investigated.

1.2.1   Does tuberculosis Lead to Diabetes?

There is growing evidence that diabetes mellitus is an important risk factor for tuberculosis and might affect disease presentation and treatment response (Dooley & Chaisson, 2009).

If diabetes can predispose a patient to tuberculosis, can infection with tuberculosis lead to diabetes mellitus? The answer is: "it is possible". Tuberculosis might induce glucose intolerance and worsen glycogenic control in people with diabetes. Some studies suggest that tuberculosis can even cause diabetes in those not previously known to be diabetic. Many studies have used oral glucose tolerance testing to show that patients with tuberculosis have higher rates of glucose intolerance than community controls. (Nichols, 1957; Zack *et al.*, 1973; Abbras, 1991). Whereas the high incidence of abnormal oral glucose tolerance found in tuberculosis patients is of concern, it is unclear whether glucose intolerance or diabetes mellitus was truly incident, or whether prevalent diabetes mellitus was being newly diagnosed in patients receiving expanded medical services related to tuberculosis treatment. Also, the implications of these findings depend on whether diabetes mellitus persists in these patients, and whether its presence is substantially more common with tuberculosis than with other infectious diseases.

In a study carried out in Nigeria, tuberculosis patients with impaired glucose tolerance had normal tests after 3 months of tuberculosis treatment (Oluboyo & Erasmus, 1990). In Turkey, oral glucose tolerance tests were given to 58 patients with active tuberculosis and 23 patients with community-acquired pneumonia (Basoglu *et al.*, 1999). Of those with tuberculosis, 10% were glucose intolerant and 9% had diabetes; of patients with community-acquired pneumonia, none had glucose intolerance and 17% were diabetic. All patients had normal tests 3 months and 2 years after the start of treatment. The latter two studies suggest that infection causes reversible glucose intolerance and that this effect is not specific to tuberculosis. In Indonesia, 13% (60 of 454) of patients with tuberculosis had diabetes, compared with 31% (18 of 556) of age-matched and sex-matched controls from the same residential unit; for 60% of these patients, diabetes was a new diagnosis. Whereas impairment of glucose metabolism probably preceded tuberculosis in these patients rather than the reverse, these data underscore the importance of screening tuberculosis patients for diabetes.

Another recently discovered bacterial risk factor maybe *Mycobacterium avium* subspecies *paratuberculosis* (*MAP*).

2   *Mycobacterium Avium* Subsp. *Paratuberculosis*: Zoonotic Potential

Recently, *Mycobacterium avium* subsp. *paratuberculosis* (*MAP*) has been postulated as the infectious agent that triggers human Type 1 (insulin-dependent) diabetes mellitus (T1D) (Dow, 2006; Sechi *et al.*, 2008; Rani *et al.*, 2010). Moreover, an association between *MAP* infection and Crohn's Disease (CD) human patients has been suggested.

Who is it *MAP*? *MAP* is the member of the *Mycobacterium avium* complex and it is the causative pathogen of the chronic, granulomatous degenerative enteritis known as Paratuberculosis or Johne's disease (JD) that mainly affects domestic and wild ruminants (Chiodini *et al.*, 1984; Buergelt *et al.*, 2000). This bacterial pathogen is also incriminated in the infection of many monogastric animals, including humans (Beard *et al.*, 2001; Hermon-Taylor *et al.*, 2000; Ghadiali *et al.*, 2004). The degree of occurrence of JD is increasing worldwide (Manning & Collins, 2001) with a significant economic impact on the livestock industry (Harris & Barletta, 2001). The disease represents a sanitary and zootechnical problem of remarkable proportions because of its incidence, the lack of a valid therapeutic and preventive strategies to curtail its spread, and the economic losses it incur due to complications from the clinical and subclinical disease (Cocito *et al.*, 1994; Ott *et al.*, 1999; Pavlik *et al.*, 2009). The infection of animals in early life occurs mostly via the faecal-oral route (Sweeney, 1996). Nevertheless, the intrauterine route of transmission has been observed in sheep and in the fetuses of cows with advanced forms of JD (Sweeney, 1996; Lambeth *et al.*, 2004). Granulomatous lesions in the intestine and the involvement of the neighbouring lymph nodes are some hallmark characteristics of *MAP* infection, and the composition of cell types within the lesions is correlated with stage of infection (Momotani *et al.*, 1988; Chiodini, 1996). As the disease progresses, the tuberculoid or TH1 response handover to a lepromatous or TH2 response which is characterised by the production of IL-4, IL-5, IL-6 and IL-10 cytokines and an influx of inflammatory cells to the infection site. The intestinal wall becomes thickened as a result of the intestine inflammation leading to poor nutrient absorption in the affected animals (Williams *et al.*, 1979; Shulaw *et al.*, 1993). The TH2 response is responsible for the activation and sustainability of the humoral immune response characterized by antibody production. Clinical symptoms, such as diarrhea and severe emaciation or wasting, are often observed at this stage of the disease.

The manifestation of the clinical disease which is typically characterized by loss of weight, diarrhea and decreased milk production in dairy herds (Chiodini *et al.*, 1984), and the high shedding of the bacteria in feces and milk is commonly noticeable as from 2 years of age and above, both in clinically and subclinically affected animals (Streeter *et al.*, 1995; Olsen *et al.*, 2002). The affected animals are emaciated and produce less milk despite having a ravenous appetite and are often a-febrile. And as the disease become chronic, death results following severe wasting and diarrhea.

Some studies (Sherman *et al.*, 1990; Singh *et al.*, 2007) have observed that high mortality rates and reduced reproductive performance of infected females are common occurrence in infected dairy herds than in the beef or mixed herds. The fastidious growth pattern of *MAP* and the absurd response of the host animal immune system to infection have reckoned the diagnosis of JD to be an uphill task. Diagnosis of subclinical infection with *MAP* in ruminant species remains one of the greatest challenges to JD control, both at the individual-animal (Collins, 1996; Manning & Collins, 2001) and herd-level (Jordan, 1996). High shedders of *MAP* and animal with clinical signs of JD are responsible for the greater part of the contamination of their environment, the economic damage in infected herds and the presence of bacteria in milk (Grant, 2003). To monitor the progression of a control programme the herds need to be tested. Serology is the most practical method used for this purpose. The enzyme-linked immunosorbent assay (ELISA) is a suitable diagnostic tool to detect serum antibodies against *MAP* on a large scale, because it is possible to test large numbers of samples with a high reproducibility (Collins, 1996; Van Maanen *et al.*, 2003; Attili *et al.*, 2011). As at now, no effective treatment of this serious infectious bacterial disease is available, and the long-term effect of vaccination, though it reduces the incidence of clinical disease and bacterial shedding, is controversial and fails to eliminate or eradicate the disease in a herd (Rosseels and Huygen, 2008). Thus, the spread of the disease can only be stop through the implementation of rigorous control programmes whereby animals that tested positive for JD are kept separate from other animals or even culled.

Ruminant milk has been described as a potential source through which humans could be infected with *MAP* (Chiodini & Hermon-Taylor, 1993; Grant, 2003; Ayele *et al.*, 2005; Favila-Humara *et al.*, 2010). The milk could be contaminated with *MAP* by either direct shedding of the organisms or fecal contamination during or after milking (Grant *et al.*, 2002). Humans are exposed to *MAP* by direct contact with infected material and in retail milk supplies (Ellingson *et al.*, 2005). Viable *MAP* has been isolated from milk and colostrum of clinically and subclinically infected cows and ewes (Sweeney *et al.*, 1992) and direct and indirect infection of the mammary gland has been documented in small ruminants (Stehman, 1996; Ngu Ngwa *et al.*, 2010; Attili *et al.*, 2012). *MAP* has been demonstrated by PCR in goats' milk from bulk tanks in farms in the UK (Grant *et al.*, 2001) and has a thick, relatively impermeable complex cell wall that is rich in lipids. This confers acid-fast properties and enhances its survival in water and in the environment for long periods thus complicating the eradication of the disease (Whittington *et al.*, 2005). Also, the complex cell wall has been observed to increased *MAP* resistance to high temperatures when pasteurizing milk (Grant *et al.*, 2005), and this is another virulence factor which may be important in the transmission of *MAP* to humans. Although, some researchers have demonstrated that effective pasteurization should kill all *MAP* organisms (Stabel, 2001), viable *MAP* has been reported in retail pasteurized milk (Grant *et al.*, 2002; Ayele *et al.*, 2005). The bacterium can survive pasteurisation. Sub pasteurization temperature of milk for cheese production may not be sufficient for complete inactivation of *MAP* (Pearce *et al.*, 2001; Gao *et al.*, 2002; Stabel & Lambertz, 2004; McDonald *et al.*, 2005; Rademaker *et al.*, 2007) showed that *MAP* is not completely destroyed in milk artificially contaminated with a high inoculum even after a combination of high pressure (600 MPa) and pasteurization. Cheese production processes have been shown to have little effect on the viability of *MAP* (Chiodini & Hermon-Taylor, 1993; Sung & Collins, 2000). Furthermore, viable bacteria have been demonstrated in hard and semi-hard cheese 120 days after production (Spahr & Schafroth, 2001). In another dimension, meat products may also serve as a source of *MAP* transmission to humans (Grant, 2006). The meat products may be contaminated following the dissemination of *MAP* within the tissues of the infected animals. Of recent, *MAP* genome was found on beef carcasses after flaying and dressing (Meadus *et al.*, 2008).

2.1   *MAP* and Crohn's Disease

MAP has been associated with Crohn's disease (CD) in humans, a chronic inflammatory bowel disease of human gastrointestinal tract, which is characterized by general malaise, chronic weight loss, abdominal pain, and diarrhea (Bull *et al.*, 2003; Abubakar *et al.*, 2007; Feller *et al.*, 2007). Although the distal ileum is most commonly involved, CD may affect any part of the gastrointestinal tract. It is a life-long disease that has no known cure and sufferers may have a poor quality of life because of pain and, in extreme cases, uncontrolled discharge of intestinal content (Hermon-Taylor & Bull 2002). It is believed that CD has a complex and multifactorial etiology.

Crohn's disease could be due to: - a persistent infection, possibly involving mycobacteria (specifically *MAP*); - a defective mucosal barrier (leaky gut) which allows uptake of bacterial, dietary and other immunogenic macromolecules; - dysregulation of the host immune response with loss of tolerance, aggressive cellular activations and disorders of apoptosis; - genetic susceptibility factors; - a combination of some, or all, of the above (Shanahan *et al.*, 2002). Mutations in a gene on chromosome 16, known as NOD2/CARD15, are associated with Crohn's disease (Hugot *et al.*, 2001). Three major mutations of this gene are most commonly encountered in Crohn's patients – R702W, G908R and L1007 fsinsC (Lesage *et al.*, 2002). The proportion of cases of Crohn's disease that can be attributed to NOD2/CARD15 mutations has been estimated at 15%-30%, which would be consistent with roles for a number of other factors, both genetic and environmental, in the pathogenesis of Crohn's disease. Those data provides compelling evidence to support the hypothesis that Crohn's disease results from bacterial insult in genetically susceptible individuals. NOD2/CARD15 serves a role in bacterial recognition, activating the nuclear factor (NF) κB pathway. Cellular studies have documented that NOD2/CARD15 is a cytosolic protein activated by muramyl dipeptide, a degradation product of bacterial peptidoglycan (Sechi *et al.*, 2005). Since the initial isolations (Chiodini *et al.*, 1986), *MAP* has been successfully cultured from resected tissue of Crohn's patients in various parts of the world: USA, UK, The Netherlands, Australia, France, Italy and the Czech Republic (Chamberlin *et al.*, 2001; Hermon-Taylor & Bull, 2002; Bull *et al.*, 2003; Naser *et al.*, 2004; Sechi *et al.* 2005, Feller *et al.*, 2007; Singh *et al.*, 2008); and also from breast milk of Crohn's Disease suffering mothers. This can expose infants to *MAP* very early in life, a significant concern if they are genetically susceptible to developing Crohn's Disease (Naser *et al.*, 2000). *MAP* has as well been cultured from the blood of CD patients (Naser *et al.*, 2004). It is also concerning that *MAP* has been found in milk and meat taken from infected cattle (Mutharia *et al.*, 2010).

However, the zoonotic potential of the organism remains controversial (Chiodini & Rossiter, 1996; Sechi *et al.*, 2005), and the etiology of CD still a mystery despite the significant medical debate that has taken place over the past years. In a short note, the clinical and histopathological similarities between human chronic granulomatous enteritis, intestinal tuberculosis, and JD obtained from literatures have led to the unsubstantiated belief that *MAP* has an important role in the etiology of CD. Furthermore, there is a broad unanimity that CD results from a sustained immune response that arise from an environmental stimulus in a susceptible host (Shanahan, 2002), and *MAP* has been postulated to be a potential stimulus at least in a subset of patients (Hermon-Taylor & El-Zaatari, 2004).

2.2 *MAP* and Diabetes

Evidence supporting a link between *MAP* and T1D includes: higher detection rates of *MAP* by IS 900 specific PCR in samples from T1D patients compared with controls; demonstration of a serological response to *MAP* antigens and whole cell lysates in T1D patients (Rosu *et al.*, 2008). Moreover the founding of a relevant SLC11A1 (ex NRAMP1) gene polymorphisms in T1D patients (Paccagnini *et al.*, 2009) previously reported in Crohn's patients (Sechi *et al.*, 2006), suggests indeed that there is a strong possibility for *MAP* to be involved with autoimmune responses in T1D just in the same manner as it did in Crohn's. NRAMP1 (Natural Resistance-Associated Macrophage Protein) is an iron transporter associated with macrophage activation. This gene has multiple pleiotropic effects on macrophage function, including regulation of cytokine production, TNF-α, Il-1 b, iNOS and regulation of MHC-II expression and antigen presentation functions (Blackwell *et al.*, 1999; Dai *et al.*, 2009). All of these activities are not only essential for protection against mycobacterial infection (innate defenses), but also critically involved in the induction and progression of autoimmune diseases. Since *MAP* persists within macrophages and it is processed by dendritic cells (DC), mutant forms of SLC11A1 may alter the processing or presentation of *MAP* antigens leading to diabetogenic responses (Dai *et al.*, 2009).

Although evidence for a cause-effect relationship is lacking, *MAP* transmission to humans has long been associated with Crohn's disease both in Italian people from Sardinia region (Sechi *et al.*, 2005; Di Sabatino *et al.*, 2011) and elsewhere (Naser *et al.*, 2004). The hypothesis stating that *MAP* infection may be a potential candidate environmental trigger also for T1D is based on these key findings: - *MAP* infection is highly prevalent in Sardinian T1D patients; - *MAP* DNA can be evidenced from blood in 63% of Sardinian T1D patients, but only in 16% of healthy controls (Sechi *et al.*, 2008); - *MAP* envelope protein MptD can be detected in the blood of 47.3% Sardinian T1D patients, but in a smaller proportion of T2D patients (7.7%) and healthy controls (12.6%) (Rosu *et al.*, 2009); - *MAP* can be cultured from blood (Rosu *et al.*, 2009); - *MAP* infections triggers a specific humoral response, as Sardinian T1D patients display high frequencies of antibodies (Abs) reacting against mycobacterial proteins (heparin-binding hemagglutinin, glycosyl transferase, whole *MAP* lysates (70% Ab+ T1D patients *vs* 7.6% Ab+ healthy controls) and the *MAP*-specific proteins MptD like MAP3738c when compared to T2D and healthy controls (Sechi *et al.*, 2008).

The linkage between *MAP* and T1D comes from the concept of molecular mimicry: cross-reactive immune responses because of significant structural homologies shared by molecules encoded by dissimilar genes. Either linear amino acid sequences of the molecules or their conformational epitopes may be shared, even though their origins are separate. The disease pathogenesis may involve multiple factors including genetics of the host, *MAP* strain, activation status of the autoreactive T cells, upregulation of pancreatic MHC class I antigens, molecular mimicry between *MAP* and β cell epitopes and T-cell mediated β-cells destruction by cytotoxic mechanism (Davies, 1997). *MAP*, as one of the environmental factors affecting the induction of T1D, may act as triggering agents of autoimmunity or (less probably) as primary injurious agents, which directly damage pancreatic β cells. Immune responses against a determinant shared by host cells (β- cells) and *MAP* could cause a tissue-specific immune response by generation of cytotoxic cross-reactive effector lymphocytes or Abs that recognize self-proteins located on the target cells (van Halteren et al., 2002; Dow, 2006). Notably, it has already been reported as a case of cross-recognition between the mycobacterial heat shock protein 65 (hsp65) and the self auto-antigen, glutamic acid decarboxylase (GAD65), involved in T1D patients (Scheinin *et al.*, 1996). Here it was demonstrated that Abs against *MAP* 3865c are capable of cross-reacting with host determinants.

It was shown that Sardinian T1D patients specifically mount anti-*MAP*3865c Abs responses. Two Abs epitopes were identified in the *MAP*3865c sequence and shown to be homologous to the β-cell anti-gen zinc transporter 8 (ZnT8) (Chimienti *et al.*, 2004) targeted by auto-Abs in T1D patients (Wenzlau *et al.*, 2007). Anti-*MAP* Abs recognizing these regions was found to be cross-reactive with the homologous ZnT8 sequences, raising the possibility of a molecular mimicry between mycobacterial and β-cell epitopes. It was successfully demonstrated the presence of *MAP*'s DNA in T1D Sardinian cases, this goal was achieved through PCR based detection of IS900 insertion element, a specific signature locus of *MAP* (Sechi *et al.*, 2008). After identifying *MAP* in the blood of T1D and aiming to understand the host im-mune responses to *MAP*, it was designed an immunoassays (indirect ELISA) for the detection of anti-*MAP* Abs in diabetic patients. ELISA tests, employing sensitive antigenic targets such as HbHa (heparin binding hemagglutinin) and Gsd (glycosyl transferase) proteins, gave encouraging results (Sechi *et al.*, 2008). However, anti-*MAP* humoral responses corresponding to HbHa and Gsd could not be indicative of an active infection and also since these proteins are encoded by wider range of mycobacteria, this raised an issue of cross-reactivity with tubercle bacilli which could be an issue to deal with the BCG vaccinated individuals. This prompted Sechi *et al.* (2008) to set up immunoassays including a *MAP* specific protein, MptD into the battery of antigens. The detection of anti-*MAP* Abs revealed extremely significant humoral immune responses in T1D patients when compared to T2D and healthy controls (Rosu *et al.*, 2009, Cossu A. *et al.*, 2011).

Final evidence supporting a link between *MAP* and T1D was presented in terms of culture of *MAP* bacilli from the blood of two of the T1D patients from Sardinia (Rosu *et al.*, 2009). Summing up, differ-ent *MAP* proteins were shown to be highly recognized in T1D patients and even if some of them were specific of *MAP* (*MAP*3738c and MptD) none of them were homologous to human proteins. It was blast-ed the whole *MAP* genome against the human genome and it was identified a protein (*MAP*3865c) not only homologus to human proteins but also specific to β-cells (Znt8). Building up on the above reports documenting a high prevalence of *MAP* infection and seroreactivity in Sardinian T1D patients (Sechi *et al.*, 2008; Rosu *et al.*, 2008; Paccagnini *et al.*, 2009; Cossu *et al.*, 2011) it was demonstrated that the *MAP*3865c protein is a target of Ab responses that cross-react with homologous ZnT8 sequences. *MAP*3865c is a 298 aminoacid 6-membrane-spanning channel which endows *MAP* with the ability to transport cations through the membrane, an important feature associated with intracellular survival of mycobacteria (Riccardi *et al.*, 2008). ZnT8 is a 369 aminoacid protein which belongs to the cation diffu-sion facilitator family of highly homologous ZnT (Slc30) proteins. It displays a remarkably similar struc-ture and function, allowing Zn(2+) to accumulate in the insulin granules of pancreatic β-cells. Zn(2+) cat-ions are essential to form hexavalent insulin storage crystals and, eventually, for effective insulin secre-tion (Wijesekara *et al.*, 2010). The intestinal localization of *MAP* infection may also favor cross-reactivity with Abs and T cells recognizing ZnT8.

The primary route of *MAP* infection is fecal-oral and once ingested, the bacterium lodges in to the mucosa associated lymphoid tissue (MALT) of the small intestine. It is then endocytosed by the M cells of Peyer's patches, which are further phagocytized by intra epithelial macrophages. Indeed, the first encounter with beta-cell antigens takes place in pancreatic lymph nodes (Gagneraul *et al.*, 2002), which also drain intestinal tissues (Turley *et al.*, 2005). The intestinal localization of *MAP* infection may also give reason for the lack of correlation between *MAP* IS900 DNA and Ab detection. Not all *MAP*-infected individuals may mount systemic Ab responses detectable in blood, or they may develop Abs against other *MAP* antigens.

Recently, an important linkage was found between *MAP* and T1D patients who were free of tuberculosis and CD based on *MAP* specific DNA and antibody detection analyses (Sechi *et al.*, 2008). On the other hand, T2D has become an epidemic and is extending in the young adult population, adolescents and even, occasionally, in children (Sturnvoll *et al.*, 2005). A number of studies have associated T2D with mycobacteria (Child *et al.*, 1995; Liu *et al.*, 2006). However, the work carried out by Rosu *et al* (2008) unequivocally refute such speculations through a robust assay that used three different antigen preparations which were shown to have acceptable sensitivity and specificity in case of T1D. They demonstrated that T2D patients do not have significant levels of anti *MAP* antibodies in contrast to their T1D counterparts and thus put to rest the long driven speculation that *MAP* is an infectious trigger of T2D. *MAP* has been isolated from the blood of Sardinian patients affected by T1D but not in those with T2D (Rosu *et al.*, 2009).

2.3   Conclusions

Just because *MAP* is detected more often in the blood of T1D patients by culture, PCR or ELISA than in control subjects does not necessarily mean that *MAP* causes T1D. This is certainly evidence of an association (the occurrence at the same time and in the same patient of *MAP* T1D) but not necessarily of causation (the organism has directly initiated the disease in the patient). There are several possible explanations for the presence of *MAP* in the blood of T1D patients: it could be an innocent bystander that has merely colonized the host; it could be a secondary infection agent but not causing the disease; or it could be the primary infectious agent and the cause of T1D. Definitive evidence proving a causal relationship between *MAP* and T1D is not available at present, perhaps it may never be. However, there is evidence suggesting some kind of association between *MAP* and at least some cases of T1D, so much that the robustness of the link is undeniable.

The most likely candidates as vehicles of transmission of *MAP* from cattle to humans are milk (and potentially other dairy products), beef and water. It is supposed that the detection of *MAP* in ruminants' milk and by-products represents the potential public health risks associated with this pathogen. Thus, the establishment of policies that will aid in curtailing the spread/transmission of *MAP* and the effects of its persistence in individuals should be encouraged. *MAP* has been shown to pass into human breast milk (Naser *et al.*, 2000). However, the consumption of infected ruminant's milk early in life has been an acknowledged risk factor in the occurrence of this disease (Gerstein, 1994; Gimeno & de Souza, 1997). This was based on the observation that children at risk for T1D who were breast fed exclusively for more than six months were less likely to have T1D later in life than similar risk children who were weaned onto cow's milk-based formula at an earlier age. Behind these studies is the postulate that there is something about ruminant's milk protein that is an immunologic trigger for T1D and that hydrolysis of the protein will eliminate the trigger phenomenon. Also, the triggering of autoimmune responses in genetically susceptible individuals is believed to be initiated by environmental microorganisms (Knip *et al.*, 2005; Dow, 2006). Furthermore, other potential routes of exposures to this organism such as water, meat, and the environment should be thoroughly investigated and associated risks and preventive measures evaluated and communicated with the public.

To conclude, T1D has only recently been included to the controversy regarding *MAP* and human disease that has been lingering for close to a century. In regards to the human toll to individuals with T1D, a quick sense of urgency to the *MAP*/T1D connection should be given an utmost importance.

References

Abbras, C. K. (1991). Fc receptor-mediated phagocytosis: abnormalities associated with diabetes mellitus. Clinical Immunology and Immunopathology, 58, 1-17.

Abubakar, I., Myhill, D. J., Hart, A. R., Lake, I., Harvey, I., Rhodes, J. M., Robinson, R., Lobo, A. J., Probes, C. S., & Hunter, P. R. (2007). A case-control study of drinking water and dairy products in Crohn's disease further investigation of the possible role of Mycobacterium avium subsp. paratuberculosis. American Journal of Epidemiology, 165, 776-783.

Achenbach, P., Lampasona, V., Landherr, U., Koczwara, K., Krause, S., Grallert, H., Winkler, C., Pflüger, M., Illig, T., Bonifacio, E., & Ziegler, A. G. (2009). Autoantibodies to zinc transporter 8 and SLC30A8 genotype stratify type 1 diabetes risk. Diabetologia, 52, 1881-1888.

Adams, S. F. (1926). The seasonal variation in the onset of acute diabetes. Archives Internal Medicine, 37, 861-862.

Akerblom, H. K. & Knip, M. (1998). Putative environmental factors in type 1 diabetes. Diabetes Metabolism Reviews, 14(1), 31-67.

Albaker, W. I. (2011). Helicobacter pylori Infection and its Relationship to Metabolic Syndrome: Is it a Myth or Fact? Saudi Journal of Gastroenterology, 17(3), 165-169.

Allison, M. E. D., Wreghitt, T., Palmer, C. R., & Alexander, G. J. M. (1994). Evidence for a link between hepatitis C virus infection and diabetes mellitus in a cirrhotic population. Journal of Hepatology, 21, 1135-1139.

Andreoletti, L., Hober, D., Hunter-Vandenberghe, C., Belaich, S., Vantyghem, M. C., Lefebvre, J., & Wattre, P. (1997). Detection of coxsackie B virus RNA sequences in whole blood samples from adult patients at the onset of type I diabetes mellitus. Journal of Medical Virology, 52, 121-127.

Atkinson, M. A., Bowman, M. A., Campbell, L., Darrow. B. L., Kaufman. D. L., & Maclaren, N. K. (1994). Cellular immunity to a determinant common to glutamate decarboxylase and coxsackie virus in insulin-dependent diabetes. Journal of Clinical Investigations, 94,2125-2129.

Attili, A. R., Ngu Ngwa, V., Pacifici, L., Preziuso, S., Domesi, A., & Cuteri, V. (2012). Mycobacterium avium subsp. paratuberculosis as an emergent pathogen in raw milk produced in Central Italy. Veterinary Research Communications (In press).

Attili, A. R., Ngu Ngwa, V., Preziuso, S., Pacifici, L., Domesi, A., & Cuteri, V. (2011). Ovine paratuberculosis: a seroprevalence study in dairy flocks reared in Central Italy. Veterinary Medicine International, ID 782875, doi:10.4061/2011/782875.

Ayele, W. Y., Svastova, P., Roubal, P., Bartos, M., & Pavlik, I. (2005). Mycobacterium avium subspecies paratuberculosis cultured from locally and commercially pasteurized cow's milk in the Czech Republic. Applied Environmental Microbiology, 71(3), 1210-1214.

Baek, H. S. & Yoon, J. W. (1990). Role of macrophages in the pathogenesis of encephalomyocarditis virus-induced diabetes in mice. Journal of Virology, 64, 5708-5715.

Baek, H. S. & Yoon, J. W. (1991). Direct involvement of macrophages in destruction of β cells leading to the development of diabetes in virus-infected mice. Diabetes, 40, 269-274.

Banatvala, J. E., Bryant, J., Schernthaner, G., Borkenstein, M., Schober, E., Brown, D., De Silva, L. M., Menser, M. A., & Silink, M. (1985). Coxsackie B, mumps, rubella and cytomegalovirus specific IgM responses in patients with juvenile-onset insulin-dependent diabetes mellitus in Britain, Austria and Australia. Lancet, 1, 1409-1412.

Barboni, E., Manocchio, I., & Asdrubali, G. (1966). Observations on diabetes mellitus associated with experimental foot-and-mouth disease in cattle. Veterinaria Italiana, 17, 362-368.

Basoglu, O. K., Bacakoglu, F., Cok, G., Sayiner, A., & Ates, M. (1999). The oral glucose tolerance test in patients with respiratory infections. Monaldi Archives for Chest Diseases, 54, 307-310.

Beard, P. M., Daniels, M. J., Henderson, D., Pirie, A., Rudge, K., Buxton, D., Rhind, S., Greig, A., Hutchings, M. R., McKendrick, I., Stevenson, K., & Sharp, J. M. (2001). Paratuberculosis infection of non-ruminant wildlife in Scotland. Journal of Clinical Microbiology, 39, 1517-1521.

Blackwell, J. M., Black, G. F., Sharples, C., Soo, S. S., Peacock, C. S., & Miller, N. (1999). Roles of Nramp1, HLA, and a gene(s) in allelic association with IL-4, in determining T helper subset differentiation. Microbes and Infection, 1(1), 95-102.

Bodansky, H. J., Staines, A., Stephenson, C., Haigh, D., & Cartwright, R. (1992). Evidence for an environmental effect in the etiology of insulin dependent diabetes in a transmigratory population. British Medical Journal, 304, 1020-1022.

Brookes, S. M., Pandolfino, Y. A., Mitchell, T. J., Venables, T. J., Shattles, W. G., Clark, D. A., Entwistle, A., & Maini, R. N. (1992). The immune response to and expression of cross-reactive retroviral gag sequences in autoimmune disease. British Journal of Rheumatology, 31, 735-742.

Brown, D. W., Welsh, R. M., & Like, A. A. (1993). Infection of peripancreatic lymph nodes but not islets precedes Kilham's rat virus-induced diabetes in BB/Wor rats. Journal of Virology, 67, 5873-5878.

Brugman, S., Klatter, F. A., Visser, J. T. J., Wildeboire-Velo, A. C. M., Harmsen, H. J. M., Rozing, J., & Bos, N. A. (2006). Antibiotic treatment partially protects against type 1 diabetes in the Bio-Breeding diabetes-prone rat. Is the gut flora involved in the development of type 1 diabetes? Diabetologia, 49, 2105-2108.

Buergelt, C. D., Layton, A. W., Ginn, P. E., Taylor, M., King, J. M., Habecker, P. L., Mauldin, E., Whitlock, R., Rossiter, C. & Collins, M. T. (2000). The pathology of spontaneous paratuberculosis in the North American bison (Bison bison). Veterinary Pathology, 3, 428-438.

Bull, T. J., McMinn, E. J., Sidi-Boumedine, K., Skull, A., Durkin, D., Neild, P., Rhodes, G., Pickup, R., & Hermon-Taylor, J. (2003). Detection and verification of Mycobacterium avium subsp. paratuberculosis in fresh ileocolonic mucosal biopsy specimens from individuals with and without Crohn's disease. Journal of Clinical Microbiology, 41(7), 2915-2923.

Calcinaro, F., Dionisi, S., Marinaro, M., Candeloro, P., Bonato, V., Marzotti, S., Corneli, R. B., Ferretti, E., Gulino, A., Grasso, F., De Simone, C., Di Mario, U., Falorni, A., Boirivant, M., & Dotta, F. (2005). Oral probiotic administration induces interleukin-10 production and prevents spontaneous autoimmune diabetes in the non-obese diabetic mouse. Diabetologia, 48, 1565-1575.

Cavallo, M. G., Baroni, M. G., Toto, A., Gearing, A. J. H., Forsey, T., Andreani, D., Thorpe, R., & Pozzilli, P. (1992). Viral infection induces cytokine release by beta islet cells. Immunology, 75, 664-668.

Chamberlin, W., Graham, D. Y., Hulten, K., El-Zimaity, H. M., Schwartz, M. R., Naser, S., Shafran, I. & El-Zaatari, F. A. (2001). Review article: Mycobacterium avium subsp. paratuberculosis as one cause of Crohn's disease. Ailment Pharmacology Therapeutics, 15, 337-346.

Champsaur, H., Bottazzo, G., Bertrams, J., Assan, R., & Bach, C. (1982). Virologic, immunologic and genetic factors in insulin-dependent diabetes mellitus. The Journal of Pediatrics, 100, 15-20.

Chapman, N. M., Kim, K. S., Drescher, K. M., Oka, K., & Tracy, S. (2008). 5' terminal deletions in the genome of a coxsackievirus B2 strain occurred naturally in human heart. Virology, 375. 480-491.

Charlton, B., Bacelj, A., & Mandel, T. E. (1988). Administration of silica particles or anti-Lyt2 antibody prevents β-cell destruction in NOD mice given cyclophosphamide. Diabetes, 37, 930-935.

Chatenoud, L., You, S., Okada, H., Kuhn, C., Michaud, B., & Bach, J. F. (2010). New opportunities based on the hygiene hypothesis. In: 99th Dahlem conference on infection, inflammation and chronic inflammatory disorders: immune therapies of type 1 diabetes. Clinical and Experimental Immunology, 160, 106-112.

Chatterjee, N. K., Hou, J., Dockstader, P., & Charbonnau, T. (1992). Coxsackievirus B4 infection alters thymic, splenic and peripheral repertoire preceding onset of hyperglycemia in mice. *Journal of Medical Virology, 38, 124-131.*

Chehadeh, W., Weill, J., Vantyghem, M. C., Alm, G., Lèfebvre, J., Wattré, P., & Hober, D. (2000). *Increased level of interferon-alpha in blood of patients with insulin-dependent diabetes mellitus: relationship with coxsackie B infection. The Journal of Infectious Diseases, 181, 1929-1939.*

Chikazawa, K., Okusa, H., Minakami, H., Kimura, K., Araki, S., & Tamada, T. (1985). *Acute onset of insulin-dependent diabetes mellitus caused by Epstein-Barr virus infection. Acta Obstetrics and Gynecology Japanaise, 37, 453-456.*

Child, D. F., William, C. P., Jones, R. P., Hudson, P. R., Jones, M., & Smith, C. J. (1995). *Heat shock protein studies in type 1 and type 2 diabetes and human islet cell culture. Diabetic Medicine, 12, 595-599.*

Chimienti, F., Devergnas, S., Favier, A., & Seve, M. (2004). *Identification and cloning of a beta-cell-specific zinc transporter. ZnT-8, localized into insulin secretory granules. Diabetes, 53(9), 2330-2337.*

Chiodini, R. J. & Hermon-Taylor, J. (1993). *The thermal resistance of Mycobacterium paratuberculosis in raw milk under conditions simulating pasteurization. Journal of Veterinary Diagnostic Investigation, 5(4), 629-631.*

Chiodini, R. J. & Rossiter, C. A. (1996). *Paratuberculosis: a potential zoonosis? Veterinary Clinics of North America Food Animal Practice, 12, 457-467.*

Chiodini, R. J. (1996). *Immunology: resistance to paratuberculosis. Veterinary Clinics of North America Food Animal Practice, 12(2), 313-343.*

Chiodini, R. J., van Kruiningen, H. J., & Merkal, R. S. (1984). *Ruminant paratuberculosis (Johne's disease): the current status and future prospects. Cornell Veterinarian, 74, 218-262.*

Chiodini, R. J., Van Kruiningen, H. J., Thayer, & Coutu, J. A. (1986). *Spheroplastic phase of mycobacteria isolated from patients with Crohn's disease. Journal of Clinical Microbiology, 24, 357-363.*

Chiu, C. Y., Greninger, A. L., Kanada, K., Kwok, T., Fisher, K. F., Runckel, C., Louie, J. K., Glaser, C. A., Yagi, S., Schnurr, D. P., Haggerty, T. D., Parsonnet, J., Ganem, D., & De Risi, J. L. (2008). *Identification of cardioviruses related to Theiler's murine encephalomyelitis virus in human infections. Proceedings of The National Academy of Sciences of the United States of America, 105, 14124-14129.*

Choi, K. S., Jun, H. S., Kim, H. N., Park, H. J., Eom, Y. W., Noh, H. L., Kwon, H., Kim, H. M., & Yoon, J. W. (2001). *Role of Hck in the pathogenesis of encephalomyocarditis virus-induced diabetes in mice. Journal of Virology, 75, 1949-1957.*

Christen, U., Edelmann, K. H., McGavern, D. B., Wolfe, T., Coon, B., Teague, M. K., Miller, S. D., Oldstone, M. B. A., & von Herrath, M. G. (2004). *A viral epitope that mimics a self antigen can accelerate but not initiate autoimmune diabetes. The Journal of Clinical Investigation, 114, 1290-1298.*

Chung, Y. H., Jun, H. S., Hirasawa, K., Lee, B. R., van Rooijen, N., & Yoon, J. W. (1997). *Role of macrophages and macrophage-derived cytokines in the pathogenesis of Kilham rat virus-induced autoimmune diabetes in diabetes-resistant BB rats. Journal of Immunology, 159, 466-471.*

Chung, Y. H., Jun, H. S., Son, M., Bao, M., Bae, H. Y., Kang, Y., & Yoon, J. W. (2000). *Cellular and molecular mechanism for Kilham rat virus-induced autoimmune diabetes in DR-BB rats. Journal of Immunology, 165, 2866-2876.*

Cocito, C., Gilot, P., Coene, M., Kesel, M., Poupart, P., & Vannuffel, P. (1994). *Paratuberculosis. Clinical Microbiology Review, 7, 328-345.*

Collins, M. T. (1996). *Diagnosis of paratuberculosis. Veterinary Clinics of North America Food Animal Practice, 12(2), 357-371.*

Concannon, P., Rich, S. S., & Nepom, G. T. (2009). *Genetics of type 1A diabetes. The New England Journal of Medicine, 360, 1646-1654.*

Conrad, B., Weissmahr, R. N., Boni, J., Arcari, R., Schupbach, J., & Mach, B. (1997). *A human endogenous retroviral superantigen as candidate autoimmune gene in type I diabetes. Cell, 90, 303-313.*

Coppieters, K. T. & von Herrath, M. G. (2010). Viruses and cytotoxic T lymphocytes in Type 1 diabetes. Clinical Reviews in Allergy and Immunology, 41, 169-178.

Coppieters, K. T., Amirian, N., & von Herrath, M. G. (2011). Incidental CD8 T cell reactivity against caspase-cleaved apoptotic self-antigens from ubiquitously expressed proteins in islets from prediabetic human leucocyte antigen-A2 transgenic non-obese diabetic mice. Clinical and Experimental Immunology, 165, 155-162.

Coppieters, K. T., Wiberg, A., Tracy, S. M., & von Herrath, M. G. (2012). Immunology in the clinic review series: focus on type 1 diabetes and viruses: the role of viruses in type 1 diabetes: a difficult dilemma. Clinical and Experimental Immunology, 168(1), 5-11.

Cossu, A., Rosu, V., Paccagnini, D., Cossu, D., Pacifico, A., & Sechi, L. A. (2011). MAP3738c and MptD are specific tags of Mycobacterium avium subsp. paratuberculosis infection in type 1 diabetes mellitus. Clinical Immunology, 141(1), 49-57.

Craig, M. E., Howard, N. J., Silink, M., & Rawlinson, W. D. (2003). Reduced frequency of HLA DRB1*03-DQB1*02 in children with type 1 diabetes associated with enterovirus RNA. The Journal of Infectious Diseases, 187, 1562-1570.

Craighead, J. E. & McLane, M. F. (1968). Diabetes mellitus: induction in mice by encephalomyocarditis virus. Science, 162, 913-915.

Dai, Y. D., Marrero, I. G., Gross, P., Zaghouani, H., Wicker, L. S., & Sercarz, E. E. (2009). Slc11a1 enhances the autoimmune diabetogenic T-cell response by altering processing and presentation of pancreatic islet antigens. Diabetes, 58(1), 156-164.

Davies, J. M. (1997). Molecular mimicry: can epitope mimicry induce autoimmune disease? Immunology Cellular Biology, 75, 113-126.

De Stefano, F., Mullooly, J. P., Okoro, C. A., Chen, R. T., Marcy, S. M., Ward, J. I., Vadheim, C. M., Black, S. B., Shinefield, H. R., Davis, R. L., & Bohlke, K. (2001). Vaccine Safety Datalink Team. Childhood vaccinations, vaccination timing, and risk of type 1 diabetes mellitus. Pediatrics, 108, E112-3.

Delovitch, T. & Singh, B. (1997). The non obese diabetic mouse as a model of autoimmune disease: immune dysregulation gets the NOD. Immunity, 7, 727-738.

Demir, M., Gokturk, H. S., Ozturk, N. A., Kulaksizoglu, M., Serin, E., & Yilmaz, U. (2008). Helicobacter pylori Prevalence in Diabetes Mellitus Patients with Dyspeptic Symptoms and its Relationship to Glycemic Control and Late Complications. Digestive Diseases and Sciences, 10.1007/s10620-007-0185-7.

Di Sabatino, A., Rovedatti, L., Vidali, F., Macdonald, T. T., & Corazza, G. R. (2011). Recent advances in understanding Crohn's disease. Internal Emergency Medicine, 7(2), 103-111.

Diomedi, M., Stanzione, P., Sallustio, F., Leone, G., Renna, A., Misaggi, G., Fontana, C., Pasqualetti, P., & Pietroiusti, A. (2008). Cytotoxin-associated gene-A-positive Helicobacter pylori strains infection increases the risk of recurrent atherosclerotic stroke. Helicobacter, 13, 525-531.

Dooley, K. E. & Chaisson, R. E. (2009). Tuberculosis and diabetes mellitus: convergence of two epidemics. Lancet Infectious Diseases, 9(12), 737-746.

Dotta, F., Censini, S., van Halteren, A. G. S., Marselli, L., Masini, M., Dionisi, S., Mosca, F., Boggi, U., Onetti Muda, a., Del Prato, S., Elliott, J. F., Covacci, A., Rappuoli, R., Roep, B. O., & Marchetti, P. (2007). Coxsackie B4 virus infection of beta cells and natural killer cell insulitis in recent-onset type 1 diabetic patients. Proceedings of The National Academy of Sciences of the United States of America, 104(12), 5115-5120.

Dow, C.T. (2006). Paratuberculosis and type 1 diabetes: is this the trigger? Medical Hypotheses, 67, 782-785.

Drescher, K. M. & Tracy S. (2008). The CVB and etiology of type 1 diabetes. Current Topics in Microbiology and Immunology, 323, 259-274.

Drescher, K. M., Kono, K., Bopegamage, S., Carson, S. D., & Tracy, S. (2004). Coxsackievirus B3 infection and type 1 diabetes development in NOD mice: insulitis determines susceptibility of pancreatic islets to virus infection. Virology, 329, 381-394.

Dyrberg, T., Schwimmbeck, P. L.,& Oldstone, M. B. A. (1988). Inhibition of diabetes in BB rats by viral infection. The Journal of Clinical Investigation, 81, 928-931.

Ellerman, K. E., Richards, C. A., Guberski, D. L., Shek, W. R., & Like, A. (1996). A Kilham rat virus triggers T-cell-dependent autoimmune diabetes in multiple strains of rat. Diabetes, 45, 557-562.

Ellerman, K., Wrobleski, M., Rabinovitch, A., & Like, A. (1993). Natural killer cell depletion and diabetes mellitus in the BB/Wor rat (revisited). Diabetologia, 36, 596-601.

Ellingson, J. L., Anderson, J. L., Koziczkowski, J. J., Radcliff, R. P., Sloan, S. J., Allen, S. E., & Sullivan, N. M. (2005). Detection of viable Mycobacterium avium subsp. paratuberculosis in retail pasteurized whole milk by two culture methods and PCR. Journal of Food Protection, 68(5), 966-972.

Favila-Humara, L. C., Chavez-Gris, G. G., Carrillo-Casas, E. M., & Hernandez-Castro, R. (2010). Mycobacterium avium subsp. paratuberculosis detection in individual and bulk milk samples from bovine herds and caprine flocks. Food-borne Pathognomonic Diseases, 7(4), 351-355.

Feller, M., Huwiler, K., Stephan, R., Altpeter, E., Shang, A., Furrer, H., Pfyffer, G. E., Jemmi, T., Baumgartner, A., & Egger, M. (2007). Mycobacterium avium subspecies paratuberculosis and Crohn's disease: a systematic review and meta-analysis. Lancet Infectious Diseases, 7(9), 607-613.

Fohlman, J. & Friman, G. (1993). Is juvenile diabetes a viral disease? Annals of Medicine, 25, 569-574.

Foulis, A. K, Farquharson, M. A., & Meager, A. (1987). Immunoreactive α-interferon in insulin-producing β cells in type I diabetes mellitus. Lancet, 2, 1423-1427.

Foulis, A. K., Farquharson, M. A., Cameron, S. O., McGill, M., Schonke, H., & Kandolf, R. (1990). A search for the presence of the enteroviral capsid protein VP1 in pancreata of patients with type 1 (insulin-dependent) diabetes and pancreata and hearts of infants who died of coxsackieviral myocarditis. Diabetologia, 33, 290-298.

Friman, G., Fohlman, J., Frisk, G., Diderholm, H., Ewald, U., Kobbah, M., & Tuvemo, T. (1985). An incidence peak of juvenile diabetes. Relation to Coxsackie B virus immune response. Acta Paediatrica Scandinavica, 320(Suppl), 14-19.

Frisk, G., Friman, G., Tuvemo, T., Fohlman, J., & Diderholm, H. (1992). Coxsackie B virus IgM in children at onset of type 1 (insulin-dependent) diabetes mellitus: evidence for IgM induction by a recent or current infection. Diabetologia, 35, 249-253.

Fukino-Kurihara, H., Fujita, H., Hakura, A., Nonaka, K., & Tarui, S. (1985). Morphological aspects on pancreatic islets of non-obese diabetic (NOD) mice. Virchows Archives, 49, 107-120.

Gagnerault, M. C., Luan, J. J., Lotton, C., & Lepault, F. (2002). Pancreatic lymph nodes are required for priming of beta cell reactive T cells in NOD mice. Journal of Experimental Medicine, 196(3), 369-377.

Gamble, D. R. (1980). Relation of antecedent illness to development of diabetes in children. British Medical Journal, 2, 99-101.

Gamble, D.R. & Taylor, K. W.(1969). Seasonal incidence of diabetes mellitus. British Medical Journal, 13, 631-633.

Gao, A., Mutharia, L., Chen, S., Rahn, K., & Odumeru, J. (2002). Effect of pasteurization on survival of Mycobacterium avium ssp. paratuberculosis in milk. Journal of Dairy Sciences, 85, 3198-3205.

Garza, K. M., Chan, S. M., Suri, R., Nguyen, L. T., Odermatt, B., Schoenberger, S. P., & Ohashi, P. S. (2000). Role of antigen-presenting cells in mediating tolerance and autoimmunity. The Journal of Experimental Medicine, 191, 2021-2027.

Gasbarrini, A., Ojetti, V., Pitocco, D., De Luca, A., Franceschi, F., Candelli, M., Sanz Torre, E., Pola, P., Ghirlanda, G., & Gasparrini, G. (1998) Helicobacter pylori infection in patients affected by insulin-dependent diabetes mellitus. European Journal of Gastroenterology & Hepatology, 10, 469-472.

Gaskins, H., Prochazka, M., Hamaguchi, K., Serreze, D., & Leiter, E. (1992). Beta cell expression of endogenous xenotropic retrovirus distinguishes diabetes-susceptible NOD/Lt from resistant NON/Lt mice. Journal of Clinical Investigation, 90, 2220-2227.

Georges, J. L., Rupprecht, H. J., Blankenberg, S., Poirier, O., Bickel, C., Hafner, G., Nicaud, V., Meyer, J., Camien, F., Tiret, L., & AtheroGene Group (2003). Impact of pathogen burden in patients with coronary artery disease in relation to systemic inflammation and variation in genes encoding cytokines. American Journal of Cardiology, 92, 515-521.

Gerstein, H. C. (1994). Cow's milk exposure and type I diabetes mellitus. A critical overview of the clinical literature. Diabetes Care, 17(1), 13-19.

Getts, M. T. & Miller, S. D. (2010).Triggering of autoimmune diseases by infections. In: 99th Dahlem conference on infection, inflammation and chronic inflammatory disorders. Clinical and Experimental Immunology, 160, 15-21.

Ghadiali, A. H., Strother, M., Naser, S. A., Manning, E. J., & Sreevatsan, S. (2004). Mycobacterium avium subsp. paratuberculosis strains isolated from Crohn's disease patients and animal species exhibit similar polymorphic locus patterns. Journal of Clinical Microbiology, 42(11), 5345-5348.

Gibbon, C., Smith, T., Egger, P. Betts, P., & Phillips, D. (1997). Early infection and subsequent insulin dependent diabetes. Archives of Disease in Childhood, 77, 384-385.

Gillespie, K. M., Bain, S. C., Barnett, A. H., Bingley, P. J., Christie, M. R., Gill, G. V., & Gale, E. A.(2004). The rising incidence of childhood type 1 diabetes and reduced contribution of high-risk HLA haplotypes. Lancet, 364, 1699-1700.

Gimeno, S. G. & de Souza, J. M. (1997). IDDM and milk consumption. A case-control study in Sao Paulo, Brazil. Diabetes Care, 20(8), 1256-1260.

Ginsberg-Fellner, F., Fedun, B., Cooper, L. Z., Witt, M. E., Franklin, B. H., Roman, S. H., Rubenstein, P., & McEvoy, R. C. (1986). Interrelationships of congenital rubella, type 1 insulin-dependent diabetes mellitus: The Immunology of Diabetes Mellitus. Jaworski, M. A., Molnar, G. D., Rajotte, R. V., Singh, B. (eds). Elsevier: Amsterdam, 279-286.

Ginsberg-Fellner, F., Witt, M. E., & Yagihaski, S. (1984). Congenital rubella-syndrome as a model for type 1 (insulin-dependent) diabetes mellitus: increased prevalence of islet cell surface antibodies. Diabetologia, 27, 87-89.

Grant, I. R. (2003). Mycobacterium paratuberculosis and milk. Acta Veterinaria Scandinavica, 44(3-4), 261-266.

Grant, I. R. (2006). Mycobacterium avium subsp. paratuberculosis in foods: current evidence and potential consequences. International Journal of Dairy Technology, 59, 112–117.

Grant, I. R., Ball, H. J., & Rowe, M. T. (2002). Incidence of Mycobacterium paratuberculosis in bulk raw and commercially pasteurized cows' milk from approved dairy processing establishments in the United Kingdom. Applied Environmental Microbiology, 68(5), 2428-2435.

Gray, A.,Wreghitt, T., Stratton, I. M., Alexander, G. J. M., Turner, R. C., & O'Rahilly, S. (1995). High prevalence of hepatitis C infection in Afro-Caribbean patients with type 2 diabetes and abnormal liver function tests. Diabetic Medicine, 12, 244-249.

Green, J., Casabonne, D., & Newton, R. (2004). Coxsackie B virus serology and Type 1 diabetes mellitus: a systematic review of published case–control studies. Diabetic Medicine, 21, 507-514.

Guberski, D. L., Thomas, V. A., Shek, W. R., Like, A. A., Handler, E. S., Rossini, A. A., Wallace, J. E., & Welsh, R. M. (1991). Induction of type I diabetes by Kilham's rat virus in diabetes-resistant BB/Wor rats. Science, 254, 1010-1013.

Gulcelik, N. E., Kaya, E., Demirbas, B., Culha, C., Koc, G., Ozkaya, M., Cakal, E., Serter, R., & Aral, Y. (2005). Helicobacter pylori prevalence in diabetic patients and its relationship with dyspepsia and autonomic neuropathy. Journal of Endocrinological Investigation, 28(3), 214-217.

Hamed, S. A., Amine, N. F., Galal, G. M., Helal, S. R., Tag El-Din, L. M., Shawky, O. A., Ahmed, E. A., & Abdel Rahman, M. S. (2008). Vascular risks and complications in diabetes mellitus: the role of helicobacter pylori infection. Journal of Stroke and Cerebrovascular Diseases,17, 86-94.

Hanafusa, T. & Imagawa, A. (2007). Fulminant type 1 diabetes: a novel clinical entity requiring special attention by all medical practitioners. Nature Clinical Practice Endocrinology & Metabolism, 3, 36-45.

Hao, W., Serreze, D. V., McCulloch, D. K., Neifing, J. L., & Palmer, J. P. (1993). *Insulin (auto) antibodies from human IDDM cross-react with retroviral antigen p73. Journal of Autoimmunity, 6, 787-798.*

Harris, H. F. (1898). *A case of diabetes mellitus quickly following mumps on the pathological alterations of salivary glands, closely resembling those found in pancreas, in a case of diabetes mellitus. The Boston Medical and Surgical Journal, CXL, 465.*

Hayashi, T., Morimoto, M., Iwata, H., & Onodera, T. (2001). *Possible involvement of IL-12 in reovirus type-2-induced diabetes in newborn DBA/1 mice. Scandinavian Journal of Immunology, 53, 572-578.*

Helmke, K., Otten, A., & Willems, W. (1980). *Islet cell antibodies in children with mumps infection. Lancet, 2, 211-212.*

Hermann, R., Knip, M., Veijola, R., Simell, O., Laine, A. P., Åkerblom, H. K., Groop, P. H., Forsblom, C., Pettersson-Fernholm, K., & Ilonen, J., FinnDiane Study Group. (2003). *Temporal changes in the frequencies of HLA genotypes in patients with Type 1 diabetes-indication of an increased environmental pressure? Diabetologia, 46(3), 420-425.*

Hermon-Taylor, J. & Bull, T. (2002). *Crohn's disease caused by Mycobacterium avium spp. paratuberculosis: a public health tragedy whose resolution is long overdue. Journal of Medical Microbiology, 51, 3-6.*

Hermon-Taylor, J. & El-Zaatari, F. A. K. (2004). *The Mycobacterium avium subspecies paratuberculosis problem and its relation to the causation of Crohn disease. In: Bartram, J., Dufour, J. C., Rees, G., Pedley, S., eds. Pathogenic Mycobacteria in Water: A Guide to Public Health Consequences, Monitoring and Management. London: IWA Publishing (pp. 74-94).*

Hermon-Taylor, J., Bull, T. J., Sheridan, J. M., Cheng, J., Stellakis, M. L., & Sumar, N. (2000). *Causation of Crohn's disease by Mycobacterium avium subspecies paratuberculosis. Canadian Journal of Gastroenterology, 14, 521-539.*

Hia, H. H., Talley, N. J., Kam, E. P., Young, L. J., Hammer, J., & Horowitz, M. (2001). *Helicobacter pylori infection is not associated with diabetes mellitus, nor with upper gastrointestinal symptoms in diabetes mellitus. The American Journal of Gastroenterology, 96(4), 1039-1046.*

Hiemstra, H. S., Schloot, N. C., van Veelen, P. A., Willemen, S. J. M., Franken, K. L. M. C., van Rood, J. J., de Vries, R. R. P., Chaudhuri, A., Behan, P. O., Drijfhout, J. W., & Roep, B. O. (2001). *Cytomegalovirus in autoimmunity: T cell cross reactivity to viral antigen and autoantigen glutamic acid decarboxylase. Proceedings of The National Academy of Sciences of the United States of America, 98, 3988-3991.*

Hiltunen, M., Hyöty, H., Knip, M., Ilonen, J., Reijonen, H., Vähäsalo, P., Roivainen, R., Lonrot, M., Leinikki, P., Hovi, T., & Åkerblom, H. K. (1997). *Islet cell antibody seroconversion in children is temporally associated with enterovirus infections. The Journal of Infectious Diseases, 175, 554-560.*

Hirasawa, K., Jun, H. S., Han, H. S., Zhang, M. L., Hollenberg, M., & Yoon, J. W. (1999). *Prevention of encephalomyocarditis virus-induced diabetes in mice by inhibition of the tyrosine signalling pathway and suppression of nitric oxide production in macrophages. Journal of Virology, 73, 8541-8548.*

Hirasawa, K., Jun, H. S., Maeda, K., Kawaguchi, Y., Itagaki, S., Mikami, T., Baek, H. S., Doi, K., & Yoon, J. W. (1997). *Possible role of macrophage-derived soluble mediators in the pathogenesis of encephalomyocarditis virus-induced diabetes in mice. Journal of Virology, 71, 4024-4031.*

Hober, D., Sane, F., Jaïdane, H., Riedweg, K., Goffard, A., & Desailloud, H. (2012). *Immunology in the clinic review series; focus on type 1 diabetes and viruses: role of antibodies enhancing the infection with Coxsackievirus-B in the pathogenesis of type 1 diabetes. Clinical & Experimental Immunology, 168, 47-51.*

Holz, A., Brett, K., & Oldstone, M. B. (2001). *Constitutive beta cell expression of IL-12 does not perturb self-tolerance but intensifies established autoimmune diabetes. The Journal of Clinical Investigation, 108, 1749-1758.*

Honeyman, M. C., Coulson, B. S., Stone, N. L., Gellert, S. A., Goldwater, P. N., Steele, C. E., Couper, J. J., Tait, B. D., Colman, P. G., & Harrison, L. C. (2000). *Association between rotavirus infection and pancreatic islet autoimmunity in children at risk of developing type 1 diabetes. Diabetes, 49, 1319-1324.*

Horn, G., Bugawan, T., Long, C., & Erlich, H. (1988). *Allelic sequence of the HLA-DQ loci: relationship to serology and to insulin-dependent diabetes susceptibility. Proceedings of The National Academy of Sciences of the United States of America, 85, 6012-6016.*

Horwitz, M. S., Bradley, L. M., Harbertson, J., Krahl, T., Lee, J., & Sarvetnick, N. (1998). Diabetes induced by Coxsackie virus: initiation by bystander damage and not molecular mimicry. Nature Medicine, 4, 781-785.

Hou, J., Sheikh, S., Martin, D. L., & Chatterjee, N. K. (1993). Coxsackie virus B4 alters pancreatic glutamic decarboxylase expression in mice soon after infection. Journal of Autoimmunity, 6, 529-542.

Hugot, J. P., Chamaillard, M., Zouali, H., Lesage. S., Cézard, J. P., Belaiche, J., Almer, S., Tysk, C., O'Morain, C. A., Gassul, M., Binder, V., Finkel, Y., Cortot, A., Modigliani, R., Laurent-Puig, P., Gower-Rousseau, C., Macri, J., Colombel, J. F., Sahbatou, M., & Thomas, G. (2001). Association of NOD2 leucine-rich repeat variants with susceptibility to Crohn's disease. Nature, 411, 599-603.

Hummel, M., Fuchtenbusch, M., Schenker, M., & Ziegler, A. G. (2000). No major association of breast-feeding, vaccinations, and childhood viral diseases with early islet autoimmunity in the German BABYDIAB study. Diabetes Care, 24, 969-974.

Hyöty, H., Hiltunen, M., Knip, M., Laakkonen, M., Vähäsalo, P., Karjalainen, J., Koskela, P., Roivainen, M., Leinikki, P., Hovi, T., & al. (1995). A prospective study of the role of coxsackie B and other enterovirus infections in the pathogenesis of IDDM. Childhood Diabetes in Finland (DiMe) Study Group. Diabetes, 44, 652.

Hyöty, H., Hiltunen, M., Reunanen, A., Leinikki, P., Vesikari, T., Lounamaa, R., Tuomilehto, J., & Åkerblom, H. K. (1993). Childhood Diabetes in Finland Study Group. Decline of mumps antibodies in type 1 (insulin-dependent) diabetic children and a plateau in the rising incidence of type 1 diabetes after introduction of the mumps-measles-rubella vaccine in Finland. Diabetologia, 36, 1303-1308.

Hyöty, H., Rasanen, L., Hiltunen, M., Lehtinen, M., Huupponen, T., & Leinikki, P. (1991). Decreased antibody reactivity to Epstein-Barr virus capsid antigen in type 1 (insulin-dependent) diabetes mellitus. Acta Patologica,Microbiologica et Immunologica Scandinavica, 99, 359-363.

Ivarsson, S. A., Lindberg, B., Nilsson, K. O., Ahlfors, K., & Svanberg, L. (1993). The prevalence of type 1 diabetes mellitus at follow-up of Swedish infants congenitally infected with cytomegalovirus. Diabetic Medicine, 10, 521-523.

Jaïdane, H., Sané, F., Hiar, R., Goffard, A., Gharbi, J., Geenen, V., & Hober, D. (2012). Immunology in the clinic review series; focus on type 1 diabetes and viruses: enterovirus, thymus and type 1 diabetes pathogenesis. Clinical & Experimental Immunology, 168, 39-46.

Jali, M. V. & Shankar, P. S. (1990). Transient diabetes following chicken pox. Journal of the Association of Physicians of India, 38, 663-664.

Jensen, A., Rosenberg, H., & Notkins, A. L. (1980). Virus-induced diabetes mellitus XVII: pancreatic islet cell damage in children with fatal viral infections. Lancet, 2, 354-358.

Jeon, C. Y., Haan, M. N., Cheng, C., Clayton, E. R., Mayeda, E. R., Miller, J. W., & Aiello, A. E. (2012). Helicobacter pylori Infection Is Associated With an Increased Rate of Diabetes. Diabetes Care, 35(6), 520-525.

Jordan, D. (1996). Aggregate testing for the evaluation of Johne's disease herd status. Australian Veterinary Journal, 73(1), 16-19.

Juhela, S., Hyöty, H., Roivainen, M., Harkonen, T., Putto-Laurila, A., Simell, O., & Ilonen J. (2000). T-cell responses to enterovirus antigens in children with type 1 diabetes. Diabetes, 49, 1308-1313.

Jun HS & Yoon JW. (2001). The role of viruses in type I diabetes: two distinct cellular and molecular pathogenic mechanisms of virus-induced diabetes in animals. Diabetologia, 44, 271-285.

Jun, H. S. & Yoon, J. W. (2003). A new look at viruses in type 1 diabetes. Diabetes/Metabolism Research and Reviews, 19(1), 8-31.

Jun, H. S., Yoon, C. S., Zbytnuik, L., van Rooijen, N., & Yoon, J. W. (1999). The role of macrophages in T cell-mediated autoimmune diabetes in nonobese diabetic mice. The Journal of Experimental Medicine, 189, 347-358.

Kang, Y. & Yoon, J. W. (1993). A genetically determined host factor controlling susceptibility to encephalomyocarditis virus-induced diabetes in mice. Journal of General Virology, 74, 1203-1213.

Karounos, D. G., Wolinsky, J. S., & Thomas, J. W. (1993). Monoclonal antibody to rubella virus capsid protein recognizes a beta-cell antigen. The Journal of Immunology, 150, 3080-3085.

Kaufman, D. L., Erlander, M. G., Clare-Salzler, M., Atkinson, M. A., Maclaren, N. K., & Tobin, A. J. (1992). Autoimmunity to two forms of glutamate decarboxylase in insulin-dependent diabetes mellitus. The Journal of Clinical Investigation, 89, 283-292.

Kim, A., Jun, H. S., Wong, L., Stephure, D., Pacaud, D., Trussell, R. A., & Yoon J. W. (1999). Human endogenous retrovirus with a high genomic sequence homology with IDDMK(1,2)22 is not specific for type I (insulin-dependent) diabetic patients but ubiquitous. Diabetologia, 42, 413-418.

Kim, K. S., Tracy, S., Tapprich, W., Bailey, J., Lee, C. K., Kim, K., Barry, W. H., & Chapman, N. M. (2005). 5'-Terminal deletions occur in coxsackievirus B3 during replication in murine hearts and cardiac myocyte cultures and correlate with encapsidation of negative-strand viral RNA. Journal of Virology, 79, 7024-7041.

Knip, M., Veijola, R., Virtanen, S. M., Hyoty, H., Vaarala, O., & Åkerblom, A. K.(2005). Environmental triggers and determinants of type-1diabetes. Diabetes, 54, 125-136.

Ko, G. T., Chan, W. B., Sung, J. J., Tsoi, C. L., Lai, C. W., & Cockram, C. S. (2001). Helicobacter pylori infection in Chinese subjects with type 2 diabetes. Endocrine Research, 27(1-2), 171-177.

Kondrashova, A., Viskari, H., Kulmala, P., Romanov, A., Ilonen, J., Hyőty, H., & Knip, M. (2007). Signs of beta-cell autoimmunity in nondiabetic schoolchildren: a comparison between Russian Karelia with a low incidence of type 1 diabetes and Finland with a high incidence rate. Diabetes Care, 30, 95-100.

Lambeth, C., Reddacliff, L. A., Windsor, P., Abbott, K. A., McGregor, H., & Whittington, R. J. (2004). Intrauterine and transmammary transmission of Mycobacterium avium subsp paratuberculosis in sheep. Australian Veterinary Journal, 82, 504-508.

Lee, K. U., Amano, K., & Yoon, J. W. (1988). Evidence for initial involvement of macrophages in development of insulitis in NOD mice. Diabetes, 37, 1989-1991.

Lesage, S., Zouali, H., Cézard, J. P., the EPWG-IBD group, Colombel, J. F., the IPEMAD group, Belaiche, J., the GETAID group, Almer, S., Tysk, C., O'Morain, C. A., Gassul, M., Binder, V., Finkel, Y., Modigliani, R., Gower-Rousseau, C., Macri, J., Merlin, F., Chamaillard, M., Jannot, A. S., Thomas, G., & Hugot, J. P. (2002). CARD15/NOD2 mutational analysis and phenotype-genotype correlation in 612 patients with inflammatory bowel disease. The American Journal of Human Genetics, 70, 845-857.

Liblau, R. S., Singer, S. M., & McDevitt, H. O. (1995). Th1 and Th2 CD4+ T cells in the pathogenesis of organ-specific autoimmune disease. Immunology Today, 16, 34-38.

Liu, P. T., Stenger, S., Li, H., Wenzel, L., Tan, B. H., Krutzik, S. R., Ochoa, M. T., Schauber, J., Wu, K., Meinken, C., Kamen, D. L., Wagner, M., Bals, R., Steinmeyer, A., Zügel, U., Gallo, R. L., Eisenberg, D., Hewison, M., Hollis, B. W., Adams, J. S., Bloom, B. R., & Modlin, R. L. (2006). Toll-like receptor triggering of a vitamin D-mediated human antimicrobial response. Science, 311, 1770-1773.

Lönnrot, M., Korpela, K., Knip, M., Ilonen, J., Simell, O., Korhonen, S., Savola, K., Muona, P., Simell, T., Koskela, P., & al. (2000). Enterovirus infection as a risk factor for beta-cell autoimmunity in a prospectively observed birth cohort: the Finnish Diabetes Prediction and Prevention Study. Diabetes, 49, 1314.

Lower, R., Tonjes, R. R., Boller, K., Denner, J., Kaiser, B., Phelps, R. C., & al. (1998). Development of insulin-dependent diabetes mellitus does not depend on specific expression of the human endogenous retrovirus HERV-K. Cell, 95, 11-14.

Ludvigsson, J. (2006). Why diabetes incidence increases-a unifying theory. Annals of the New York Academy of Sciences, 1079, 374-382.

Lutsey, P. L., Pankow, J. S., Bertoni, A. G., Szklo, M., & Folsom, A. R. (2009). Serological evidence of infections and type 2 diabetes: the MultiEthnic Study of Atherosclerosis. Diabetic Medicine, 26, 149-152.

Malecki, M., Bien, A. I., Galicka-Latala, D., Stachura, J., & Sieradzki, I. (1996). The prevalence of Helicobacter pylori infection and types of gastritis in diabetic patients. The Krakow study. Experimental and Clinical Endocrinology & Diabetes, 104, 365-369.

Manco, M., Putignani, L., & Bottazzo, G. F. (2010). Gut microbiota, lipopolysaccharides, and innate immunity in the pathogenesis of obesity and cardiovascular risk. Endocrines Reviews, 31, 817-844.

Marliss, E. B. (1983). The juvenile diabetes foundation workshop on spontaneously diabetic BB rat as potential for insight into human juvenile diabetes. Metabolism Clinical and Experimental, 32(Suppl 1), 1-166.

Marttila, J., Juhela, S., Vaarala, O., Hyöty, H., Roivainen, M., Hinkkanen, A., Vilja, P., Simell, O., & Ilonen, J. (2001). Responses of coxsackievirus B4-specific T-cell lines to 2C protein-characterization of epitopes with special reference to the GAD65 homology region. Virology, 284, 131-141.

Mason, A. L., Lau J. Y. N., Hoang, N., Qian, K., Alexander, G. J. M., Xu, L., Guo, L., Jacob, S., Regenstein, F. G., Zimmerman, R., Everhart, J. E., Wasserfall, C., MacLaren, N. K., & Perrillo, R. P. (1999). Association of Diabetes Mellitus and Chronic Hepatitis C Virus Infection. Hepatology, 29(2), 328-333.

Matsuzaki, T., Nagata, Y., Kado, S., Uchida, K., kato, I., Hashimoto, S., & Yokokura, T. (1997). Prevention of onset in an insulin-dependent diabetes mellitus model, NOD mice, by oral feeding of Lactobacillus casei. APMIS, 105, 643-649.

McDonald, W. L., O'Riley, K. J., Schroen, C. J., & Condron, R. J. (2005). Heat inactivation of Mycobacterium avium ssp. paratuberculosis in milk. Applied Environmental Microbiology, 71, 1785-1789.

McEvoy, R., Cooper, L., Rubinstein, P., Fedun, B., & Ginsberg-Feliner, F. (1986). Type I diabetes mellitus (IDDM) and autoimmunity in patients with congenital rubella syndrome (CRS): increased incidence of insulin autoantibodies. Diabetes, 35, 187A.

Meadus, W. J., Gill, C. O., Duff, P., Badoni, M., & Saucier, L. (2008). Prevalence on beef carcasses of Mycobacterium avium subsp. paratuberculosis DNA. International Journal of Food Microbiology, 124, 291-294.

Menser, M. A., Forrest, J. M., & Bransby, R. D. (1978). Rubella infection and diabetes mellitus. Lancet, 1, 57-60.

Momotani, E., Whipple, D. L., Thiermann, A. B., & Cheville, N. F. (1988). Role of M cells and macrophages in the entrance of Mycobacterium paratuberculosis into domes of ileal Peyer's patches in calves. Veterinary Pathology, 25(2), 131-137.

Morishima, T., McClintock, P. R., Auklakh, G. S., Billups, L. C., & Notkins, A. L. (1982). Genomic and receptor attachment difference between mengovirus and encephalomyocarditis virus. Virology, 122, 461-465.

Mutharia, L. M., Klassen, M. D., Fairles, J., Sarbut, S., & Gill, C. O. (2010). Mycobacterium avium subsp. paratuberculosis in muscle, lymphatic and organ tissues from cows with advanced Johne's disease. International Journal of Food Microbiology, 136, 340-344.

Muting, D., Wohlgemuth, D., & Dorsett, R. (1969). Liver cirrhosis and diabetes mellitus. Geriatrics, 24, 91-99.

Nabipour, I., Vahdat, K., Jafari, S. M., Pazoki, R., & Sanjdideh, Z. (2006). The association of metabolic syndrome and Chlamydia pneumoniae, Helicobacter pylori, cytomegalovirus, and herpes simplex virus type 1: the Persian Gulf Healthy Heart Study. Cardiovascular Diabetology, 5, 25.

Nakagawa, C., Hanafusa, T., Miyagawa, J., Yutsudo, M., Nakajima, H., Yamamoto, K., Tomita, K., Kono, N., Hakura, A., & Tarui, S. (1992). Retrovirus gag protein p30 in the islets of nonobese diabetic mice: relevance for pathogenesis of diabetes mellitus. Diabetologia, 35, 614-618.

Naser, S. A., Ghobrial, G., Romero, C., & Valentine, J. F. (2004). Culture of Mycobacterium avium subspecies paratuberculosis from the blood of patients with Crohn's disease. Lancet, 364, 1039-1044.

Naser, S. A., Schwartz, D., & Shafran, I. (2000). Isolation of Mycobacterium avium subsp paratuberculosis from breast milk of Crohn's disease patients. American Journal of Gastroenterology, 95(4), 1094-1095.

Ngu Ngwa, V., Attili, A. R., Preziuso, S., Valente. C., & Cuteri, V. (2010). A comparative study of serum and milk ELISAs for the diagnosis of Ovine Paratuberculosis (Ovine Johne's Disease – OJD). In The Acts of XVIII International Congress of FeMeSPRum (pp. 32-37).

Nichols, G. P. (1957). *Diabetes among young tuberculous patients; a review of the association of the two diseases. American Review of Tuberculosis, 76, 1016-1030.*

Nicoletti, F., Scalia, G., Lunetta, M., Condorelli, F., Di Mauro, M., Barcellini, W., Stracuzzi, S., Pagano, M., & Meroni, P. L. (1990). *Correlation between islet cell antibodies and anti-cytomegalovirus IgM and IgG antibodies in healthy first-degree relatives of type 1 (insulin-dependent) diabetic patient. Clinical Immunology and Immunopathology, 55, 139-147.*

Niedereau, C., Fischer, R., Sonnenberg, A., Stremmel, W., Trampisch, H., & Strohmeyer, G. (1985). *Survival and causes of death in cirrhotic and noncirrhotic patients with primary hemochromatosis. The New England Journal of Medicine, 313, 1256-1262.*

Nigro, G., Pacella, M. E., Patane, E., & Midulla, M. (1986). *Multi-system Coxsackievirus B-6 infection with findings suggestive of diabetes mellitus. European Journal of Paediatrics, 145, 557-559.*

Numazaki, K., Goldman, H., Seemayer, T. A., Wong, I., & Wainberg, M. A. (1990). *Infection by human cytomegalovirus and rubella virus of cultured human fetal islets of Langerhans. In Vivo, 4, 49-54.*

Numazaki, K., Goldman, H., Wong, I., & Wainberg, M. A. (1989). *Infection of cultured human fetal pancreatic islet cells by rubella virus. American Journal of Clinical Pathology, 91, 446-451.*

Nyman, U., Lundberg, I., Hedfors, E., & Pettersson, I. (1990). *Recombinant 70-kD protein used for determination of auto-antigenic epitopes recognized by anti-RNP sera. Clinical & Experimental Immunology, 81,52-58.*

Ohashi, P. S., Oehen, S., Buerki, K., Pircher, H., Ohashi, C. T., Odermatt, B., Malissen, B., Zinkernagel, R. M., & Hengartner, H. (1991). *Ablation of 'tolerance' and induction of diabetes by virus infection in viral antigen transgenic mice. Cell, 65, 305-317.*

Ojetti, V., Pellicano, R., Fagoonee, S., Migneco, A., Berrutti, M., & Gasbarrini, A. (2010). *Helicobacter pylori infection and diabetes. Minerva Medica, 101, 115-119.*

Okada, H., Kuhn, C., Feillet, H.,& Bach, J. F. (2010). *The 'hygiene hypothesis' for autoimmune and allergic diseases: an update. Clinical & Experimental Immunology, 160, 1-9.*

Oldensbury, B., Diepersloot, R. J. A., & Hoekstra, J. B. L. (1996). *High seroprevalence of Helicobacter pylori in diabetes mellitus patients. Digestive Diseases and Sciences, 41, 458-461.*

Oldstone, M. B. A, Nerenberg, M., Southern, P., Price, J., & Lewicki, H. (1991). *Virus infection triggers insulin-dependent diabetes mellitus in a transgenic model: role of anti-self (virus) immune response. Cell, 65, 319-331.*

Oldstone, M. B. A. (1988). *Prevention of type 1 diabetes in NOD mice by virus infection. Science, 239, 500-502.*

Olsen, I., Sigurgardottir G., & Djonne, B. (2002). *Paratuberculosis with special reference to cattle. Veterinary Quarterly, 24, 12-28.*

Oluboyo, P. O. & Erasmus, R. T. (1990). *The significance of glucose intolerance in pulmonary tuberculosis. Tubercle, 71, 135-138.*

Onodera, T., Jenson, A. B., Yoon, J. W., & Notkins, A. L. (1978). *Virus-induced diabetes mellitus: reovirus infection of pancreatic beta cells in mice. Science, 301, 529-531.*

Onodera, T., Toniolo, A., Ray, U. R., Jenson, A. B., Knazek, R. A., & Notkins, A. L. (1981). *Virus-induced diabetes mellitus. The Journal of Experimental Medicine, 153, 1457-1465.*

Ott, S. L., Well, S. J., & Wagner, B. A. (1999). *Herd- level economic losses associated with Johne's disease on U.S. dairy operations. Preventive Veterinary Medicine, 40, 179-192.*

Ou, D., Mitchell, L. A., Metzger, D. L., Gillam, S., & Tingle, A. J. (2000). *Cross-reactive rubella virus and glutamic acid decarboxylase (65 and 67) protein determinants recognized by T cells of patients with type 1 diabetes mellitus. Diabetologia, 43, 750-762.*

Ozyilkan, E. & Arslan, M. (1996). *Increased prevalence of diabetes mellitus in patients with chronic hepatitis C virus infection. The American Journal of Gastroenterology, 91, 1480-1481.*

Ozylikan, E., Erbas, T., Simsek, H., Telatar, F., Kayhan, B., & Telatar, H. (1994). Increased prevalence of hepatitis C virus antibodies in patients with diabetes mellitus [Letter]. Journal of Internal Medicine, 235, 283-285.

Paccagnini, D., Sieswerda, L., Rosu, V., Masala, S., Pacifico, A., Gazouli, M., Ikonomopoulos, J., Ahmed, N., Zanetti, S., & Sechi, L. A. (2009). Linking chronic infection and autoimmune diseases: Mycobacterium avium subspecies paratuberculosis, SLC11A1 polymorphisms and type-1 diabetes mellitus. PLoS One, 4(9), e7109.

Pak, C. Y., Cha, C. Y., Rajotte, R. V., McArthur, R. G., & Yoon, J. W. (1990). Human pancreatic islet cell-specific 38 kDa autoantigen identified by cytomegalovirus-induced monoclonal islet cell autoantibody. Diabetologia, 33, 569-572.

Pak, C. Y., Jun, H. S., Lee, M., & Yoon, J. W. (1995). Beta cell-specific expression of retroviral mRNAs and group-specific antigen and the development of beta cell-specific autoimmunity in non-obese diabetic mice. Autoimmunity, 20, 19-24.

Pak, C.Y., Eun, H. M., McArthur, R.G., & Yoon, J. W. (1988). Association of cytomegalovirus infection with autoimmune type 1 diabetes. Lancet, 2, 1-4.

Parkkonen, F., Hyöty, H., Ilonen, J., Reijonen, H., Yla-Herttuala, S., & Leinikki, P. (1994). Antibody reactivity to an Epstein-Barr virus BERF4- encoded epitope occurring also in Asp-57 region of HLA-DQ8 β chain. Clinical & Experimental Immunology, 95, 287-293.

Parkkonen, P., Hyöty, H., Koskinen, L., & Leinikki, P. (1992). Mumps virus infects beta cells in human fetal islet cell cultures upregulating the expression of HLA class I molecules. Diabetologia, 35, 63-69.

Pato, E., Cour, M. I., Gonzalez-Cuadrado, S., Gonzalez-Gomez, C., Munoz, J. J., & Figueredo, A. (1992). Coxsackie B4 and cytomegalovirus in patients with insulin-dependent diabetes. Anales de Medicina Interna, 9, 30-32.

Patterson, C. C., Dahlquist, G. G., Gyurus, E., Green, A., & Soltész, G. (2009). Incidence trends for childhood type 1 diabetes in Europe during 1989-2003 and predicted new cases 2005-20: a multicentre prospective registration study. Lancet, 373, 2027-2033.

Pavlik, I., Falkinham III, J. O., & Kazda, J. (2009). Environments providing favourable conditions for the multiplication and transmission of mycobacteria, 89-197. In: Kazda J., Pavlik I., Falkinham III J.O., Hruska K. (eds.): The Ecology of Mycobacteria: Impact on Animal's and Human's Health. 2nd ed. Springer, (pp. 522).

Pearce, L. E., Truong, H. T., Crawford, R. A., Yates, G. F., Cavaignac, S., & de Lisle, G. W. (2001). Effect of turbulent-flow pasteurization on survival of Mycobacterium avium ssp. paratuberculosis added to raw milk. Applied Environmental Microbiology, 67, 3964-3969.

Petrides, A. S. (1994). Liver disease and diabetes mellitus. Diabetes Rev, 2, 2-18.

Prabhakar, B. S., Haspel, M. V., McClintock, P. R., & Notkins, A. L. (1982). High frequency of antigenic variants among naturally occurring human Coxsackie B4 virus isolates identified by monoclonal antibodies. Nature, 300, 374-376.

Prince, G., Jenson, A. B., Billups, L., Notkins, A. L. (1978). Infection of human pancreatic beta cell cultures with mumps virus. Nature, 27, 158-161.

Pundziute-Lycka, A., Urbonaite, B., & Dahlquist, G. (2000). Infections and risk of Type I (insulin-dependent) diabetes mellitus in Lithuanian children. Diabetologia, 43, 1229-1234.

Query, C. C. & Keene, J. D. (1987). A human autoimmune protein associated with U_1 RNA contains a region of homology that is crossreactive with retroviral $p30^{gag}$ antigen. Cell, 51, 211-220.

Rabinovitch, A. (1994). Immunoregulatory and cytokine imbalances in the pathogenesis of IDDM: therapeutic intervention by immunostimulation? Diabetes, 43, 613-621.

Rademaker, J. L., Vissers, M. M., & Te Giffel, M. C. (2007). Effective heat inactivation of Mycobacterium avium subsp. paratuberculosis in raw milk contaminated with naturally infected feces. Applied Environmental Microbiology, 73(13), 4185-4190.

Rani, P. S., Sechi, L. A., & Ahmed, N. (2010). Mycobacterium avium subspecies paratuberculosis is a trigger of type-1 diabetes: destination Sardinia, or beyond? Gut Pathogens, 2(1), 1-6.

Rayfield, E., Kelly, K., & Yoon, J. W. (1986). Rubella virus-induced diabetes in hamsters. Diabetes, 35, 1276-1281.

Redondo, M. J., Jeffrey, J., Fain, P. R., Eisenbarth, G. S., & Davis, B. (2008). Concordance for islet autoimmunity among monozygotic twins. The New England Journal of Medicine, 359, 2849-2850.

Riccardi, G., Rivellese, A. A., & Giacco, R. (2008). Role of glycemic index and glycemic load in the healthy state, in prediabetes, and in diabetes. American Journal of Clinical Nutrition, 87(1), 269S-274S.

Richardson, S. J., Willcox, A., Bone, A. J., Foulis, A. K., & Morgan, N. G. (2009). The prevalence of enteroviral capsid protein vp1 immunostaining in pancreatic islets in human type 1 diabetes. Diabetologia, 52, 1143-1151.

Richter, W., Mertens, T., Schoel, B., Muir, P., Ritzkowsky, A., Scherbaum, W. A., & Boehm, B. O. (1994). Sequence homology of the diabetes-associated autoantigen glutamate decarboxylase with coxsackie B4-2C protein and heat shock protein 60 mediates no molecular mimicry of autoantibodies. The Journal of Experimental Medicine, 180, 721-726.

Rosseels, V. & Huygen, K. (2008). Vaccination against paratuberculosis. Expert Review Vaccines, 7(6), 817-832.

Rosu, V., Ahmed, N., Paccagnini, D., Gerlach, G., Fadda, G., Seyed, E. H., Zanetti, S., & Sechi, L.A. (2009). Specific immunoassays confirm association of Mycobacterium avium subsp. paratuberculosis with type-1 but not type-2 diabetes mellitus. PLos One, 4(2), e4386.

Rosu, V., Ahmed, N., Paccagnini, D., Pacifico, A., Zanetti, S., & Sechi, L. A. (2008). Mycobacterium avium subspecies paratuberculosis is not associated with Type-2 Diabetes Mellitus. Annal of Clinical Microbiological Antimicrobials, 7, 7-9.

Sairenji, T., Daibata, M., Sorli, C. H., Qvistbäck, H., Humphreys, R. E., Ludwigsson, J., Palmer, J., Landin-Olsson, M., Sundkvist, G., Michelsen, B., & al. (1991). Relating homology between the Epstein-Barr virus BOLF1 molecule and HLA-DQw8 beta chain to recent onset type 1 (insulin-dependent) diabetes mellitus. Diabetologia, 34, 33-39.

Salminen, K., Sadeharju, K., Lönnrot, M., Vähäsalo, P., Kupila, A., Korhonen, S., Ilonen, J., Simell, O., Knip, M., & Hyöty, H. (2003). Enterovirus infections are associated with the induction of beta-cell autoimmunity in a prospective birth cohort study. Journal of Medical Virology, 69, 91-98.

Sarmiento, L., Cabrera-Rode, E., Lekuleni, L., Cuba, I., Molina, G., Fonseca, M., Heng-Hung, L., Borroto, A. D., Gonzalez, P., Mas-Lago, P., & Diaz-Horta, O. (2007). Occurrence of enterovirus RNA in serum of children with newly diagnosed type 1 diabetes and islet cell autoantibody-positive subjects in a population with a low incidence of type 1 diabetes. Autoimmunity, 40, 540-545.

Schattner, A. & Rager-Zisman, B. (1990). Virus-induced autoimmunity. Reviews of Infectious Diseases, 12, 204-222.

Scheinin, T., Tran Minh, N. N., Tuomi, T., Miettinen, A., & Kontiainen, S. (1996). Islet cell and glutamic acid decarboxylase antibodies and heat-shock protein 65 responses in children with newly diagnosed insulin-dependent diabetes mellitus. Immunology Letters, 49(1-2), 123-126.

Schloot, N. C., Willemen, S. J., Duinkerken, G., Drijfhout, J. W., de Vries, R. R., & Roep, B. O. (2001). Molecular mimicry in type 1 diabetes mellitus revisited: T-cell clones to GAD65 peptides with sequence homology to Coxsackie or proinsulin peptides do not crossreact with homologous counterpart. Human Immunology, 62, 299-309.

Schwartz, D., Shafran, I., Romero, C., Piromalli, C., Biggerstaff, J., Naser, N., Chamberlin, W., & Naser, S. A. (2000). Use of short-term culture for identification of Mycobacterium avium subsp. paratuberculosis in tissue from Crohn's disease patients. Clinical Microbiology and Infectious, 6, 303-307.

Sechi, L. A., Ahmed, N., Felis, G. E., Duprè, I., Cannas, C., Fadda, G., Bua, A., & Zanetti, S. (2006). Immunogenicity and cytoadherence of recombinant Heparin Binding Haemagglutinin (HBHA) of Mycobacterium avium subsp. paratuberculosis: Functional promiscuity or a role in virulence? Vaccine, 24, 236-243.

Sechi, L. A., Paccagnini, D., Salza, S., Pacifico, A., Ahmed, N., & Zanetti, S. (2008). Mycobacterium avium subspecies paratuberculosis bacteremia in type-1 diabetes mellitus: an infectious trigger? Clinical Infectious Diseases, 46, 148-149.

Sechi, L. A., Scanu, A. M., Molicotti, P., Cannas, S., Mura, M., Dettori, G., Fadda, G., & Zanetti, S. (2005). Detection and isolation of Mycobacterium avium subspecies paratuberculosis from intestinal mucosal biopsies of patients with and without Crohn's disease in Sardinia. American Journal of Gastroenterology, 100, 1529-1536.

Seewaldt, S., Thomas, H. E., Ejrnaes, M., Christen, U., Wolfe, T., Rodrigo, E., Coon, B., Michelsen, B., Kay, T. W., & von Herrath, M. G. (2000). Virus-induced autoimmune diabetes: most beta-cells die through inflammatory cytokines and not perforin from autoreactive (anti-viral) cytotoxic T-lymphocytes. Diabetes, 49, 1801-1809.

Serreze, D. V., Ottendorfer, E. W., Ellis, T. M., Gauntt, C. J., & Atkinson, M. A. (2000). Acceleration of type 1 diabetes by a coxsackievirus infection requires a preexisting critical mass of autoreactive T-cells in pancreatic islets. Diabetes, 49, 708-711.

Shanahan, F. (2002). Crohn's disease. Lancet, 359, 62-69.

Sherman, D. M., Gay, J. M., & Bouley, D. S. (1990). Comparison of the complement fixation and agar gel immunodiffusion tests for the diagnosis of subclinical bovine paratuberculosis. American Journal of Veterinary Research, 51, 461-465.

Shulaw, W. P., Bech-Nielsen, S., Rings, D. M., Getzy, D. M., & Woodruff, T. S. (1993). Serodiagnosis of paratuberculosis in sheep by use of agar gel immunodiffusion. American Journal of Veterinary Research, 54, 13-19.

Simo, R., Hernandez, C., Genesca, J., Jardi, R., & Mesa, J. (1996). High prevalence of hepatitis C virus infection in diabetic patients. Diabetes Care, 19, 998-1000.

Singh, A. V., Singh, S. V., Makharia, G. K., Singh, P. K., & Sohal, J. S. (2008). Presence and characterization of Mycobacterium avium subspecies paratuberculosis from clinical and suspected cases of Crohn's disease and in the healthy human population in India. International Journal of Infectious Diseases, 12(2), 190-197.

Singh, U. P., Singh, S., Singh, R., Karls, R. K., Quinn, F. D., Potter, M. E., & Lillard, J. W., Jr. (2007). Influence of Mycobacterium avium subsp. paratuberculosis on colitis development and specific immune responses during disease. Infectious Immunology, 75, 3722-3728.

So, W. Y., Tong, P. C., Ko, G. T., Ma, R. C., Ozaki, R., Kong, A. P., Yang, X., Ho, C. S., Lam, C. C., & Chan, J. C. (2009). Low plasma adiponectin level, white blood cell count and Helicobacter pylori titre independently predict abnormal pancreatic beta-cell function. Diabetes Research and Clinical Practice, 86, 89-95.

Spahr, U. & Schafroth, K. (2001). Fate of Mycobacterium avium subsp. paratuberculosis in Swiss Hard and Semihard Cheese Manufactured from raw milk. Applied and Environmental Microbiology, 67(9), 4199-4205.

Stabel, J. R. & Lambertz, A. (2004). Efficacy of pasteurization conditions for the inactivation of Mycobacterium avium subsp. paratuberculosis in milk. Journal of Food Protection, 67, 2719-2726.

Stabel, J. R. (2001). On-farm batch pasteurisation destroys Mycobacterium paratuberculosis in waste milk. Journal of Dairy Sciences, 84, 524-527.

Stauffer, Y., Marguerat, S., Meylan, F., Ucla, C., Sutkowski, N., Huber, B., Pelet, T., & Conrad, B. (2001). Interferon-alpha-induced endogenous superantigen: a model linking environment and autoimmunity. Immunity, 15, 591-601.

Stefan, Y., Malaisse-Lagae, F., Yoon, J. W., Notkins, A. L., & Orci, L. (1978). Virus-induced diabetes in mice: a quantitative evaluation of islet cell population by immunofluorescence technique. Diabetologia, 15, 395-401.

Stehman, S. M. (1996). Paratuberculosis in Sheep, Goats, Deer and South American Camelids in Paratuberculosis (Johne's Disease), ed. RW Sweeney; Veterinary Clinics of North America Food Animal Practice, 12(2), 441-455.

Stene, L.C. & Rewers, M. (2012). Immunology in the clinic review series; focus on type 1 diabetes and viruses: the enterovirus link to type 1 diabetes: critical review of human studies. Clinical & Experimental Immunology, 168, 12-23.

Streeter, R. N., Hoffsis, G. F., Bech-Nielsen, S., Shulaw, W. P., & Rings, D. M. (1995). Isolation of Mycobacterium paratuberculosis from colostrums and milk of subclinically infected cows. American Journal of Veterinary Research, 56, 1322-1324.

Stumvoll, M., Goldstein, B. J., & van Haeften, T. W. (2005). Type 2 diabetes: principles of pathogenesis and therapy. Lancet, 365, 1333-1346.

Suenaga, K. & Yoon, J. W. (1988). Association of beta cell-specific expression of endogenous retrovirus with the development of insulitis and diabetes in NOD mice. Diabetes, 37, 1722-1726.

Sung, N. & Collins, M. (2000). Effect of three factors in cheese production (pH, salt, and heat) on Map viability. Applied and Environmental Microbiology, 66, 1334-1339.

Surcel, H. M., Ilonen, J., Kaar, M. L., Hyöty, H., & Leinikki, P. (1988). Infection by multiple viruses and lymphocyte abnormalities at the diagnosis of diabetes. Acta Paediatrica Scandinavica, 77, 471-474.

Sweeney, R. W., Whitlock, R. H., & Rosenberger, A. E. (1992). Mycobacterium paratuberculosis cultured from milk and supramammary lymph nodes of infected asymptomatic cows. Journal of Clinical Microbiology, 30(1), 166-171.

Sweeney, R.W. (1996). Transmission of paratuberculosis. Veterinary Clinics of North America Food Animal Practice, 12, 305-312.

Szopa, T. M., Titchener, P. A., Portwood, N. D., & Taylor, K. W. (1993). Diabetes mellitus due to viruses-some recent developments. Diabetologia, 36, 687-695.

Szopa, T. M., Ward, T., & Taylor, K. W. (1986). Impaired metabolic functions in human pancreatic islets following infection with Coxsackie B4 virus in vitro. Diabetologia, 30, 587A.

Tajima, M., Yazawa, T., Hagiwara, K., Kurosawa, T., & Takahashi, K. (1992). Diabetes mellitus in cattle infected with bovine viral diarrhea mucosal disease virus. Journal of Veterinary Medicine A, 39, 616-620.

Tajima, M., Yuasa, M., Kawanabe, M., Taniyama, H., Yamato, O., Maede, Y. (1999). Possible causes of diabetes mellitus in cattle infected with bovine diarrhoea virus. Zentralblatt fur Veterinarmedizin Reihe B, 46, 207-215.

Talal, N., Flescher, E., & Dang, H. (1992). Are endogenous retroviruses involved in human autoimmune disease? Journal of Autoimmunity, 5(A), 61-66.

Tanaka, S., Nishida, Y., Aida, K., Maruyama, T., Shimada, A., Suzuki, M., Shimura, H., Takizawa, S., Takahashi, M., Akiyama, D., Arai-Yamashita, S., Furuya, F., Kawaguchi, A., Kaneshige, M., Katoh, R., Endo, T., & Kobayashi, T. (2009). Enterovirus infection, CXC chemokine ligand 10 (CXCL10), and CXCR3 circuit: a mechanism of accelerated beta-cell failure in fulminant type 1 diabetes. Diabetes, 58, 2285-2291.

Tian, J., Lehmann, P. V.,& Kaufman, D. L. (1994). T cell cross-reactivity between Coxsackie virus and glutamate decarboxylase is associated with a murine diabetes susceptibility allele. The Journal of Experimental Medicine, 180, 1979-1984.

Tiittanen, M., Westerholm-Ormio, M., Verkasalo, M., Savilahti, E., & Vaarala, O. (2008). Infiltration of forkhead box P3-expressing cells in small intestinal mucosa in coeliac disease but not in type 1 diabetes. Clinical & Experimental Immunology, 152, 498-507.

Toniolo, A., Onodera, T., Jordan, G., Yoon, J. W., & Notkins, A. L. (1982). Virus induced diabetes mellitus: glucose abnormalities produced in mice by all six members of the Coxsackie B virus group. Diabetes, 31, 496-499.

Tracy, S., Drescher, K. M., Chapman, N. M., Kim, K. S., Carson, S. D., Pirruccello, S., Lane, P. H., Romero, J. R., & Leser, J. S. (2002). Toward testing the hypothesis that group B coxsackieviruses (CVB) trigger insulin-dependent diabetes: inoculating nonobese diabetic mice with CVB markedly lowers diabetes incidence. Journal of Virology, 76, 12097-12111.

Tracy, S., Drescher, K. M., Jackson, J. D., Kim, K., & Kono, K. (2010). Enteroviruses, type 1 diabetes and hygiene: a complicated relationship. Reviews in Medical Virology, 20, 106-116.

Turley, S. J., Lee, J. W., Dutton-Swain, N., Mathis, D., & Benoist, C. (2005). Endocrine self and gut nonself intersect in the pancreatic lymph nodes. Proceedings of the National Academic of Sciences of the United States of America, 102, 17729-17733.

Tuvemo, T., Dahlquist, G., Frisk, G., Blom, L., Friman, G., Landin-Olsson, M., & Diderholm, H. (1989). The Swedish childhood diabetes study III: IgM against Coxsackie B viruses in newly diagnosed type 1 (insulin-dependent) diabetic children - no evidence of increased antibody frequency. Diabetologia, 32, 745-747.

Vaarala, O., Atkinson, M. A., & Neu, J. (2008). The Perfect Storm' for type 1 diabetes. The complex interplay between intestinal microbiota, gut permeability, and mucosal immunity. Diabetes, 57, 2555-2562.

van Halteren, A. G., Roep, B. O., Gregori, S., Cooke, A., van Eden, W., Kraal, G., & Wauben, M. H. (2002). Cross-reactive mycobacterial and self hsp60 epitope recognition in I-A(g7) expressing NOD, NOD-asp and Biozzi AB/H mice. Journal of Autoimmunity, 18, 139-147.

van Maanen, C., Koster, C., van Veen, B., Kalis, C. H. J., & Collins, M. T. (2003). Validation of Mycobacterium avium subsp. paratuberculosis antibody detecting ELISA's. In: R. A. Juste, M. V. Geijo, J. M. Garrido (Eds.), Proceedings of the 7th International Colloquium on Paratuberculosis, Bilbao, Spain, (pp 182).

von Herrath, M. & Holz, A. (1997). Pathological changes in the islet milieu precede infiltration of islets and destruction of beta-cells by autoreactive lymphocytes in a transgenic model of virus-induced IDDM. Journal of Autoimmunity, 10, 231-238.

von Herrath, M. G., Allison, J., Miller, J. F., & Oldstone, M. B. (1995). Focal expression of interleukin-2 does not break unresponsiveness to 'self' (viral) antigen expressed in beta cells but enhances development of autoimmune disease (diabetes) after initiation of an anti-self immune response. The Journal of Clinical Investigation, 95, 477-485.

von Herrath, M. G., Fujinami, R. S., & Whitton, J. L. (2003). Microorganisms and autoimmunity: making the barren field fertile? Nature Reviews Microbiology, 1, 151-157.

Vuorinen, T., Nikolakaros, G., Simell, O., Hyypia, T., & Vainionpaa, R. (1992). Mumps and Coxsackie B3 virus infection of human fetal pancreatic islet-like cell clusters. Pancreas, 7, 460-464.

Wang, D., Coscoy, L., Zylberberg, M., Avila, P. C., Boushey, H. A., Ganem, D., & De Risi, J. L. (2002). Microarray-based detection and genotyping of viral pathogens. Proceedings of The National Academy of Sciences of the United States of America, 99, 15687-15692.

Ward, K.P., Galloway, W. H., & Auchterlonie, I. A. (1979). Congenital cytomegalovirus infection and diabetes. Lancet, 1, 497.

Wellen, K. E. & Hotamisligil, G. S. (2005). Inflammation, stress, and diabetes. The Journal of Clinical Investigation, 115, 1111-1119.

Wen, L., Ley, RE., Volchkov, P. Y., Stranges, P. B., Avanesyan, L., Stonebraker, A. C., Hu, C., Wong, F. S., Szot, G. L., Bluestone, J. A., Gordon, J. I., & Chervonsky, A. V. (2008). Innate immunity and intestinal microbiota in the development of Type 1 diabetes. Nature, 455, 1109-1113.

Wenzlau, J. M., Juhl, K., Yu, L., Moua, O., Sarkar, S. A., Gottlieb, P., Rewers, M., Eisenbarth, G. S., Jensen, J., Davidson, H. W., & Hutton, J. C. (2007). The cation efflux transporter ZnT8 (Slc30A8) is a major autoantigen in human type 1 diabetes. Proceedings of the National Academic of Sciences of the United States of America, 104(43), 17040-17045.

Westerholm-Ormio, M., Vaarala, O., Pihkala, P., Ilonen, J., & Savilahti, E. (2003). Immunologic activity in the small intestinal mucosa of pediatric patients with type 1 diabetes. Diabetes, 52, 2287-2295.

Whittington, R. J., Marsh, I. B., & Reddacliff, L. A. (2005). Survival of Mycobacterium avium subsp. paratuberculosis in dam water and sediment. Applied Environmental Microbiology, 71(9), 5304-5308.

Wijesekara, N., Dai, F. F., Hardy, A. B., Giglou, P. R., Bhattacharjee, A., Koshkin, V., Chimienti, F., Gaisano, H. Y., Rutter, G. A., & Wheeler, M. B. (2010). Beta cell-specific Znt8 deletion in mice causes marked defects in insulin processing, crystallisation and secretion. Diabetologia, 53(8), 1656-1668.

Wilberz, S., Partke, H. J., Dagnaes-Hansen, F., & Herberg, L. (1991). Persistent MHV (mouse hepatitis virus) infection reduces the incidence of diabetes mellitus in non-obese diabetic mice. Diabetologia, 34, 2-5.

Williams, E. S., Spraker, T. R., & Schoonveld, G. G. (1979). Paratuberculosis (Johne's disease) in bighorn sheep and a Rocky Mountain goat in Colorado. Journal of Wildlife Diseases, 15, 221-227.

Woodward, M., Morrison, C., & Mccoll, K. (2000). An investigation into factors associated with Helicobacter pylori infection. Journal of Clinical Epidemiology, 53, 175-181.

Yadav, H., Jain, S., & Sinha, P. R. (2007). Antidiabetic effect of probiotic dahi containing Lactobacillusacidophilus and Lactobacillus casei in high fructose fed rats. Nutrition, 23, 62-68.

Yasumoto, N., Hara, M., Kitamoto, Y.U., Nakayama, M., & Sato, T. (1992). Cytomegalovirus infection associated with acute pancreatitis, rhabdomyolysis and renal failure. Internal Medicine, 31, 426-430.

Yeung, W. C., Rawlinson, W. D., & Craig, M. E. (2011). Enterovirus infection and type 1 diabetes mellitus: systematic review and meta-analysis of observational molecular studies. British Medical Journal, 342, d35.

Yoon, J. W. & Kominek, H. I. (1996). Role of Coxsackie B viruses in the pathogenesis of diabetes mellitus: Microorganisms, Autoimmune Diseases, Rose, N. R., Friedman, H. (eds). Plenum Press: New York, 129-158.

Yoon, J. W., Austin, M., Onodera, T., & Notkins, A. L. (1979). Virus-induced diabetes mellitus: isolation of a virus from the pancreas of a child with diabetic ketoacidosis. The New England Journal of Medicine, 300, 1173-1179.

Yoon, J. W., Bachurski, C. J., & McArthur, R. G. (1986). Concept of virus as an etiological agent in the development of IDDM. Diabetes Research and Clinical Practice, 2, 365-366.

Yoon, J. W., London, W. T., Curfman, B. L., Brown, R. L., & Notkins, A. L. (1986). Coxsackie virus B4 produces transient diabetes in nonhuman primates. Diabetes, 35, 712-716.

Yoon, J. W., McClintock, P. R., Onodera, T., & Notkins, A. L. (1980). Virus-induced diabetes mellitus XVIII. Inhibition by a nondiabetogenic variant of encephalomyocarditis virus. The Journal of Experimental Medicine, 152, 878-892.

Yoon, J. W., Morishima, T., McClintock, P. R., Austin, M., & Notkins, A. L. (1984). Virus-induced diabetes mellitus: mengovirus infects pancreatic beta cells in strains of mice resistant to encephalomyocarditis virus. Journal of Virology, 50, 684-690.

Yoon, J. W., Onodera, T., & Notkins, A. L. (1978). Virus-induced diabetes mellitus. XV. Beta cell damage and insulin-dependent hyperglycemia in mice infected with Coxsackie virus B4. The Journal of Experimental Medicine, 148, 1068-1080.

Yoon, J. W., Selvaggio S., Onodera, T., Wheeler, J., & Jenson, AB. (1981). Infection of cultured human pancreatic β cell with reovirus type 3. Diabetologia, 20, 462-467.

Zack, M. B., Fulkerson, L. L., & Stein, E. (1973). Glucose intolerance in pulmonary tuberculosis. American Review of Respiratory Disease Journal, 108, 1164-1169.

Zoll, J., Erkens Hulshof, S., Lanke, K., Verduyn Lunen, F., Melchers, W. J. G., Schoondermark-van de Ven, E., Roivainen, M., Galama, J. M. D., & van Kuppeveld, F. J. M. (2009). Saffold virus, a human Theiler's-like cardiovirus, is ubiquitous and causes infection early in life. PLoS Pathogens, 5, e1000416.

Neuroimmune Alterations in Diabetes: Implications to Molecular Pathomechanisms of Complications

Anna Boyajyan, Meri Hovsepyan, Elina Arakelova, Gohar Tsakanova

Institute of Molecular Biology

National Academy of Sciences of the Republic of Armenia, Armenia

1   Introduction

Diabetes mellitus (DM) is a group of metabolic diseases characterized by hyperglycemia resulting from defects in insulin secretion, insulin action, or both. The chronic hyperglycemia of diabetes is associated with long-term damage, dysfunction, and failure of different organs, especially the eyes, kidneys, nerves, heart, and blood vessels (Bonow & Gheorghiade, 2004).

The number of patients with DM is steadily increasing due to population growth, aging, urbanization, and increasing prevalence of obesity and physical inactivity (Bonow & Gheorghiade, 2004; Wild *et al.*, 2004; Shaw *et al.*, 2010). It was estimated that there were 171 million people suffering from diabetes mellitus in 2000 and in 2030 the number of diabetes-affected people will increase to 439 million (Bonow & Gheorghiade, 2004; Wild *et al.*, 2004; Shaw *et al.*, 2010). The expected rise in the number of diabetic patients will lead to an enormous increase in the socioeconomic burden.

DM is characterized by multiple vascular complications. Endothelial and vascular smooth muscle cell dysfunction inflammation and hypercoagubility are the key factors in diabetic arteriopathy (Huysman & Mathieu, 2009). Beside the severe microvascular complications, diabetic nephropathy, retinopathy or neuropathy, macrovascular complications including diabetic cardiomyopathy are frequent among diabetic patients (Marshall & Flyvbjerg, 2006; Huysman & Mathieu, 2009; Keymel *et al.*, 2011). DM leads to premature and accelerated atherosclerosis with an increased risk of cardiovascular and cerebrovascular events (Wingard *et al.*, 1993; Grundy *et al.*, 1999; Fox *et al.*, 2004; Booth *et al.*, 2006). Thus, coronary artery disease (Devine *et al.*, 1981; Cuocolo *et al.*, 2009), myocardial ischemia (Ambepityia *et al.*, 1990), infarction (Weitzman *et al.*, 1982; Kapur & De Palma, 2007) and ischemic stroke (Oppenheimer *et al.*, 1985; Olsson *et al.*, 1990; Jorgensen *et al.*, 1994; Laing *et al.*, 2003; Idris *et al.*, 2006) commonly occurs and represent the ultimate cause of death in patients with DM (Weitzman *et al.*, 1982; Kapur & De Palma, 2007; Oppenheimer *et al.*, 1985; Olsson *et al.*, 1990; Jorgensen *et al.*, 1994; Laing *et al.*, 2003).

Research efforts aim to elucidate pathophysiological mechanisms contributing to the disease process, progression and complications. However, the complexicity of molecular events and pathways involved in etiopathomechanisms of DM and responsible for diabetic complications creates big obstacles in understanding the real consequence of DM and related complications. This highly limits the development of the efficient measures on early diagnosis, prevention, and treatment of DM and its complications.

In the present chapter we summarize the results of our studies of neuroimmune state of patients with long-term diabetes and also provide brief overview of the related data obtained by other research groups. These findings suggest that DM is characterized by neuroimmune dysfunction, which underlies the development and progression of diabetic complications and is responsible for high frequency of cerebrovascular and cardiovascular pathologies in DM patients, as well as for association of diabetic stroke with high severity and mortality, and poor clinical outcome.

2   Alterations in the Immune Response in DM

Patients with DM have infections more often than those without DM. The course of the infections is also more complicated in this patient group. One of the possible causes of this increased prevalence of infections is defects in immunity. Both type 1 and type 2 DM (DM1 and DM2, respectively), two main forms of DM, are characterized by the immune system disturbances mainly related to the innate immunity (Moutschen *et al.*, 1992; Geerlings & Hoepelman, 1999).

DM1, or juvenile-onset diabetes, results from a cellular-mediated autoimmune destruction of the β-cells of the pancreas Langerhans islet. Markers of the immune destruction, the β-cell including autoantibodies to Langerhans islet cells, insulin, glutamic acid decarboxylase (GAD65), and tyrosine phosphatase-like protein (islet antigen-2 and islet antigen-2b) are detected in the blood of DM1 patients. In addition, DM1 is often accompanied by other autoimmune disorders including Graves' disease, Hashimoto's thyroiditis, Addison disease, pernicious anemia, and diffuse toxic goiter. Onset of DM1 is often accompanied by insulitis, an inflammation of the islets of Langerhans islets of the pancreas (Kukreja *et al.*, 2002). Interestingly, that at the same time in DM1 patients the reduced primary antibody response to T-cell dependent antigens as well as the T-cell response to primary protein antigens was shown (Eibl *et al.*, 2002).

It is well known, that early disability and mortality of DM2 patients are mainly conditioned by macrovascular complications (atherosclerosis, coronary artery disease, acute myocardial infarction, stroke, etc), provoking the development of inflammatory response (Huysman & Mathieu, 2009; Barış *et al.*, 2009). On the other hand, hyperactivation of the immune response triggered by oxidative stress or other factors, results in the dysfunction of the insulin producing β-cells and to insulin resistance (Kaneto *et al.*, 2005; Solinas *et al.*, 2007), thus promoting DM2. There are probably many different causes of DM2. Although the specific etiologies are not known, autoimmune destruction of β-cells does not occur. It is proposed that immune mediated acute phase reactions that are part of the innate immune response are involved in DM2 pathogenesis. This suggestion is supported by a large number of experimental data showing elevated levels of serum amyloid A, C-reactive protein, and cytokines in the blood of DM2 patients (Crook *et al.*, 1993; Pickup & Crook, 1998; Crook, 2004; Donath & Shoelson, 2011). Regarding cytokines, in early stage of DM2 the increase in interleukin (IL)-1 and tumor necrosis factor-α (TNF-α) was observed (Ozer *et al.*, 2003), whereas in long-term DM2 the decreases production of IL-1β and IL-2 by monocytes and T lymphocytes was detected (Geerlings & Hoepelman, 1999). Furthermore, it was shown that poorly controlled diabetics have reduced lymphocyte proliferation in response to different stimuli (Geerlings & Hoepelman, 1999). Long-term DM2 is also characterized by a decreased chemotaxis of polymorphonuclear lymphocytes and monocytes (Delamaire *et al.*, 1997), impaired monocyte adhesion to vascular endothelium (Jialal et al., 2002), and reduced phagocytic activity (Lecube *et al.*, 2012).

In long-term DM accompanied with diabetic complications the presence of antibodies against membrane phospholipids, vascular endothelium (Kluz & Adamiec, 2003), C3d opsonins and membrane attack complex (MAC) and development of the inflammatory reactions in capillary wells (Rosoklija *et al*, 2000) were detected. In addition, it was shown that CD40–CD40L interactions promote pancreatic and adipose tissue, as well as vascular inflammation in DM2 (Seijkens *et al.*, 2013). The role of the immune response abnormalities in the development of diabetic complications is unclear. Here the main question is whether the immune system disturbances are primary pathogenic factors for DM complications or not.

In our own studies we investigated the functional state of the major mediators of the immune response, immune complexes and the complement cascade, in patients withDM1 and DM2 (Hovsepyan *et al.*, 2002; Hovsepyan *et al.*, 2002; Hovsepyan *et al.*, 2004; Ovsepyan *et al.*, 2004; Hovsepyan *et al*, 2006; Arakelova *et al.*, 2011). In total, 86 patients with DM1, 110 patients with DM2, and 96 healthy subjects have been involved in the studies. Duration of the illness was 8-10 years; all patients have DM-specific complications, micro- and macroangiopathies.

Formation of immune complexes (IC) is a normal physiological reaction of organism to foreign or autoantigen. IC may interact with both humoral and cellular components of the immune recognition system, activate the complement cascade, and thus affect the immune response on multiple levels (Schifferli *et al.*, 1986; Ng *et al.*, 1988; Moulds *et al.*, 2009). In healthy conditions IC are easily eliminated from circulation through complement deposition, followed by their opsonization, phagocytosis, and further processing by proteases (Schifferli *et al.*, 1986; Ng *et al.*, 1988; *Hebert*, 1991; Thornton, 1994). In pathologic conditions inappropriate clearance or deposition of IC result in increased levels of IC in circulation. Circulating IC (CIC) may deposit in endothelial of vascular structures provoking prolonged inflammatory response by permanent activation of the complement cascade through the classical pathway, generation of cytotoxic agents and tissue damage (Theofilopoulos, 1980; McDougal & McDuffie, 1985; Konstantinova, 1996; Shmagel & Chereshnev, 2009; Burut *et al.*, 2010). Deposition of CIC is a prominent feature of many diseases characterized by altered immune response and development of inflammatory reactions (Shmagel & Chereshnev, 2009; Burut *et al.*, 2010; Theofilopoulos & Dixon, 1980), and plays a decisive role in atherogenesis (Burut *et al.*, 2010). The most aggressive sub-population of CIC is so called "pathogenic" CIC, which may originate in the excess of either antibody or antigen. Pathogenic CIC are smaller in size than classic CIC, are hardly recognized by phagocytes and removed from circulation (Konstantinova, 1996; Cavallo & Granholm, 1990; Monsalvo *et al.*, 2011).

We evaluated the total levels of CIC and the levels of their pathogenic sub-population in the blood of patients with DM1 and DM2 in comparison to healthy controls (Hovsepyan *et al.*; 2002a; Hovsepyan *et al.*, 2002b; Ovsepyan *et al.*, 2004) using earlier described procedures for isolation of CIC and spectrophotometric determination of their levels (Digeon *et al.*, 1977; Tarnacka *et al.*, 2002). According to the obtained results in both groups of patients the increased levels of both total CIC and pathogenic CIC were detected. Thus the average levels of total CIC and pathogenic CIC in the blood of DM1 patients were 1.87and 2 times, respectively, significantly higher than in controls ($p<0.05$). In case of DM2 patients the average blood levels of total CIC and their pathogenic sub-population were, respectively, 1.67and 4 times significantly higher than in controls ($p<0.05$).A positive correlation between the blood levels of total and pathogenic CIC in DM1 ($r = 0.9, p< 0.05$) and DM2 ($r = 0.85, p<0.05$) was detected indicating that elevation in the total blood CIC levels in DM mainly occurs due to increase in pathogenic species of CIC in their general population.

Further we evaluated the protein composition of total CIC isolated from the blood of DM1 and DM2 patients by sodium dodecyl sulphate (SDS)-gel electrophoresis. According to the obtained results (Figure 1) high level of specificity for protein composition of CIC was detected, when comparing DM1 and DM2 with each other or with other diseased conditions characterized by the increased blood levels of CIC and their pathogenic subpopulation. Here for comparison we include data related to schizophrenia (Hakobyan *et al.*, 2004; Hakobyan *et al.*, 2001), strokes (Boiadzhian *et al.*, 2007; Arakelian *et al.*, 2003), and familial Mediterranean fever (complicated and not complicated with renal amyloidosis) (Mkrtchyan *et al.*, 2002). In each case different distribution of the CIC proteins by molecular weights was detected.

The complement system is major effector of the immune response, which acts on the interface of innate and adaptive immunity and consists of more than 40 soluble proteins (mostly serum glycoproteins), cell surface receptors and regulators. Many of the complement soluble proteins are proenzymes (serine proteases), producing and circulating in inactive forms (zymogens), but activating when cleaved into two peptides, which represent immunoregulatory molecules and inflammatory mediators. Mostly all tissues and organs, including brain, are able to produce complement proteins, but liver is their main source. Being the first line of defense against infections and initiating a variety of cellular and humoral

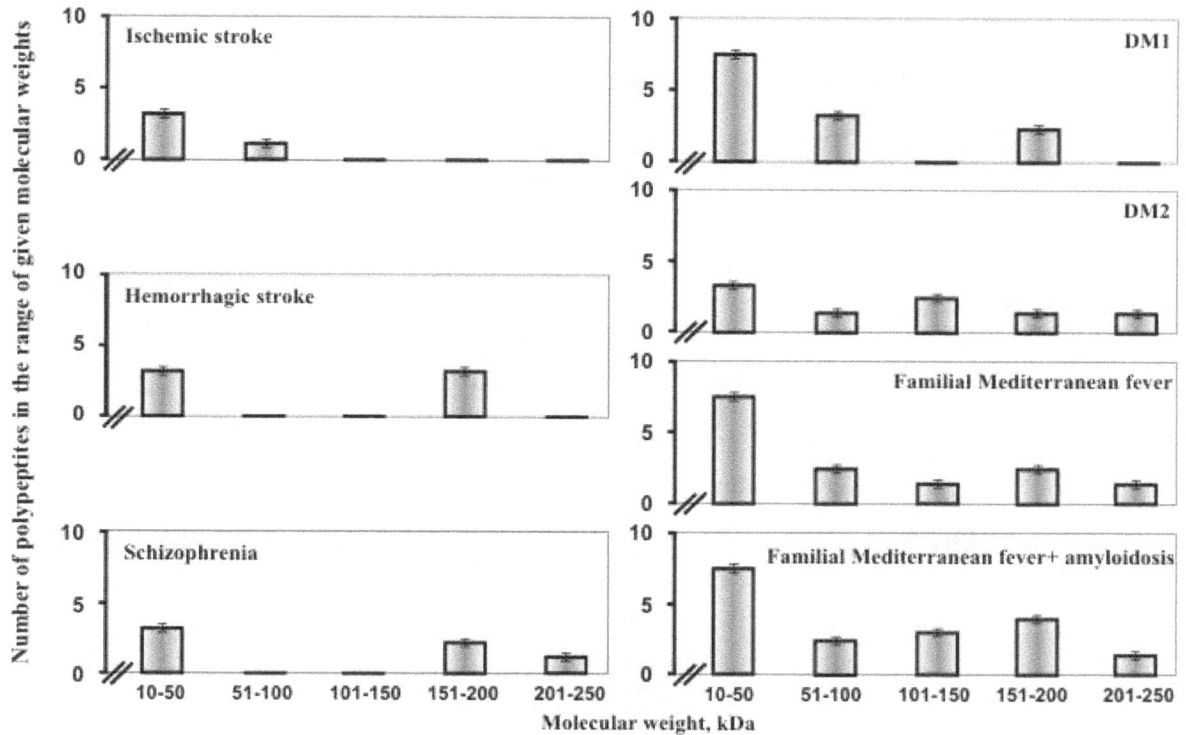

Figure 1: Composition of CIC in different diseased conditions. Data related to healthy subjects were subtracted from the patients data by computer simulation. Electrophoresis was performed in non-reduced conditions.

reactions and intermolecular interactions, complement represents a cytotoxic host defense system. Complement mediates a variety of effector functions and is a key component and trigger of many immunoregulatory mechanisms. It is a complex cascade involving proteolytic cleavage of its components, soluble proteins, often activated by cell receptors. This cascade ultimately results in induction of the antibody responses, inflammation, phagocyte chemotaxis, and opsonization of immune complexes, foreign pathogens, transformed, apoptotic and necrotic cells or cell debris, facilitating their recognition, clearance, and lysis. Complement exhibits three activation pathways - classical, alternative, and lectin, initiated via separate mechanisms and result in formation of opsonins, anaphylatoxins and chemotaxins, and a single terminal pathway that results in a formation of MAC and subsequent cell lysis (Figure 2) (Sim & Laich, 2000; Cole & Morgan, 2003; Nauta *et al.*, 2004). Changes in the functional activity of the complement cascade contribute to the pathology of many human diseases (Sakamoto *et al.*, 1998; Volankis & Frank, 1998; Mollnes *et al.*, 2002). The alterations in the complement cascade have been considered as indicator of the implication of inflammatory component in disease etiology, pathogenesis and/or progression (Sakamoto *et al.*, 1998; Volankis & Frank, 1998; Mollnes *et al.*, 2002).

   In our study we assessed functional activity of the complement cascade in DM by determining total hemolytic activities of its classical pathway and hemolytic activities of its individual components, C1, C2, C3, and C4 proteins, in the blood serum of DM1 and DM2 patients and healthy controls (Hovsepyan *et al.*, 2004; Hovsepyan *et al.*, 2006). In addition, in DM2-affected subjects total hemolytic activity of the

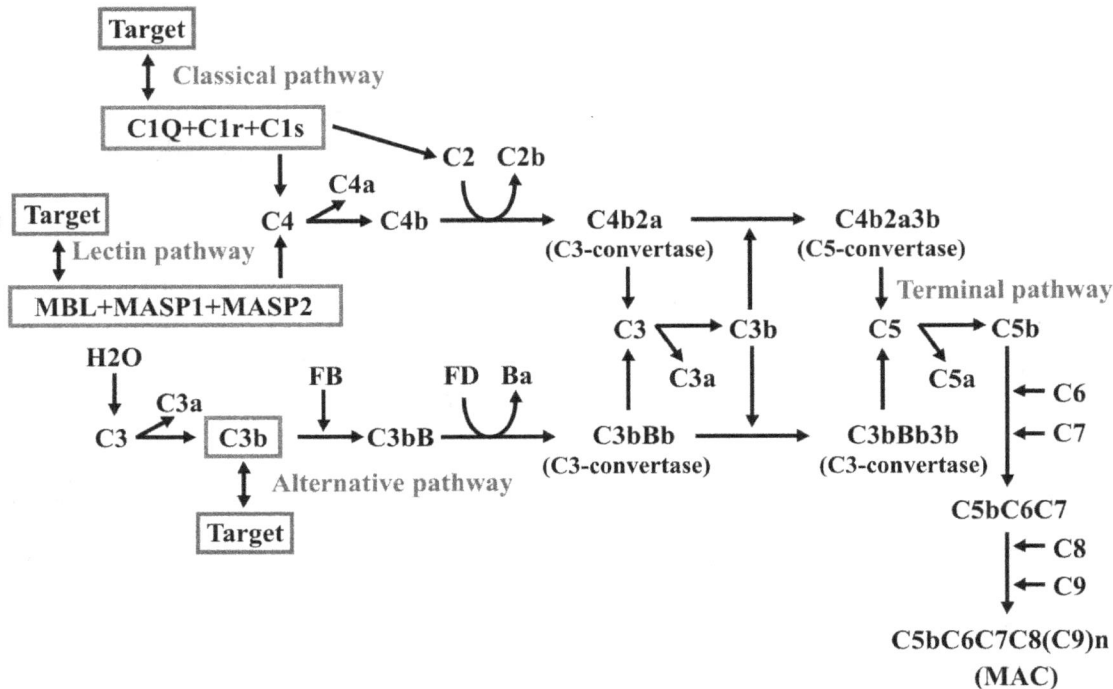

Figure 2: Complement activation pathways. C1Q, C1r, C1s - subunits of the complement C1 component; MBL - mannan-binding lectin; MASP1 - MBL-associated serine protease 1; MASP2 - MBL-associated serine protease 2; FD - factor D; FB - factor B; MAC – membrane attack complex.

complement alternative pathway, and the levels of MAC, final product of the complement activation, were determined (Hovsepyan *et al.*, 2006; Arakelova *et al.*, 2011).C1, C2 and C4 are main components of the classical pathway, and C3 is the initial point for the alternative pathway and a converge point of all three complement activation pathways, starting up for the terminal pathway leading to MAC formation (Figure 2) (Sakamoto *et al.*, 1998; Volankis & Frank, 1998; Mollnes *et al.*, 2002). Hemolytic activities were measured by application of the earlier developed methods (Doods & Sim, 1997; Morgan, 2000; Watford *et al.*, 2000).

According to the obtained results presented in Table 1, mean values of the total hemolytic activity of the complement classical pathway (TC), as well as of the activities of its C1, C3 and C4 components in DM1 and DM2patients were significantly higher than in healthy controls ($p<0.05$). The detected changes were significantly more pronounced in DM2 patients, compared to DM1 ($p<0.05$). Mean value of the C2 component activity in DM2 patients was also significantly higher than in healthy controls ($p<0.05$), whereas no significant difference in this parameter between DM1 patients and healthy controls was observed ($p<0.05$).In addition, in case of DM2 patients, as compared to healthy subjects, a significantly increased mean level of the total hemolytic activity of the complement alternative pathway (TA) was detected ($p<0.05$).

Study group	Hemolytic activity, % of lysed cells*, mean±SD					
	TC	TA	C1	C2	C3	C4
DM1 patients (n=86)	56.5±9.0^a		15.4±3.8^f	43.0±8.6^i	6.8±1.5^l	10.2±2.5^o
Healthy controls (n=96)	52.1±7.9^b	68±10.9^d	9.8±1.2^g	44.9±8.9^j	4.1±0.9^m	6.2±1.5^p
DM2 patients (n=110)	79.2±12.0^c	60±9.0^e	21.5±5.0^h	50.3±10.0^k	9.0±1.9^n	11.3±2.7^q

Table 1: Functional activity of the complement pathway in patients with DM1 and DM2.
*- as a target cells, sheep erythrocytes sensitized with rabbit anti-sheep erythrocyte antibody (TC, C1, C2, C3 and C4) and rabbit erythrocytes (TA) were used. [a b] -$p<0.05$, [b c]- $p<0.01$, [a c] - $p<0.005$, [d e] - $p<0.05$, [f g] - $p<0.05$, [g h] - $p<0.002$, [f h] - $p<0.005$, [i k] - $p<0.05$, [j k] - $p<0.05$, [l m] - $p<0.05$, [m n] - $p<0.015$, [l n] - $p<0.05$, [o p] - $p<0.0004$, [o q] - $p<0.05$, [p q]- $p<0.00015$, [i j] - $p>0.05$.

We also determined the levels of MAC in the blood of DM2 patients and healthy controls by the enzyme-linked immunosorbent assay (ELISA) (Arakelova, 2011) using earlier developed method (Morgan, 1988). As it was mentioned before, the terminal cascade of the complement activation is similar for all three complement activation pathways. This terminal pathway is launched by splitting of the C3 complement protein into two active fragments and is finally leading to formation of MAC (C5b-9), the terminal product of the complement system activation (Figure 2). Insertion of MAC into plasmatic membrane results in its perforation and cell lysis. MAC may also trigger apoptosis, initiate production of inflammatory mediators, cytokines, prostaglandins, thromboxanes, leukotrienes, and active forms of oxygen as well as expression of adhesion molecules (Sim & Laich, 2000; Cole & Morgan, 2003; Nauta et al., 2004; Sakamoto et al., 1998; Volankis & Frank, 1998; Mollnes et al., 2002).

According to the obtained results, in patients with DM2 the mean level of MAC was 1.6 times significantly higher than in healthy controls (mean±SD: 11.1±3.0 µg/ml vs. 6.9±1.7µg/ml, respectively; $p<0.0007$) indicating hyperactivation of the terminal complement cascade. This data is in consistence with the results of earlier reported studies, which demonstrated accumulation of the complement activation intermediate and terminal products, C3-derived opsonins and MAC in endoneurial and retinal microvessels of DM2 patients (Rosoklija et al., 2000; Gerl et al., 2002).

Correlation between the rate of the carbohydrate metabolism compensation and the incidence of micro- and macroangiopathies in DM2 reflects a causal *relationship between* hyperglycemia and the risk for development of chronic diabetic complications. It was shown that, the risk for development of vascular pathology in DM2 significantly increases even when a slight increase (1%) in glycated hemoglobin level is observed (UKPDS Group, 1998). In this regard, it is interesting that deposition of MAC on the membranes of endothelial cells, apart from cytotoxic effects, also results in the release of the growth factors, which stimulate cell proliferation and under a long-term influence can induce hypertrophy and thrombogenicity of the vessel wall (Sim & Laich, 2000; Cole & Morgan, 2003; Nauta et al., 2004; Sakamoto et al., 1998; Volankis & Frank, 1998; Mollnes et al., 2002). Normally, the MAC production, even in the conditions of the complement system hyperactivation, is controlled by the regulatory protein CD59 capable to inhibit a formation of MAC (Acosta et al., 2004; Huang et al., 2005). However, the experimental data demonstrate that, the glycated CD59 loses its ability to inhibit formation of MAC (Acosta et al., 2000; Qin et al., 2004; Cheng & Gao, 2005). This fact represents particular interest in the light of our

findings, since, as it is well known, the enhanced smooth muscle cell and retinal endothelial cell proliferation and, as a result, the hypertrophy and thrombogenicity of vascular wall lead to disruption of vascular permeability and development of angiopathies (Huysman & Mathieu, 2009; McMillan, 1997).

Besides that, it was also demonstrated that the DM2 is characterized by intensifications of apoptotic activity in neuronal and vessel cells that stimulates development of retinopathies (Barber *et al.*, 2011;
Park *et al.*, 2003). In this regard, taking into consideration our own data, it can be proposed that the products of proteolytic activation of the complement C3 and C4 proteins (C3b, C4b, iC3b and C3dg), which
are known triggers of apoptosis (Sim & Laich, 2000; Cole & Morgan, 2003; Nauta *et al.*, 2004; Sakamoto
et al., 1998; Volankis & Frank, 1998; Mollnes *et al.*, 2002), can contribute to this pathologic process.

Thus, based on the results of our investigations we concluded that one of the mechanisms of DM2-
associated hyperglycemia-induced complications may include glycosylation and subsequent inactivation
of the inhibitor of MAC formation.

In summary, it is obvious that long-term DM accompanied with diabetic complications is characterized by hyperactivation of the complement cascade that may be induced by the complex of hormonal,
metabolic and genetic alterations observed in DM. On the other hand, the accumulation of the complement activation products may in turn provoke further progressing of DM and development of diabetic
complications by damaging vascular walls and affecting platelet-vascular and humoral components of
hemostasis. This will change the antigenic and functional characteristics of vessels, alter permeability and
resistance of their walls, induce development of the immunopathological reactions and finally lead to the
narrowing of vessel lumen and reduction of the inner vessel surface, development of edema and endothelial dystrophy. Hyperproduction of chemotactic agents, opsonins, anaphylatoxins and MAC as a result of
hyperactivation of the complement system, along with other factors, may, to a large extent, force the progressing of these pathogenic changes.

3   Neuronal Changes in DM

In addition to abnormalities in the immune response DM1 and DM2 are also accompanied by neuropsy-
chological alterations (Ryan *et al.*, 1984; Skenazy *et al.*, 1984; Perlmuter *et al.*, 1984; Ryan *et al.*, 1985;
Mooradian, 1988; Perlmuter *et al.*, 1989). The neurologic manifestations most frequently described in
association with DM are involved changes of the peripheral nerves and nerve roots and are often accompanied by delays in integrative and sensory transduction processes (Cracco *et al.*, 1980; Harkins *et al.*,
1985; Khardori *et al.*, 1986). On the other hand, it was shown that in absence of acute vascular deficiency
DM related structural changes in the central neuronal system (CN S) are not prominent (de Jong, 1977).
However, both myelopathy and encephalopathy may be part of the diabetic process (de Jong, 1977; Troisi
et al.,1999).DM has a differential effect on different subpopulations of myenteric neurons.DM-related
alterations in the enteric nervous system include changes in the inhibitory and excitatory enteric neurons,
including loss of inhibitory neurons in early DM enteric neuropathy. The functional consequences of these neuronal changes result in altered gastric emptying, diarrhea or constipation. DM can also affect gastrointestinal motility through alterations in extrinsic neuronal control. Recent research on the neuro–
immune interactions demonstrates inflammation-associated neurodegeneration which can lead to motility
related problems in DM (Chandrasekharan & Srinivasan, 2007).

According to brain imaging studies DM2 has increased incidence of small vessel disease including
white matter lesions and lacunae infarcts (Vermeer*et al.*, 2002) and increased risk of temporal lobe atro-

phy (Korf *et al.*, 2007).Reduction of hippocampus and amygdala volumes in DM2 patients compared to non diabetics was shown (Korf *et al.*, 2006; den Heijer *et al.*, 2003) as well as association of DM2 with degeneration of ganglions, demyelization and axon loss (de Jong, 1977; Moscou & Pereant, 2010).

Patients with DM1 have increased activity of hypothalamic-pituitary axis (Asfeldt, 1972; Mooradian, 1997), increased growth hormone secretion in response to exercise and stimulation of dopamine and thyrotropin releasing hormone (Mooradian, 1997; Merimee *et al.*, 1978; Ceda *et al.*, 1982).

In our investigations we determined the activity of a marker enzyme for adrenergic neurons, dopamine β-monooxygenase (DBM; EC 1.14.17.1), and a modulator of β-adrenergic receptor activity, in patients with DM1, DM2, and healthy subjects (Hovsepyan *et al.*, 2002). The enzyme is catalyzing formation of noradrenaline from dopamine, and its activity in the blood reflects central and peripheral adrenergic activity (Beliaev *et al.*, 2009). Study subjects represent the same patients and healthy controls as described in the previous section. Blood activity of DBM was measured according to earlier described spectrophotometric assay using tyramine as a substrate (Nagatsu & Udenfriend, 1972). According to the obtained results the specific activity of DBM in the blood of DM1 patients was in average 5.7 tines significantly lower than in healthy controls ($p<0.00000001$). The same applies to DM2 patients; in this case the specific activity of DBM in patients group was in average 9.5 times significantly lower than in healthy controls ($p<0.00000001$). The obtained results are presented in Figure3 and suggest that long-term DM1 and DM2 are associated with deficient adrenergic activity.

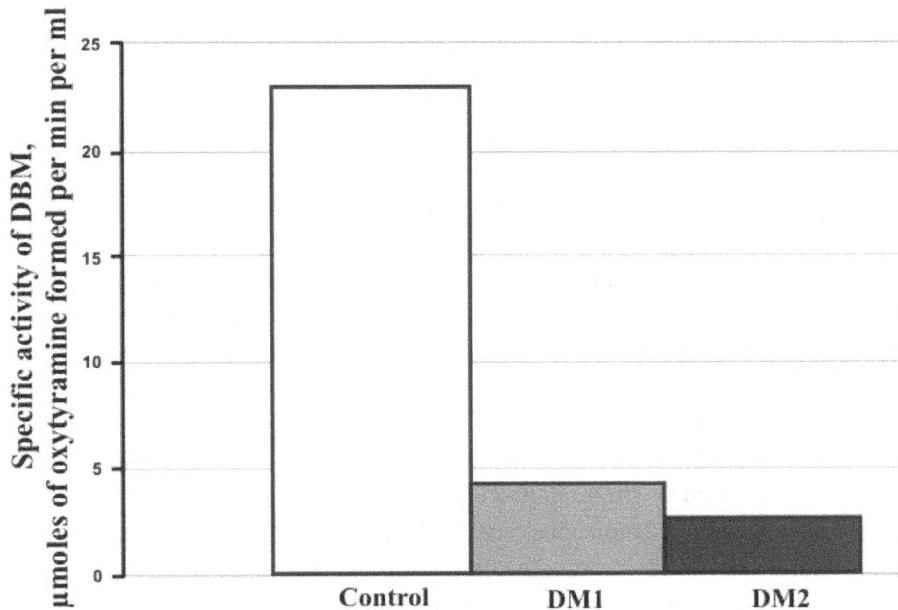

Figure 3: Specific activity of DBM (SD=±20%) in the blood of patients with DM1 (*n*=86), DM2 (*n*=110) and healthy controls (*n*=96).Control vs. DM1 - $p<0.00000001$; Control vs. DM2 –$p<0.00000001$; DM1 versus DM2 –$p<0.0005$.

Animal studies also revealed a number of neuro-humoral and related biochemical alterations in DM (Mooradian, 1988; Srinivasan & Ramarao, 2007; Islam& Loots, 2009). Experimental DM lowers glycogen levels in CNS and promotes glycogen consumption (Srinivasan & Ramarao, 2007; Islam& Loots, 2009). In addition, there were detected changes in brain amino acid patterns as well as in levels of monoamines and their metabolites (Crandall *et al.*, 1981; Crandall & Fernstrom, 1983; Glanville & Anderson, 1986; Chu *et al.*, 1986; Kwok & Juorio, 1986; Bitar*et al.*, 1986). Furthermore, the increased levels of dopamine in hippocampus and decreased levels of serotonin in hypothalamus and brain stem were observed in diabetic animals (Mooradian, 1997). Although the changes in the blood brain barrier (BBB) are readily demonstrable in animal models of DM in human subjects the changes have not been consistently demonstrable (Horani & Mooradian, 2003). To determine if clinical long-term DM is associated with disruption of the blood–brain barrier (BBB), we measured blood serum levels of antibodies to neuron-specific enolase (NSE; *EC*4.2.1.11), a peripheral marker of BBB disruption (Selakovic *et al.*, 2005); in the same cohorts of DM1 and DM2 patients using a chemiluminescent Western blot (Hovsepyan *et al.*, 2004). There was detected a significant increase in antibodies to NSE in both DM1 and DM2 subjects compared to controls. This study suggests that DM in humans may be associated with alterations in the BBB integrity that allow the emergence of antibodies against neuronal antigens.

Thus, DM in humans as well as in experimental animals leads to various structural and functional disturbances in nervous system resulting in its dysfunction and BBB damage.

The oxidative stress and production of free radicals are the main causes leading to the development of insulin resistance, β-cell dysfunction, decrease in glucose tolerance, and development of DM. The oxidative stress plays an important role in the pathophysiology of DM and is the common factor in the development of diabetic complications, micro- and macroangiopathies (Wright *et al.*, 2006) and DM-associated neuronal changes (Voukali *et al.*, 2011). We performed a comparative analysis of the functional activity of antioxidant system and intensity of lipid peroxidation process in the blood serum of acute ischemic stroke patients complicated and none-complicated with DM2 (on the first day of stroke onset), DM2 patients, and healthy controls (Tsakanova *et al.*, 2010; Tsakanova *et al.*, 2011). In particular, we determined total activity of non-enzymatic water-soluble low-molecular-weight antioxidants by photochemiluminescent analysis, ferroxidase activity of ceruloplasmin and the content of lipid hydroperoxides by spectrophotometric assays (Tsakanova *et al.*, 2010; Tsakanova *et al.*, 2011). All patients with DM2 have micro- and macroangiopathies. Duration of the illness was 9-12 years. The obtained results suggest that stroke complicated with DM2 is characterized by significantly higher intensity of the lipid peroxidation process as compared to stroke none-complicated with DM2 ($p<0.05$), that, probably, is one of the determining factors responsible for more severe clinical course of strokes in patients with DM compared to those who are not suffering from DM. Our study also demonstrated that mechanisms of the compensatory response to oxidative stress on the level of antioxidants in stroke patients complicated with DM2 differ from those detected in stroke none-complicated with DM2. On the base of the obtained results we suggested that metabolic, molecular, and cellular level alterations typical for long-term DM2 impair compensatory mechanisms protecting the body from oxidative.

On the other hand, it is known that diabetic angiopathies of cerebral arteries lead to microcirculation disturbances and contribute to the development of cerebral ischemia. DM is a risk factor for ischemic stroke, and the prevalence of stroke, its severity and frequency of deaths among patients with DM is much higher (Bonow & Gheorghiade, 2004; Tuomilehto *et al.*, 1996). In our own study we investigated the relationship between post-ischemic inflammatory response and the state of BBB in acute stroke progression in patients with acute ischemic stroke complicated and none-complicated with DM2 by measuring the levels of proinflammatory and chemotactic cytokines (IL-1β, IL-6, TNF-α and monocyte chemoattractant protein-1 (MCP-1), chemokine (C-X-C motif) ligand 1 (CXCL1), respectively), brain-specific proteins (NSE and S100b) and antibodies to these proteins in the blood serum of the study subjects on different time points of stroke onset using ELISA and Western blot (Boyajyan *et al.*, 2007; Boyajyan *et al.*, 2008). Patients with long-term DM2 and healthy controls were also involved in this study. All patients with DM2 have micro- and macroangiopathies. Duration of the illness was 9-12 years. According to the obtained results a significant increase of the levels of all the analyzed cytokines in both groups of the ischemic stroke patients was detected on days 1-5 of stroke onset, with the maximum level on day 1. Notably, the levels of cytokines in DM2-complicated patients were significantly higher than in those none-complicated with DM2 ($p < 0.05$). In all groups of patients the presence of antibodies specific to NSE and S100b was detected with highest concentration in case of ischemic stroke patients complicated with DM2. According to the obtained results, significantly increased levels of NSE and S100b were detected on days 1-7 of stroke onset with the maximum level on day 3. As in case of cytokines, here also the levels of NSE and S100b in DM2-complicated patients were significantly higher than in those none-complicated with DM2 ($p < 0.05$). In addition, a positive correlation between the levels of analyzed cytokines, on the one hand, and the levels of NSE and S100b, on the other hand, in ischemic stroke patients, both complicated and none-complicated with DM2, was detected suggesting about the relationship between the intensity of postischemic inflammatory response and BBB disruption.

Therefore, the results of our study suggest that in ischemic stroke complicated with DM2 the systemic inflammatory reactions are more intense than in case of stroke none-complicated with DM2. That may be a result of the initial BBB destruction detected by us in long-term DM2 (Hovsepyan *et al.*, 2004), since our data presented above indicated the presence of positive correlation between the intensity of postischemic inflammatory response and BBB disruption (Boyajyan *et al.*, 2007; Boyajyan *et al.*, 2008). The alteration in BBB integrity may, on the one hand, promote the influx of immunomodulators to the brain and enhance the inflammatory response in the damaged areas of the brain, and, on the other hand, promote a migration of immunocompetent cells and inflammatory mediators from the brain to the peripheral circulation through the brain endothelium triggering the development of the inflammatory reactions on the systemic level.

References

Acosta, J., Hettinga, J., Fluckiger, R., Krumrei, N., Goldfine, A., Angarita, L. & Halperin, J. (2000). Molecular basis for a link between complement and the vascular complications of diabetes. Proc Natl Acad Sci USA, 97(10), 5450-55.

Acosta, J., Qin, X. & Halperin, J. (2004). Complement and complement regulatory proteins as potential molecular targets for vascular diseases. Curr Pharm, 10(2), 203-11.

Ambepityia, G., Kopelman, P.G., Ingram, D., Swash, M., Mills, P.G. & Timmis, A.D. (1990). Exertional myocardial ischemia in diabetes: a quantitative analysis of anginal perceptual threshold and the influence of autonomic function. J Am Coll Cardiol, 15(1), 72-7.

Arakelian, A., Boiadzhian, A., Pogosian, A., Bakunts, G., Silvanian, G. & Egiian, L. (2003). Circulating immune complexes in ischemic and hemorrhagic strokes. Zh Nevrol Psikhiatr Im S S Korsakova, 8, 44-7.

Arakelova, E.A., Ovsepyan, M.R., Boyadzhyan, A.S., Arakelyan, A.A., Gevorkyan, A.A. & Mamikonyan, A.A. (2011). The membrane attack complex as an indicator of complement hyperactivation in type 2 diabetes mellitus. Diabetes Mellitus (Mosc), 52(3), 17-20.

Asfeldt, V.H. (1972). Hypophyseo-adrenocortical function in diabetes mellitus. Acta Med Scand, 191, 349-54.

Barber, A.J., Gardner, T.W. & Abcouwer, S.F. (2011). The significance of vascular and neural apoptosis to the pathology of diabetic retinopathy.Invest Ophthalmol Vis Sci, 52(2), 1156-1163.

Bariş, N., Erdoğan, M., Sezer, E., Saygili, F., Ozgönül, A., Turgan, N. & Ersöz, B. (2009). Alterations in L-arginine and inflammatory markers in type 2 diabetic patients with and without microalbuminuria. Acta Diabetol 46(4), 309-16.

Beliaev, A., Ferreira, H., Learmonth, D. A. & Soares-da-Silva, P. (2009). Dopamine β-monooxygenase: mechanism, substrates and inhibitors. Current Enz Inhib, 5, 27-43.

Bitar, M., Koulu, M., Rapoport, S.I. & Linnoila, M. (1986) Diabetes induced alteration in brain monoamine metabolism in rats. J Pharmac Exp Ther, 236, 432-37.

Boiadzhian, A.S., Arakelova, E.A., Arakelian, A.A., Avetisian, G.V., Aivazian, V.A., Manucharian, G.G., Mkrtchian, G.M., Sim, R. B. & Willis, A. K. (2007). Circulating immune complexes in families with positive history of ischemic stroke. Zh Nevrol Psikhiatr Im S S Korsakova,21, 43-6.

Bonow, R.O. & Gheorghiade, M. (2004). The diabetes epidemic: a national and global crisis. Am J Med, 116(Suppl. 5A): 2S-10S.

Booth, G.L., Kapral, M.K., Fung, K. & Tu, J.V. (2006). Relation between age and cardiovascular disease in men and women with diabetes compared with non-diabetic people: a population-based retrospective cohort study. Lancet, 368, 29-36.

Boyajyan, A.S., Arakelova, E.A., Ayvazyan, V.A., & Manukyan, L.A. (2008) Interleukins and chemokines in acute ischemic stroke complicated and non-complicated with diabetes. Cytokines and Inflammation (St. Petersburg), 7(1), 40-3.

Boyajyan, A.S., Arakelova, E. A., Ayvazyan, V.A., Mktrchyan, G.M., Tsakanova, G.V., Avetisyan, G.V., Hovhannisyan, L. P., Khoyetsyan, A.G., Manukyan, L.A., Arakelyan, A.A., Hovsepyan, M.R., Mayilyan, K.R. & Hakobyan, S.S. (2007). Relationships between postischemic inflammatory response and alterations in blood brain barrier integrity. Blood (Yerevan), 1(5), 45-54.

Burut, D.F., Karim, Y. & Ferns, G.A. (2010). The role of immune complexes in atherogenesis. Angiology 61(7), 679-89.

Cavallo, T. & Granholm, N.A. (1990). Repeated exposure to bacterial lipopolysaccharide interferes with disposal of pathogenic immune complexes in mice. Clin Exp Immunol, 79(2), 253-9.

Ceda, G.P., Speroni, G., Dall'Aglio, E., Valenti, G. & Butturini, U. (1982).Non-specific growth hormone responses to thyrotropin releasing horone in insulin-dependent diabetes. Sex and age-related pituitary responsiveness. J Clin Endocr Metab, 55, 170-4.

Chandrasekharan, B. & Srinivasan, S. (2007). Diabetes and the enteric nervous system. Neurogastroenterol Motil, 19, 951-60.

Cheng, Y. & Gao, M. (2005). The effect of glycation of CD59 on complement-mediated cytolysis.Cell Mol Immunol, 2(4), 313-17.

Chu, P.C., Lin, M.T., Shian, L.R. & Leu, S.Y. (1986). Alterations in physiologic functions and in brain monoamine content in streptozotocine-diabetic rats. Diabetes, 35, 481-5.

Cole, D.S. & Morgan, B. P. (2003). Beyond lysis: how complement influences cell fate. Clin Sci, 104(5), 455-66.

Cracco, J.B., Castors, S. & Mark, E. (1980). Conduction velocity in peripheral nerve and spinal afferent pathways in juvenile diabetics. Neurology, 30, 370-1.

Crandall, E.A, Gillis, M.A. & Fernstrom, J.D. (1981). Reduction in brain serotonin synthesis rate in streptozotocin-diabetic rats. Endocrinology, 109(1), 310-2.

Crandall, E.A. & Fernstrom, J.D. (1983).Effects of experimental diabetes on the levels of aromatic and branched-chain amino acids in rat blood and brain. Diabetes, 32, 222-30.

Crook, M. (2004). Type 2 diabetes mellitus: a disease of the innate immune system? An update. Diabet Med 21(3), 203-7.

Crook, M.A., Tutt P., Simpson, H. & Pickup, J.C. (1993). Serum sialic acid and acute phase proteins in type 1 and type 2 diabetes mellitus. Clin Chim Acta, 219 (1-2), 131-8.

Cuocolo, A., Concilio, C., Acampa, W., Ferro, A., Evangelista, L., Daniele, S. & Petretta, M. (2009). Cardiovascular risk stratification of diabetic patients. Minerva Endocrinol 34(3), 205-21.

de Jong, R.N. (1977). CNS manifestation in diabetes mellitus. Postgrad Med J, 61, 101-7.

Delamaire, M., Maugendre, D., Moreno, M., Le Goff, M.C., Allannic, H. & Genetet, B. (1997). Impaired leucocyte functions in diabetic patients. Diabet Med 14(1), 29-34.

den Heijer, T., Vermeer, S.E., van Dijk, E.J., Prins, N. D., Koudstaal, P. J., Hofman, A. & Breteler, M. M. (2003). Type 2 diabetes and atrophy of medial temporal lobe structures on brain MRI. Diabetologia, 46(12), 1604-10.

Devine, S.M., Liedtke, A.J. & Zelis, R. (1981). Coronary artery disease in diabetic patients. In: Clinical Cardiology and Diabetes. NY: Futura Publishing Co 2, 1-87

Digeon, M., Laver, M., Riza, J. & Bach, J. F. (1977). Detection of circulating immune complexes in human aorta by simplified assays with polyethylene glycol. J. Immunol. Methods, 16(2), 165-83

Donath, M.Y. & Shoelson, S.E. (2011). Type 2 diabetes as an inflammatory disease. Nat Rev Immunol, 11(2), 98-107.

Doods, A. W. & Sim, R. B. (1997). Complement. A practical approach. Practical Approach series. Oxford: Oxford University Press Inc.

Eibl, N., Spatz, M., Fischer, G.F., Mayr, W.R., Samstag, A., Wolf, H.M., Schernthaner, G. & Eibl MM. (2002). Impaired primary immune response in type-1 diabetes: results from a controlled vaccination study. Clin Immunol, 103(3 Pt 1), 249-59.

Fox, C.S., Coady, S., Sorlie, P.D., Levy, D., Meigs, J.B., D'Agostino, R.B.Sr., Wilson, P.W. & Savage, P.J. (2004). Trends in cardiovascular complications of diabetes. JAMA, 292(20), 2495-9.

Geerlings, S.E. & Hoepelman, A.I. (1999). Immune dysfunction in patients with diabetes mellitus (DM). FEMS Immunol Med Microbiol, 26(3-4), 259-65.

Geerlings, S.E. & Hoepelman, A.I. (1999). Immune dysfunction in patients with diabetes mellitus (DM). FEMS Immunol Med Microbiol, 26(3-4), 259-65.

Gerl, V.B., Bohl, J., Pitz, S., Stoffelns, B., Pfeiffer, N. & Bhakdi, S. (2002). Extensive deposits of complement C3d and C5b-9 in the choriocapillaris of eyes of patients with diabetic retinopathy. Invest Ophthalmol Vis Sci, 43(4), 1104-8.

Glanville, N.T. & Anderson, G.H. (1986). Hypothalamic catecholamine metabolism in diabetic rats. The effects of insulin deficiency and meal ingestion. J Neurochem, 46, 753-9.

Grundy, S.M., Benjamin, I.J., Burke, G.L., Chait, A., Eckel, R.H., Howard, B.V., Mitch, W., Smith, S.C.Jr. & Sowers, J.R. (1999). Diabetes and cardiovascular disease: a statement for healthcare professionals from the American Heart Association. Circulation, 100(10), 1134-46.

Hakobyan, S., Avetisyan, G., Boyajyan, A., Torosyan, S., Khachatryan, G. & Tatevosyan, S. (2001). Circulating immune complexes in blood of patients with positive family history of schizophrenia. Dokl Biochem Biophys, 380, 343-4.

Hakobyan, S.S. & Boyajyan, A.S. (2004). Immune complexes in patients with schizophrenia. Psychopharmacol Biol Narcol, 4 (2-3), 687-8.

Harkins, S.W., Gardner, D.F. & Anderson, R.A. (1985). Auditory and somatosensory far field evoked potentials in diabetes mellitus. Int J Neurosci, 28, 41-7.

Hebert, L.A. (1991). The clearance of immune complexes from the circulation of man and other primates. Am J Kidney Dis, 17, 352-61.

Horani, M. & Mooradian, A.D. (2003). Diabetes and the blood-brain barrier. Curr Pharm Des, 9, 833-40.

Hovsepyan, M.R., Haas, M.J., Boyajyan, A. S., Guevorkyan, A.A,. Mamikonyan, A.A., Myers S. & Mooradian, A.D. (2004). Astrocytic and neuronal biochemical markers in the sera of subjects with diabetes mellitus. Neurosci Lett, 369, 224-7.

Hovsepyan, M., Boyajyan, A., Aivazyan, V., Mayilyan, K., Guevorkyan, A. & Mamikonyan, A. (2002a).Concentration of circulating immune complexes and dopamine-β-hydroxylase activity in the blood of patients with diabetes mellitus type 1 at the late stages of the disease progression. Diabetes Mellitus (Mosc), 17 (4), 44-5.

Hovsepyan, M., Boyajyan, A., Manukyan, L., Gevorgyan, A. & Mamikonyan, A. (2004). Activation of complement by classical pathway in diabetes mellitus. Gitutiun ev tekhnika (Yerevan), 2, 14-7.

Hovsepyan, M.R., Boyajyan, A.S. & Hovhannisyan, L.P. (2006).Activation of the complement system by the classical and alternative pathways in prolonged type 2 diabetes mellitus. Probl Endokrinol (Mosk), 6, 14-7.

Hovsepyan, M.R., Boyajyan, A.S., Haroutiunyan, V.M., Hakobyan, G.S. & Guevorkyan, A.A. (2002b). Protein composition of circulating immune complexes in late stages of diabetes mellitus. Vestnik MANEB (St. Petersburg), 7(6/54), 169-72.

Huang, Y., Smith, C. A, Song, H., Morgan, B. P., Abagyan, R. & Tomlinson, S. (2005). Insights into the human CD59 complement binding interface toward engineering new therapeutics. J Biol Chem, 280(40), 34073-79.

Huysman, E. & Mathieu, C. (2009). Diabetes and peripheral vascular disease. Acta Chir Belg, 109(5), 587-94.

Idris, I., Thomson, G.A. & Sharma, J.C. (2006). Diabetes mellitus and stroke. Int J Clin Pract, 60(1), 48-56.

Islam, M.S. & Loots, D.T. (2009). Experimental rodent models of type 2 diabetes: a review.Methods Find Exp Clin Pharmacol, 31(4), 249-61.

Jialal, I., Devaraj, S. & Venugopal, S.K. (2002). Oxidative stress, inflammation, and diabetic vasculopathies: the role of alpha tocopherol therapy. Free Radic Res, 36(12), 1331-6.

Jorgensen, H., Nakayama, H., Raaschou, H.O. & Olsen, T.S. (1994). Stroke in patients with diabetes. The Copenhagen stroke study. Stroke, 25, 1977-84.

Kaneto, H., Matsuoka, T.A., Nakatani, Y., Kawamori, D., Miyatsuka, T., Matsuhisa, M. & Yamasaki, Y. (2005). Oxidative stress, ER stress, and the JNK pathway in type 2 diabetes. J Mol Med (Berl), 83(6), 429-39.

Kapur, A. & De Palma, R. (2007). Mortality after myocardial infarction in patients with diabetes mellitus. Heart, 93(12), 1504-6.

Khardori, R., Soler, N.G., Good, D.-C., Devles-Howard, A.B, Broughton, D. & Walbert, J. (1986). Brainstem auditory and visual evoked potentials in type I (insulin-dependent) diabetic patients. Diabetologia, 29, 362-5.

Kluz, J. & Adamiec, R. (2003). The role of anti-endothelial cell antibodies in the pathogenesis of atherosclerosis and diabetic angiopathy. Przegl Lek, 60(11), 751-54.

Konstantinova, N.A. (1996). Immune complexes and tissue injury. Moscow: Medicine.

Korf, E.S., van Straaten, E.C., de Leeuw, F.E., van der Flier, W.M., Barkhof, F., Pantoni, L., Basile, A.M., Inzitari, D., Erkinjuntti, T., Wahlund, L.O., Rostrup, E., Schmidt, R., Fazekas, F. & Scheltens, P. (2007). Diabetes mellitus, hypertension and medial temporal lobe atrophy: the LADIS study. Diabet Med, 24(2), 166-71.

Korf, E.S., White, L.R., Scheltens, P. & Launer, L.J. (2006). Brain aging in very old men with type 2 diabetes: the Honolulu-Asia Aging Study. Diabetes Care, 29(10), 2268-74.

Kukreja, A., Cost, G., Marker, J., Zhang, C., Sun, Z., Lin-Su, K., Ten, S., Sanz, M., Exley, M., Wilson, B., Porcelli, S. & Maclaren, N. (2002). Multiple immuno-regulatory defects in type-1 diabetes. J Clin Invest, 109, 131-40.

Kwok, R.P.S & Juorio, A.V. (1986). Concentration of striatal tyramine and dophamine metabolism in diabetic rats and effect of insulin administration. Neuroendocrinology, 43, 590-6.

Laing, S.P., Swerdlow, A.J., Carpenter, L.M., Slater, S.D., Burden, A.C., Botha, J.L., Morris, A.D., Waugh, N.R., Gatling, W., Gale, E.A., Patterson, C.C., Qiao, Z., & Keen, H. (2003). Mortality from cerebrovascular disease in a cohort of 23000 patients with insulin-treated diabetes. Stroke, 34(2), 418-21.

Lecube, A., Pachón, G., Petriz, J., Hernández, C. & Simó, R. (2011). Phagocytic activity is impaired in type 2 diabetes mellitus and increases after metabolic improvement. PLoS ONE, 6(8), e23366.

Marshall, S.M. & Flyvbjerg, A. (2006). Prevention and early detection of vascular complications of diabetes. BMJ, 333(7566), 475-80.

McDougal, J.S. & McDuffie, F.C. (1985). Immune complexes in man: detection and clinical significance. Adv Clin Chem, 241-60.

McMillan, D.E. (1997). Development of vascular complications in diabetes. Vasc Med, 2(2), 132-42.

Merimee, T.J., Fitsgerald, C.R., Gold, L.A. & McCort, J. (1978). Characteristics of GH secretion in clinically stable diabetes. Diabetes, 28, 308-12.

Mkrtchyan, G.M., Boyajyan, A.S., Karageuzyan, K.G., Aivazyan, A.A., Pashinyan, S.A. & Nazaretyan, E.E. (2002). Protein composition of circulating immune complexes in patients with periodic disease complicated or not complicated by renal amyloidosis. Dokl Biol Sci, 385, 329-30.

Mollnes, T.E., Song, W.C. & Lambris, J.D. (2002). Complement in inflammatory tissue damage and disease. Trends Immunol Today, 23(2), 61-6.

Monsalvo, A.C., Batalle, J.P., Lopez, M.F., Krause, J.C., Klemenc, J., Hernandez, Z., Maskin, B., Bugna, J., Rubinstein, C., Aguilar, L., Dalurzo, L., Libster, R., Savy, V., Baumeister, E., Aguilar, L., Cabral, G., Font, J., Solari, L., Weller, K.P., Johnson, J., Echavarria, M., Edwards, K.M., Chappell, J.D., Crowe, J.E.Jr., Williams, J.V., Melendi, G.A. & Polack, F.P. (2011). Severe pandemic 2009 H1N1 influenza disease due to pathogenic immune complexes. Nat Med, 17(2), 195-9.

Mooradian, A.D. (1988). Diabetic complications of the central nervous system. Endocrin Rev, 9, 346-56.

Mooradian, A.D. (1997). Pathophysiology of central nervous system complications in diabetes mellitus. Clin Neurosci, 4(6), 322-6.

Morgan, B.P., Daniels, R.H. & Williams, B.D. (1988). Measurement of terminal complement complexes in rheumatoid arthritis. Clin Exp Immunol, 73, 473-8.

Morgan, P. (2000). Complement methods and protocols. Methods of Molecular Biology series. Totowa, New Jersey: Humana Press Inc.

Moscou, B. & Pereant, M. (2010). Pathological features of diabetic neuropathy. AMT, 2(4), 262-4.

Moulds, J.M. (2009). Introduction to antibodies and complement. Transfus Apher Sci, 40(3), 185-8.

Moutschen, M.P., Scheen, A.J., & Lefebvre, P.J. (1992). Impaired immune responses in diabetes mellitus: analysis of the factors and mechanisms involved. Relevance to the increased susceptibility of diabetic patients to specific infections. Diabete Metab, 18(3), 187-201.

Nagatsu, T. & Udenfriend, S. (1972). Photometric assay of dopamine β-hydroxylase activity in human blood. Clin Chem, 18(9), 980-3.

Nauta, A.J., Roos, A. & Daha, M.R. (2004). A regulatory role for complement in innate immunity and autoimmunity. Int Arch Allergy Immunol, 134(4), 310-23.

Ng, Y.C., Schifferli, J.A. & Walport, M.J. (1988). Immune complexes and erythrocyte CR1 (complement receptor type 1): effect of CR1 numbers on binding and release reactions. Clin Exp Immunol, 71, 481-5.

Olsson, T., Vitanen, M., Asplund, K., Eriksson, S. & Hägg, E. (1990). Prognosis after stroke in diabetic patients. A controlled prospective study. Diabetologia, 33, 244-9.

Oppenheimer, S., Halfbraid, B.I., Oswald, G.A. & Yudkin, J.S. (1985). Diabetes mellitus and early mortality from stroke. Br Med J, 291(6501), 1014-5.

Ovsepyan, M.R., Boyadjyan, A.S., Mamikonyan, A.A., Gevorkyan, A.A. (2004). Circulating immune complexes at the late stages of diabetes mellitus. Immunology (Mosc), 25(6), 375-7.

Ozer, G., Teker, Z., Cetiner, S., Yilmaz, M., Topaloglu, A.K., Onenli-Mungan, N. & Yuksel, B. (2003). Serum IL-1, IL-2, TNFalpha and INFgamma levels of patients with type 1 diabetes mellitus and their siblings. J Pediatr Endocrinol Metab, 16(2), 203-10.

Park, S.H., Park, J.W., Park, S.J., Kim, K.Y., Chung, J.W., Chun, M.H. & Oh, S.J. (2003). Apoptotic death of photoreceptors in the streptozotocin-induced diabetic rat retina. Diabetologia, 46(9), 1260-68.

Perlmuter, L.C., Goldfinger, S.H., Shore, A.R. & Nathan, D.M. (1989). Cognitive function in non-insulin dependent diabetes. In: Neurophsychological and Behavioral Aspects of Insulin and Non-insulin Dependent Diabetes. NY: Spinger Verlag, 1433-638.

Perlmuter, L.C., Hakami, M.K., Hodgson-Harrington, C., Ginsberg, J., Katz, J., Singer, D.E. & Nathan, D.M. (1984). Decreased cognitive function in non-insulin dependent diabetic patients. Am J Med, 77, 1043-8.

Pickup, J.C. & Crook MA. (1998). Is type II diabetes mellitus a disease of the innate immune system? Diabetologia, 41(10), 1241-8.

Qin, X., Goldfine, A., Krumrei, N., Grubissich, L., Acosta, J., Chorev, M., Hays, A. P. & Halperin, J. A. (2004). Glycation inactivation of the complement regulatory protein CD59. A possible role in the pathogenesis of the vascular complications of human diabetes. Diabetes, 53, 2653-61.

Rosoklija, G.B., Dwork, A.J., Younger, D.S., Karlikaya, G., Latov, N. & Hays, A.P. (2000). Local activation of the complement system in endoneurial microvessels of diabetic neuropathy. Acta Neuropathol (Berl), 99(1), 55-62.

Ryan, C., Vega, A. & Drash, A. (1985). Cognitive deficits in adolescents who developed diabetes early in life. Pediatrics, 5, 921-7.

Ryan, C., Vega, A., Longstreet, C. & Drash, A. (1984). Neurophsychological changes in adolescents with insulin-dependent diabates. J Consult Clin Psychol, 52, 335-42.

Sakamoto, M., Fujisawa, Y. & Nishioka, K. (1998). Physiologic role of the complement system in host defense, disease, and malnutrition. Nutrition, 14(4), 391-8.

Schifferli, J.A., Ng, Y.C. & Peters, D.K. (1986). The role of complement and its receptor in the elimination of immune complexes. N Eng J Med, 315, 488-95.

Seijkens, T., Kusters, P., Engel, D. & Lutgens, E. (2013). CD40-CD40L: Linking pancreatic, adipose tissue and vascular inflammation in type 2 diabetes and its complications. Diab Vasc Dis Res, 10(2), 115-22.

Selakovic, V., Raicevic, R. & Radenovic, L. (2005). The increase of neuron-specific enolase in cerebrospinal fluid and plasma as a marker of neuronal damage in patients with acute brain infarction. J Clin Neurosci, 12, 542–7.

Shaw, J.E., Sicree, R.A. & Zimmet, P.Z. (2010). Global estimates of the prevalence of diabetes for 2010 and 2030. Diabetes Res Clin Pract, 87(1), 4-14.

Shmagel, K.V. & Chereshnev, V.A. (2009). Molecular bases of immune complex pathology. Biochemistry (Mosc), 74(5), 469-79.

Sim, R.B. & Laich, A. (2000). Serine proteases of the complement system. Biochem Soc Trans, 28, 545-50.

Skenazy, J.A. & Bigler, E.D. (1984). Neurophsychological findings in diabetes mellitus. J Clin Psycol, 40, 246-58.

Solinas, G., Vilcu, C., Neels, J.G., Bandyopadhyay, G.K., Luo, J.L., Naugler, W., Grivennikov, S., Wynshaw-Boris, A., Scadeng, M., Olefsky, J.M. & Karin, M. (2007). JNK1 in hematopoietically derived cells contributes to diet-induced inflammation and insulin resistance without affecting obesity. Cell Metab, 6(5), 386-97.

Srinivasan, K. & Ramarao, P. (2007). Animal models in type 2 diabetes research: an overview. Indian J Med Res, 125(3), 451-72.

Keymel, S., Heinen, Y., Balzer, J., Rassaf, T., Kelm, M., Lauer, T. & Heiss, C. (2011). Characterization of macro- and microvascular function and structure in patients with type 2 diabetes mellitus. Am J Cardiovasc Dis, 1(1), 68-77.

Tarnacka, B., Gromadzka, G. & Czlonkowska, A. (2002). Increased circulating immune complexes in acute stroke: the triggering role of Chlamydia pneumoniae and cytomegalovirus. Stroke, 33(4), 936-40.

Theofilopoulos, A.N. (1980). Evaluation and clinical significance of circulating immune complexes. Prog Clin Immunol, 4, 63-106.

Theofilopoulos, A.N. & Dixon F.J. (1980). Immune complexes in human diseases. Am J Pathol, 100(2), 529-94.

Thornton, B.P., Větvicka, V. & Ross, G.D. (1994). Natural antibody and complement-mediated antigen processing and presentation by B lymphocytes. J Immunol, 152(4), 1727-1737.

Troisi, R., Debruyne, J. & de Hemptinne, B. (1999). Improvement of hepatic myelopathy after liver transplantation. N Engl J Med, 340, 151.

Tsakanova, G.V., Ayvazyan V.A., Boyajyan, A.S., Arakelova, E.A. & Grigoryan, G.S. (2010). State of antioxidant and pro-oxidant systems in acute ischemic stroke complicated and none-complicated with diabetes mellitus. Medical Science of Armenia, 50(1), 74-8.

Tsakanova, G.V., Ayvazyan, V.A., Boyajyan, A.S., Arakelova, E.A., Grigoryan, G.S., Guevorkyan, A.A. & Mamikonyan, A.A. (2011). A comparative study of antioxidant system and intensity of lipid peroxidation in type 2 diabetes mellitus and ischemic stroke aggravated and not aggravated by type 2 diabetes mellitus. Bull Exp Biol Med, 151(5), 564-6.

Tuomilehto, J., Rastenyte, D., Jousilahti, P., Sarti, C. & Vartiainen, E. (1996). Diabetes mellitus as a risk factor for death from stroke. Prospective study of the middle-aged Finnish population. Stroke, 27(2), 210-5.

UKPDS Group. (1998). Intensive blood glucose control with sulphonylureas or insulin compared with conventional treatment and risk of complications in patients with type 2 diabetes. Lancet, 352, 837-53.

Vermeer, S.E., Koudstaal, P.J., Oudkerk, M., Hofman, A. & Breteler, M.M. (2002). Prevalence and risk factors of silent brain infarcts in the population-based Rotterdam Scan Study. Stroke, 33, 21-5, 2002.

Volankis, J.E. & Frank, M.M. (1998). The human complement system in health and disease. New York: Mircel Dekker Inc.

Voukali, E., Shotton, H.R. & Lincoln, J. (2011). Selective responses of myenteric neurons to oxidative stress and diabetic stimuli. Neurogastroenterol Motil, 23(10), 964-e411.

Watford, W.T., Ghio, A.J. & Wright, J.R. (2000). Complement-mediated host defense in the lung. Physiol Lung Cell Mol Physiol, 279 (5), 790-8.

Weitzman, S., Wagner, G.S., Heiss, G., Haney, T.L. & Slomen, G. (1982). Myocardial infarction site and mortality in diabetes. Diabetes Care, 5, 31-5.

Wild, S., Roglic, G., Green, A., Sicree, R. & King, H. (2004). Global prevalence of diabetes: estimates for the year 2000 and projections for 2030. Diabetes Care, 27(5), 1047-53.

Wingard, D.L., Barrett-Connor, E.L., Scheidt-Nave, C. & McPhillips, J.B. (1993). Prevalence of cardiovascular and renal complications in older adults withnormal or impaired glucose tolerance or NIDDM. A population-based study. Diabetes Care, 16(7), 1022-5.

Wright, E., Scism-Bacon, J.L. & Glass, L.C. (2006). Oxidative stress in type 2 diabetes: the role of fasting and postprandial glycaemia. Int J Clin Pract, 60(3), 308-14.